FOURTH EDITION

CLINICAL
KINESIOLOGY
and ANATOMY

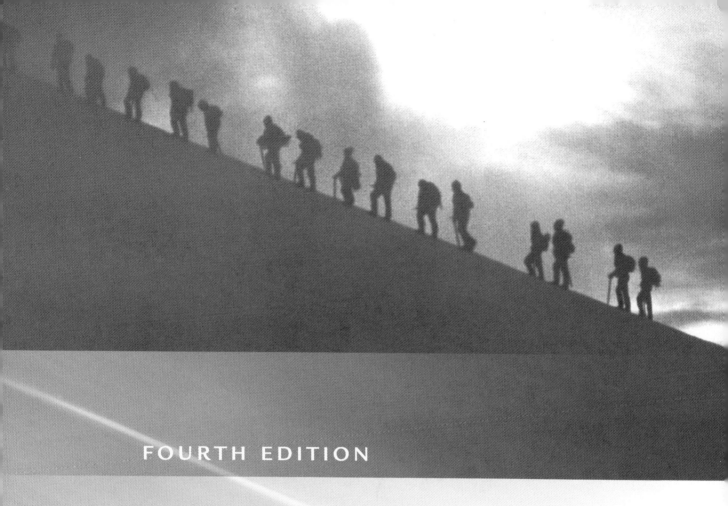

FOURTH EDITION

CLINICAL KINESIOLOGY
and ANATOMY

Lynn S. Lippert, MS, PT

Program Director, Retired
Physical Therapist Assistant Program
Mount Hood Community College
Gresham, Oregon

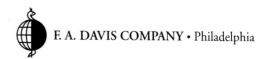

F. A. DAVIS COMPANY • Philadelphia

F. A. Davis Company
1915 Arch Street
Philadelphia, PA 19103
www.fadavis.com

Printed in the United States of America

Last digit indicates print number: 10 9 8 7 6 5 4

Acquisitions Editor: Margaret M. Biblis
Manager of Content Development: Deborah J. Thorp
Developmental Editor: Peg Waltner
Design Manager: Carolyn O'Brien

As new scientific information becomes available through basic and clinical research, recommended treatments and drug therapies undergo changes. The author(s) and publisher have done everything possible to make this book accurate, up to date, and in accord with accepted standards at the time of publication. The author(s), editors, and publisher are not responsible for errors or omissions or for consequences from application of the book, and make no warranty, expressed or implied, in regard to the contents of the book. Any practice described in this book should be applied by the reader in accordance with professional standards of care used in regard to the unique circumstances that may apply in each situation. The reader is advised always to check product information (package inserts) for changes and new information regarding dose and contraindications before administering any drug. Caution is especially urged when using new or infrequently ordered drugs.

Library of Congress Cataloging-in-Publication Data

Lippert, Lynn, 1942–
    Clinical kinesiology and anatomy/Lynn S. Lippert.—4th ed.
        p. ; cm.
    Rev. ed. of: Clinical kinesiology for physical therapist assistants.
    Includes bibliographical references and index.
    ISBN-13: 978-0-8036-1243-3
    ISBN-10: 0-8036-1243-5
  1. Kinesiology. 2. Physical therapy assistants.
    [DNLM: 1. Kinesiology, Applied. 2. Movement. 3. Musculoskeletal System—anatomy & histology.
  4. Physical Therapy Modalities. WE 103 L765c 2006] I. Lippert, Lynn, 1942- Clinical kinesiology for physical therapist assistants. II. Title.
    QP303.L53 2006
    612.7'6–dc22

                                        2006003745

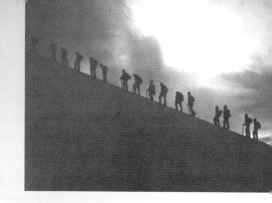

Dedication

I have been blessed by the love and support of a true friend and colleague, whose insights, knowledge, and truthfulness have been invaluable in the writing of this book. Sal Jepson dusted off her artistic talents to draw the original illustrations and helped get the original book off the "drawing board." Her continued support has made revisions of the book possible. One can have no greater friend.

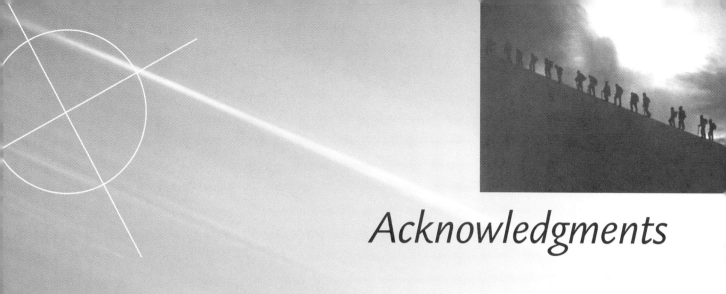

Acknowledgments

Like a child, it takes a village to create a book and see it through completion of its fourth edition. Sal Jepson drew most of the original illustrations. These illustrations continue to provide the basis for the current drawings. Don Davis, my physics guru, continues to look over my shoulder to ensure that the world of physics and biomechanics is accurately portrayed. Mimi Eick, PT helped 'brainstorm' many of the functional activities and clinical exercises, while Debbie Van Dover, Med, PT, gave helpful suggestions and allowed 'field testing' of them in her Kinesiology lab. Heather Hannam, PT, served as a resource for the TMJ chapter. The Mt. Hood Community College PT Assistant students were also most helpful with their feedback. Vanessa Gaerlan- Wang BA, PTA, gave assistance to the author and artist by demonstrating the various activities and exercises for the photo shoot.

I would like to extend my appreciation to Rob Craven, President, and the many people at F. A. Davis for their commitment to making this a textbook that will make us all proud. Margaret Biblis, Publisher, brought new energy and vision. Deborah Thorp, Content Development Manager, kept the wheels of production well oiled. The production team, consisting of Bob Butler, Production Manager, Michael Carcel, Illustration Coordinator, Carolyn O'Brien, Design Manager, Lisa Thompson, Copy Editor, have worked very hard under some rather difficult circumstances to bring this book to its highly polished state. Kim Harris, always a friendly voice, knows where everyone is at any given time and saw that my questions and phone calls were answered. A special thank-you goes to Peg Waltner, Developmental Editor. She has spent countless hours working with me to ensure the book's accuracy and success. She has also worked tirelessly with the illustrator.

My family has been most patient and understanding throughout this process. Without the support at home, I would not have had the time or energy. They did not always have an easy task.

So, to the fourth edition village, thank you one and all. Words cannot accurately express my feelings and appreciation. I couldn't have done it without you.

Reviewers

Marja P. Beaufait, MA, PT
Associate Professor
Physical Therapist Assistant Program
St. Petersburg College
St. Petersburg, Florida

Dolores B. Bertoti, MS, PT
Dean of Academic Advancement
Associate Professor
Center for Academic Advancement
Alvernia College
Reading, Pennsylvania

Wendy D. Bircher, MS, PT
Director
Physical Therapist Assistant Program
San Juan College
Farmington, New Mexico

Laurie Clute, MS, PT
Professor
Director of Physical Therapy Program
Allied Health Department
New Hampshire Community
  Technical College
Claremont, New Hampshire

Jamie Duley, MS, PT
Instructor
Health and Wellness Department
Delta College
Freeland, Michigan

Sandra Froehling, OTR/L
Instructor
Occupational Therapy Assistant Department
Anoka-Hennepin Technical College
Anoka, Minnesota

Christine Kowalski, EdD, PTA
Department Chair of Health Science
Physical Therapy Assistant Program Director
Montana State University–Great Falls
College of Technology
Cascade, Montana

Becky Robler, MEd, OTR
Instructor/Director of Health Careers
  Success Program
Occupational Therapy/Health Professions
  Department
Pueblo Community College
Pueblo, Colorado

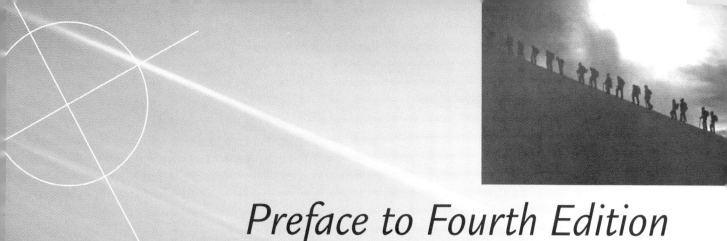

Preface to Fourth Edition

Fifteen years ago, this project began as an attempt to provide a basic Kinesiology and Anatomy text to Physical Therapist Assistant students. Jean-Francois Vilain, publisher at F.A. Davis Company recognized the need and published this as the first textbook written for the Physical Therapist Assistant. The narrow title, *Clinical Kinesiology for Physical Therapist Assistants* was chosen to try to encourage others to write much-needed books and publishers to publish them. While many books have been written, there remain content areas lacking appropriate texts, and where students would benefit if they existed. Our work here is clearly not done.

However, the publisher felt that the time had come to change the title of this text to *Clinical Kinesiology and Anatomy,* opening the market to other disciplines. However, this text remains a basic textbook. Students who want a basic understanding of kinesiology and anatomy with a clinical perspective will find this text of great value. Examples, activities, and exercises are not focused solely on physical therapy, but have been broadened to be of use to those in occupational therapy, athletic training, massage therapy, and other fields needing this basic level of understanding.

As with previous editions, the emphasis is on basic kinesiology and anatomy. Simple, easy-to-follow descriptions and explanations remain the core of this book. Clinical relevance has been increased by the addition of the following: (1) Brief definitions and descriptions of common pathologies in terms of anatomical location; (2) In addition to general anatomy review, questions involving the analysis of functional activities and clinical exercises.

Not all disciplines may need all of the information within this text. Some disciplines may not place emphasis on the arthrokinematic features, for example. The book is written so that the arthrokinematic chapter can be omitted from study. Examples and questions regarding this subject matter can also be omitted without the student being at a disadvantage in terms of understanding other subject matter. The chapters dedicated to the various joints begin with the upper extremity and proceed to the axial skeleton, and then to the lower extremity. However, because these chapters are essentially self-standing, the order in which they are read can easily be changed. One could begin with the lower extremity, or with the axial skeleton and not lose understanding.

There are several textbooks that give a more in-depth analysis of the subject matter; however, *Clinical Kinesiology and Anatomy* is intended to provide an easy-to-understand basic introduction.

Lynn S. Lippert

Preface to the Third Edition

There are some changes and several new faces in this revision, however, the depth and scope of the text remains the same. It has been satisfying and rewarding to continually hear that one of the main strengths of the book is the simple, easy-to-follow descriptions and explanations.

The muscular system has been expanded to include an explanation of open and closed kinetic chain principles. The gait chapter now includes an explanation of many common pathological gait patterns. Several illustrations have been redrawn for greater clarity.

Five new chapters have been added. A chapter on basic biomechanics provides explanations and examples of the various biomechanical principles commonly used in physical therapy. Chapters describing the temporomandibular joint and the pelvic girdle have been added for those who want a basic description of those joints' structure and function. Normal posture and arthrokinematics, which were included in the

Kinesiology Laboratory Manual for Physical Therapist Assistants, have been described and expanded upon in this revision.

There is not universal agreement within the physical therapy community regarding the scope of practice of the physical therapist assistant. It is generally felt that joint mobilization is not an entry-level skill. I do not disagree with this. However, PT assistants are exposed to and involved in patient treatments where these skills are utilized. For this reason, they need basic understanding of the terminology and principles, and this text provides them with this information.

This revision of *Clinical Kinesiology for Physical Therapist Assistants* is the result of many suggestions from educators, students, and clinicians. The profession needs good textbooks that cover many additional areas of physical therapist assistant education. I hope that by its fourth edition, this text will have its place on the bookshelf along with those yet-to-be-written texts.

Lynn S. Lippert

Preface to the Second Edition

Most of the people who write and lecture on anatomy agree on what is there and where it is, although they do not always agree on what to call it. Kinesiologists tend to agree that motion occurs, but they certainly do not agree on what muscles cause a motion or on the relative importance of each muscle's action in that motion.

In *Clinical Kinesiology for Physical Therapist Assistants,* the emphasis is on basic kinesiology. In describing joint motion and muscle action, I have focused on describing the commonly agreed-on prime movers, using the terminology most widely accepted within the discipline of physical therapy. Many textbooks exist that describe in greater detail various motions and muscles, in both normal and pathological conditions.

For more in-depth analysis, the student should consult these books.

The idea of writing a kinesiology textbook for physical therapist assistant students has been around for several years. Somehow, time constraints and the pressures of other projects always got in the way. When educators gathered to discuss issues regarding physical therapist assistant education, lack of appropriate textbooks was always high on the list of problems. It became evident that if such textbooks were to exist, the physical therapist assistant educators were the ones who needed to write them.

Clinical Kinesiology for Physical Therapist Assistants is the result of those discussions. I hope that it is only the first of many textbooks that emphasize physical therapist assistant education.

Lynn S. Lippert

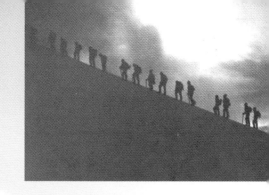

Contents

PART I
Basic Clinical Kinesiology and Anatomy

CHAPTER 1   Basic Information 3

CHAPTER 2   Skeletal System 11

CHAPTER 3   Articular System 17

CHAPTER 4   Arthrokinematics 27

CHAPTER 5   Muscular System 35

CHAPTER 6   Nervous System 49

CHAPTER 7   Basic Biomechanics 71

PART II
*Clinical Kinesiology and Anatomy
of the Upper Extremities*

CHAPTER 8   Shoulder Girdle 93

CHAPTER 9   Shoulder Joint 107

CHAPTER 10   Elbow Joint 121

CHAPTER 11   Wrist Joint 133

CHAPTER 12   Hand 143

PART III
*Clinical Kinesiology and Anatomy
of the Trunk*

CHAPTER 13   Temporomandibular Joint 169

CHAPTER 14   Neck and Trunk 183

CHAPTER 15   Respiratory System 205

CHAPTER 16   Pelvic Girdle 217

PART IV
*Clinical Kinesiology and Anatomy
of the Lower Extremities*

CHAPTER 17   Hip 231

CHAPTER 18   Knee 251

CHAPTER 19   Ankle Joint and Foot 265

PART V
*Clinical Kinesiology and Anatomy
of the Body*

CHAPTER 20   Posture 289

CHAPTER 21   Gait 299

Bibliography 317

Answers to Review Questions 321

Index 337

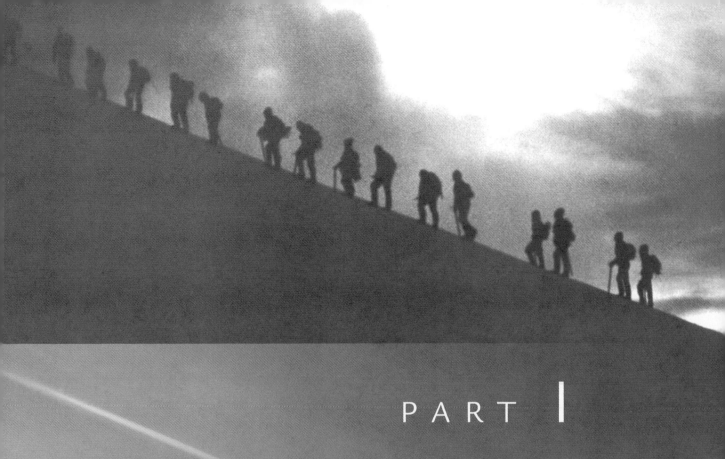

PART I

Basic Clinical Kinesiology and Anatomy

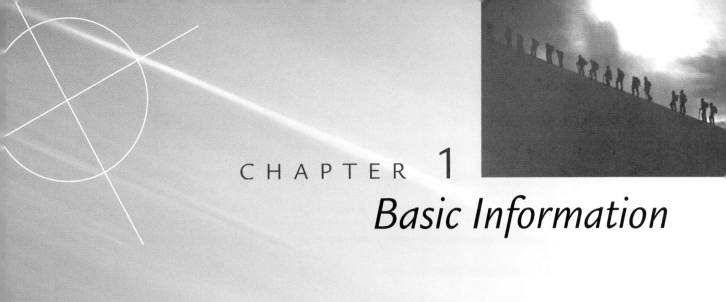

CHAPTER 1
Basic Information

Descriptive Terminology

Types of Motion

Joint Movements (Osteokinematics)

Review Questions

By definition, **kinesiology** is the study of movement. However, this definition is too general to be of much use. Kinesiology brings together the fields of anatomy, physiology, physics, and geometry, and relates them to human movement. Thus, kinesiology utilizes principles of mechanics, musculoskeletal anatomy, and neuromuscular physiology.

Mechanical principles that relate directly to the human body are used in the study of **biomechanics.** Because we may use a ball, racket, crutch, prosthesis, or some other implement, their biomechanical interaction must be considered as well. This may involve looking at the *static* (nonmoving) and/or *dynamic* (moving) *systems* associated with various activities. Dynamic systems can be divided into kinetics and kinematics. **Kinetics** are those forces causing movement, whereas **kinematics** are those time, space, and mass aspects of a moving system. These and other basic biomechanical concepts will be discussed in Chapter 7.

This text will give most emphasis to the musculoskeletal anatomy components, which are considered the key to understanding and being able to apply the other components. Many students are subject to negative thoughts at the mere mention of the word *kinesiology.* Their eyes glaze over, and their brains freeze. Perhaps, based on past experience with anatomy, they feel that their only hope is mass memorization. However, this may prove to be an overwhelming task with no long-term memory gain.

As you proceed through this text, you should keep in mind a few simple concepts. First, the human body is arranged in a very logical way. Like all aspects of life, there are exceptions. Sometimes the logic of these exceptions is apparent, and sometimes the logic may be apparent only to some higher being. Whichever is the case, you should note the exception and move on.

Second, if you have a good grasp of descriptive terminology and can visualize the concept or feature, then strict memorization is not necessary. For example, if you know generally where the patella is located and what the structures are around it, you can accurately describe its location using your own words. You do not need to memorize someone else's words to be correct.

By keeping in mind some of the basic principles affecting muscles, understanding individual muscle function need not be so mind-boggling. If you know (1) what motions a particular joint allows, (2) that a muscle must span a particular joint surface to cause a certain motion, (3) what that muscle's line of pull is, then (4) you will know the particular action(s) of a specific muscle. For example, (1) the elbow allows only flexion and extension. (2) A muscle must span the joint anteriorly to flex and posteriorly to extend. (3) The biceps brachii is a vertical muscle on the anterior surface of the arm. (4) Therefore, the biceps flexes the elbow.

Yes, kinesiology can be understood by mere mortals. Its study can even be enjoyable. There is no natural or human-made law that says otherwise. A word of caution should be given: Like exercising, it is better to study in small amounts several times a week than to study for a long period in one session before the exam.

Descriptive Terminology

The human body is active and constantly moving; therefore, it is subject to frequent changes in position. The relationship of the various body parts to each other also changes. To be able to describe the organization of the human body, it is necessary to use some arbitrary position as a starting point from which movement or location of structures can be described. This is known as the **anatomical position** (Fig. 1-1A) and is described as the human body standing in an upright position, eyes facing forward, feet parallel and close together, arms at the sides of the body with the palms facing forward. Although the position of the forearm and hands is not a natural one, it does allow for accurate description. The **fundamental position** (Fig. 1-1B) is the same as the anatomical position except that the palms face the sides of the body. This position is often used in discussing rotation of the upper extremity.

Specific terms are used to describe the location of a structure and its position relative to other structures (Fig. 1-2). **Medial** refers to a location or position toward the midline, and **lateral** refers to location or position farther from the midline. For example, the

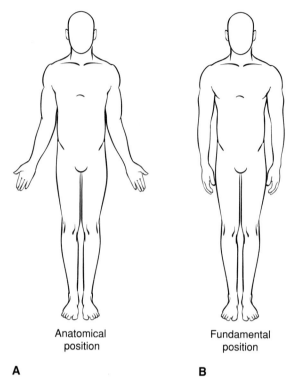

Anatomical position

Fundamental position

A   **B**

Figure 1-1. Descriptive positions.

ulna is on the medial side of the forearm, and the radius is lateral to the ulna.

Anterior refers to the front of the body or to a position closer to the front than another. **Posterior** refers to the back of the body or to a position more to the

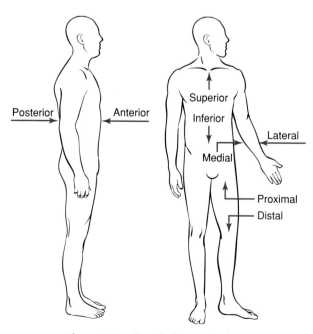

Figure 1-2. Descriptive terminology.

back. For example, the sternum is anterior on the chest wall, and the scapula is posterior. **Ventral** is a *synonym* (word with the same meaning) of anterior, and **dorsal** is a synonym of posterior; anterior and posterior are more commonly used in kinesiology. *Front* and *back* also refer to the surfaces of the body, but these are considered lay terms and are not widely used by healthcare professionals.

Distal and proximal are used to describe locations on the extremities. **Distal** means away from the trunk, and **proximal** means toward the trunk. For example, the humeral head is located on the proximal end of the humerus. The elbow is proximal to the wrist but distal to the shoulder.

Superior is used to indicate the location of a body part that is above another or to refer to the upper surface of an organ or structure. **Inferior** indicates that a body part is below another or refers to the lower surface of an organ or structure. For example, the body of the sternum is superior to the xiphoid process but inferior to the manubrium. Sometimes people use **cranial** or *cephalad* (from the word root *cephal,* meaning "head") to refer to a position or structure close to the head. **Caudal** (from the word root for "tail") refers to a position or structure closer to the feet. For example, cauda *equina,* which means "horse's tail," is the inferior end of the spinal cord. Cranial and caudal are terms like dorsal and ventral that are best used to describe positions on a quadruped (four-legged animal). Humans are bipeds or two-legged animals. You can see that if the dog in Figure 1-3 were to stand on its hind legs, dorsal would become posterior and cranial would become superior, and so on.

A structure may be described as **superficial** or **deep** depending on its relative depth. For example, in describing the layers of the abdominal muscles, the external oblique is deep to the rectus abdominis but superficial to the internal oblique. Another example is the scalp being described as superficial to the skull.

Types of Motion

Linear motion, also called *translatory motion,* occurs in more or less a straight line from one location to another. All the parts of the object move the same distance, in the same direction, and at the same time. If this movement occurs in a straight line, it is called **rectilinear motion,** such as the motion of a child sledding down a hill (Fig. 1-4). If the movement occurs not in a straight line but in a curved path, it is called **curvilinear motion.** Figure 1-5 demonstrates the path a diver takes, after leaving the diving board, until entering the water. Other examples of this type of motion are the path of a ball, a javelin thrown across a field, or the earth's orbit around the sun.

Movement of an object about a fixed point is called **angular motion,** also known as *rotatory motion* (Fig. 1-6). All the parts of the object move through the same angle, in the same direction, and at the same time. They do not move the same distance. When a person flexes the elbow, the hand travels farther through space than does the wrist or forearm.

It is not uncommon to see both types of movement occurring at the same time, the entire object moving in a linear fashion and the individual parts moving in an angular fashion. In Figure 1-7, the person's whole body

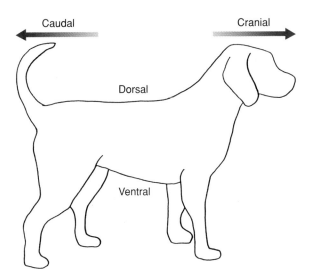

Figure 1-3. Descriptive terminology for a quadruped.

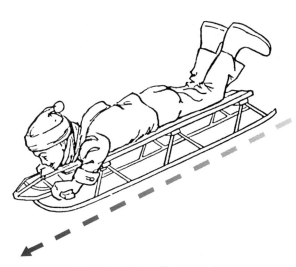

Figure 1-4. Rectilinear motion.

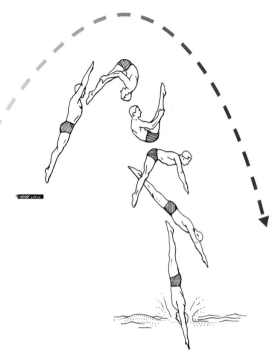

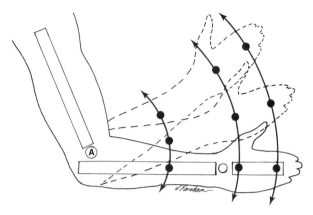

Figure 1-6. Angular motion. (From Norkin, CC, and Levangie, PK: Joint Structure and Function, ed 3. FA Davis, Philadelphia, 2001, p 3, with permission.)

Figure 1-5. Curvilinear motion. (Adapted from Jensen, CR, and Schultz, GW: Applied Kinesiology. McGraw-Hill, New York, 1970, p 200, with permission.)

attached to the scapula, is angular and gets its angular motion from the sternoclavicular joint.

moves across the room in the wheelchair (linear motion), while individual joints, such as the shoulders, elbows, and wrists, rotate about their axes (angular motion). If the individual were walking, the whole body would be exhibiting linear motion, while the hips, knees, and ankles would be exhibiting angular motion. For the ball to travel in its curvilinear path, it must be thrown. Thus, the upper extremity joints of the person throwing the ball move in an angular direction.

Generally speaking, most movement within the body is angular; movement outside the body tends to be linear. Exceptions to this statement can be found. For example, the movement of the scapula in elevation/depression and protraction/retraction is essentially linear. However, the movement of the clavicle, which is

Joint Movements (Osteokinematics)

Joints move in many different directions. As will be discussed, movement occurs around joint axes and through joint planes. The following terms are used to describe the various joints movements that occur at synovial joints (Fig. 1-8). Synovial joints are freely movable joints where most joint motion occurs. These joints are discussed in more detail in Chapter 3. This type of joint motion is also called **osteokinematics.** This deals with the relationship of the *movement of bones around a joint axis* (e.g., humerus moving on scapula), as opposed to **arthrokinematics,** which deals with the relationship of *joint surface movement* (humeral head's movement within glenoid fossa of scapula). This will be discussed in more detail in Chapter 4.

Flexion is the bending movement of one bone on another, causing a decrease in the joint angle. Usually

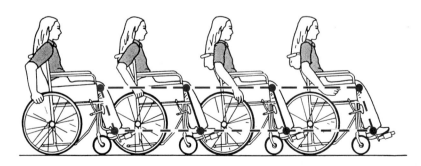

Figure 1-7. Combination of linear and angular motion. (From Hay, JG, and Reid, JG: The Anatomical and Mechanical Bases of Human Motion. Prentice-Hall, Englewood Cliffs, NJ, 1982, p 116, with permission.)

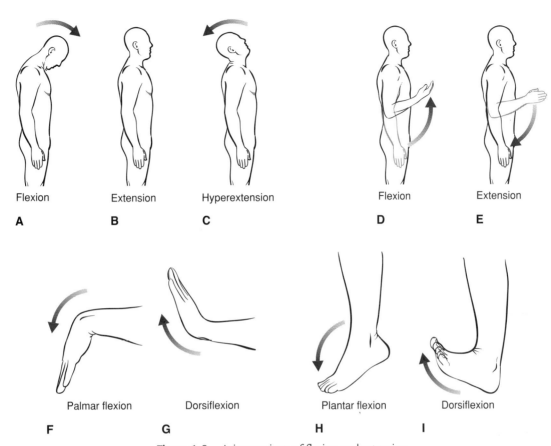

Figure 1-8.   Joint motions of flexion and extension.

this occurs between anterior surfaces of articulating bones. In the case of the neck, flexion is a "bowing down" motion (Fig. 1-8A). However, with the knee, the posterior surfaces approximate each other, causing flexion. The hip can be viewed as flexing on the trunk when the lower extremity is the moving component. When the lower extremities are fixed and the trunk becomes the moving component, the trunk flexes. Actually, whether flexion represents an increase or decrease in joint angle will depend upon your point of reference. As previously described, flexion begins at 180 degrees (full extension) and moves toward zero degrees; thus, it is a decrease in the joint angle. However, when performing a goniometric measurement of elbow flexion, one would begin in anatomical position (full extension), which is considered zero. The amount of flexion increased toward 180 degrees. In this case, flexion would represent an increase in the joint angle (Fig. 1-8D).

Conversely, **extension** is the straightening movement of one bone from another causing an increase of the joint angle. This motion usually returns the body part to the anatomical position after it has been flexed (Fig. 1-8B,E).

Hyperextension is the continuation of extension beyond the anatomical position (Fig. 1-8C). Flexion at the wrist may be called **palmar flexion** (Fig. 1-8F), and flexion at the ankle may be called **plantar flexion** (Fig. 1-8H). Extension at both wrist and ankle joints may be called **dorsiflexion** (Fig 1-8G,I).

Abduction is movement away from the midline of the body (Fig. 1-9A), and **adduction** (Fig. 1-9B) is movement toward the midline. Exceptions to this midline definition are the fingers and toes. The reference point for the fingers is the middle finger. Movement away from the middle finger is abduction. It should be noted that the middle finger abducts (to the right and to the left) but adducts only as a return movement from abduction to the midline. The point of reference for the toes is the second toe. Similar to the middle finger, the second toe abducts to the right and the left but does not adduct except as a return movement from abduction.

When the shoulder joint is abducted to 90 degrees and then moved backward, it is called **horizontal abduction** (Fig. 1-9C). If the shoulder is adducted from this 90-degree position, it is called **horizontal adduction** (Fig. 1-9D).

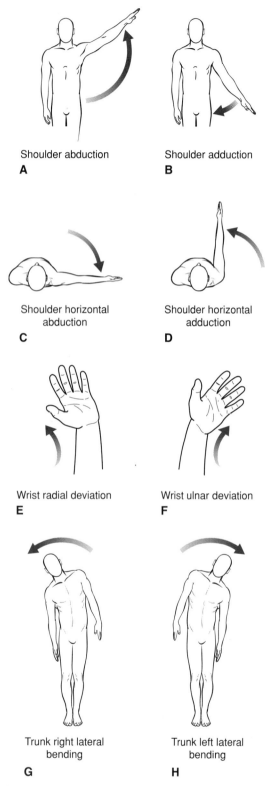

Shoulder abduction
A

Shoulder adduction
B

Shoulder horizontal abduction
C

Shoulder horizontal adduction
D

Wrist radial deviation
E

Wrist ulnar deviation
F

Trunk right lateral bending
G

Trunk left lateral bending
H

Figure 1-9.   Joint motions of abduction and adduction.

Terms more commonly used to refer to wrist abduction and adduction are *radial* and *ulnar deviation*. When the hand moves laterally, or toward the thumb side, it is **radial deviation** (Fig. 1-9E). When the hand moves medially from the anatomical position toward the little finger side at the wrist, it is **ulnar deviation** (Fig. 1-9F).

When the trunk moves sideways, the term **lateral bending** is used. The trunk can laterally bend to the right or to the left (Fig. 1-9G,H). If the right side of the trunk bends, moving the shoulder toward the right hip, it is called right lateral bending. The term *lateral flexion* is sometimes used to describe this sideward motion. However, because this term is easily confused with *flexion*, it will not be used.

Circumduction is motion that describes a circular, cone-shaped pattern. It involves a combination of four joint motions: (1) flexion, (2) abduction, (3) extension, and (4) adduction. For example, if the shoulder were to move in a circle, the hand would move in a much larger circle. The entire arm would move in a cone-shaped pattern (Fig. 1-10).

Rotation is movement of a bone or part around its longitudinal axis. If the anterior surface moves inward toward the midline, it is called **medial rotation** (Fig. 1-11A). This is sometimes referred to as *internal rotation*. Conversely, if the anterior surface moves outward away from the midline, it is called **lateral rotation** (Fig. 1-11B), or *external rotation*. The neck and trunk rotate either to the right or left side (Fig. 1-11C,D). Visualize the neck rotating as you look over your right shoulder. This would be "right neck rotation."

Rotation of the forearm is referred to as supination and pronation. In anatomical position the forearm is

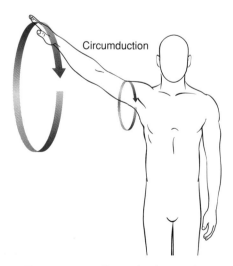

Circumduction

Figure 1-10.   Circumduction motion.

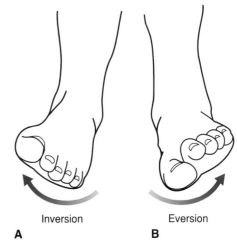

Figure 1-12.   Inversion and eversion.

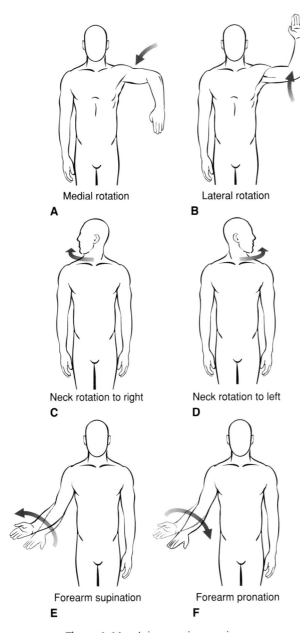

Figure 1-11.   Joint rotation motions.

is mostly a linear movement along a plane parallel to the ground and away from the midline (Fig. 1-13A), and **retraction** is mostly a linear movement in the same plane but toward the midline (Fig. 1-13B). Protraction of the shoulder girdle moves the scapula away from the midline as does protraction of the jaw, whereas retraction in both of these cases returns the body part toward the midline, or back to anatomical position.

in **supination** (Fig. 1-11E). This faces the palm of the hand forward, or anteriorly. In **pronation** (Fig. 1-11F), the palm is facing backward, or posteriorly. When the elbow is flexed, the "palm up" position refers to supination and "palm down" is pronation.

The following are terms used to describe motions specific to certain joints. **Inversion** is moving the sole of the foot inward at the ankle (Fig. 1-12A), and **eversion** is the outward movement (Fig. 1-12B). **Protraction**

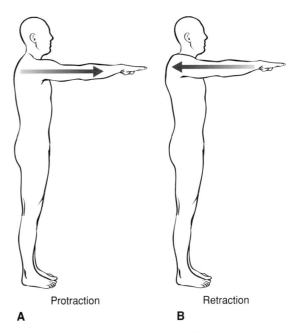

Figure 1-13.   Protraction and retraction.

Review Questions

1. Using descriptive terminology, complete the following:
   a. The sternum is _____ to the vertebral column.
   b. The calcaneus is on the _____ portion of the foot.
   c. The hip is _____ to the chest.
   d. The femur is _____ to the tibia.
   e. The radius is on the _____ side of the forearm.

2. When a football is kicked through the goal posts, what type of motion is being demonstrated by the football? By the kicker?

3. Looking at a spot on the ceiling directly over your head involves what joint motion?

4. Putting your hand in your back pocket involves what shoulder joint rotation?

5. Picking up a pencil on the floor beside your chair involves what trunk joint motion?

6. Putting your right ankle on your left knee involves what type of hip rotation?

7. What is the only difference between *anatomical* position and *fundamental* position?

8. If you place your hand on the back of a dog, that is referred to as what surface? If you place your hand on the back of a person, that is referred to as what surface?

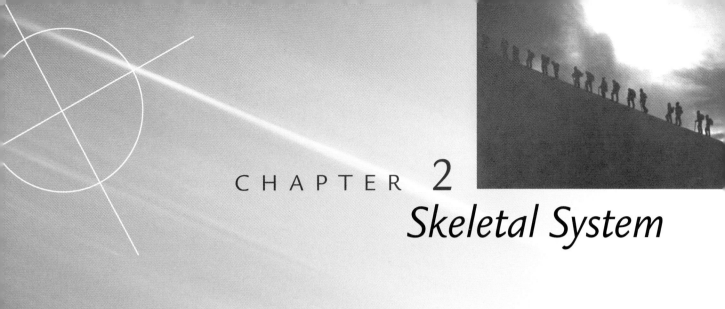

CHAPTER 2

Skeletal System

Functions of the Skeleton

Types of Skeletons

Composition of Bone

Structure of Bone

Types of Bones

Review Questions

Functions of the Skeleton

The skeletal system, which is made up of numerous bones, is the rigid framework of the human body. It gives support and shape to the body. It protects vital organs such as the brain, spinal cord, and heart. It assists in movement by providing a rigid structure for muscle attachment and leverage. The skeletal system also manufactures blood cells in various locations. The main sites of blood formation are the ilium, vertebra, sternum, and ribs. This formation occurs mostly in flat bones. Calcium and other mineral salts are stored throughout all osseous tissue of the skeletal system.

Types of Skeletons

The bones of the body are grouped into two main categories: axial and appendicular. The **axial skeleton** forms the upright part of the body. It consists of approximately 80 bones of the head, thorax, and trunk (Fig. 2-1). The **appendicular skeleton** attaches to the axial skeleton and contains the 126 bones of the extremities (Fig. 2-2). There are 206 bones in the body. Individuals may have additional sesamoid bones, such as in the flexor tendons of the great toe and of the thumb.

Table 2-1 lists the bones of the adult human body. The sacrum, coccyx, and hip bones are each made up of several bones fused together. In the hip bone, these fused bones are known as the *ilium, ischium,* and *pubis.*

Composition of Bone

Bones can be considered organs because they are made up of several different types of tissue (fibrous, cartilaginous,

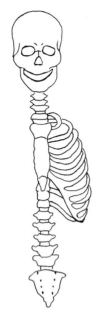

Figure 2-1.   Axial skeleton.

osseous, nervous, and vascular), and they function as integral parts of the skeletal system.

Bone is made up of one-third *organic* (living) material and two-thirds *inorganic* (nonliving) material. The organic material gives the bone elasticity, whereas the inorganic material provides hardness and strength, which makes bone opaque on an x-ray.

Compact bone makes up a hard, dense outer shell. It always completely covers bone and tends to be thick along the shaft and thin at the ends of long bones. It is also thick in the plates of the flat bones of the skull.

Cancellous bone is the porous and spongy inside portion called the *trabeculae,* which means "little beams" in Latin. They are arranged in a pattern that resists local stresses and strains. These trabeculae tend to be filled with marrow and make the bone lighter. Cancellous bone makes up most of the articular ends of bones.

Structure of Bone

The **epiphysis** is the area at each end of the diaphysis, and this area tends to be wider than the shaft (Fig. 2-3). In adult bone the epiphysis is osseous, but in growing bone the epiphysis is cartilaginous material and is called the **epiphyseal plate.** Longitudinal growth occurs here through the manufacturing of new bone.

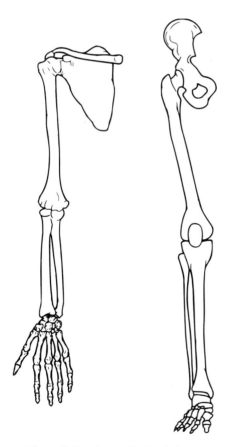

Figure 2-2.   Appendicular skeleton.

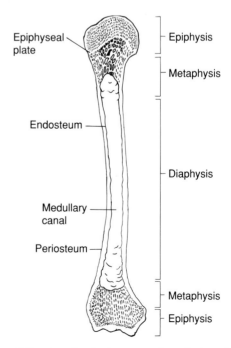

Figure 2-3.   Longitudinal cross section of a long bone.

Table 2-1	Bones of the Human Body		
	Single	**Paired**	**Multiple**
Axial Skeleton			
Cranium (8)	Frontal Sphenoid Ethmoid Occipital	Parietal Temporal	None
Face (14)	Mandible Vomer	Maxilla Zygomatic Lacrimal Inferior concha Palatine Nasal	None
Other (7)	Hyoid	Ear ossicles (3)	None
Vertebral column (26)	Sacrum (5)* Coccyx (3)*	None	Cervical (7) Thoracic (12) Lumbar (5)
Thorax (25)	Sternum	Ribs (12 Pairs) True: 7 False: 3 Floating: 2	None
Appendicular Skeleton			
Upper extremity (64)	None	Scapula Clavicle Humerus Ulna Radius	Carpals (8) Metacarpals (5) Phalanges (14)
Lower extremity (62)	None	Hip (3)* Femur Tibia Fibula Patella	Tarsals (7) Metatarsals (5) Phalanges (14)

*Denotes bones that are fused together.

The **diaphysis** is the main shaft of bone. It is made up mostly of compact bone, which gives it great strength. Its center, the **medullary canal,** is hollow, which, among other features, decreases the weight of the bone. This canal contains marrow and provides passage for nutrient arteries. The **endosteum** is a membrane that lines the medullary canal. It contains **osteoclasts,** which are mainly responsible for bone resorption.

In long bones, the flared part at each end of the diaphysis is called the **metaphysis.** It is made up mostly of cancellous bone and functions to support the epiphysis.

Periosteum is the thin fibrous membrane covering all of the bone except the articular surfaces that are covered with hyaline cartilage. The periosteum contains nerve and blood vessels that are important in providing nourishment, promoting growth in diameter of immature bone, and repairing the bone. It also serves as an attachment point for tendons and ligaments.

On an x-ray, a growing bone will show a distinct line between the epiphyseal plate and the rest of the bone (Fig. 2-4A). Because this line does not exist in the normal adult bone, its absence indicates that bone growth has stopped (Fig. 2-4B).

There are two types of epiphyses found in children whose bones are still growing (Fig. 2-5). A **pressure epiphysis** is located at the ends of long bones where they receive pressure from the opposing bone making

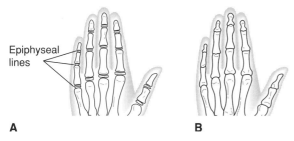

A   **B**

Figure 2-4.   Epiphyseal lines in the hand bones of a child *(A)* and an adult *(B)*.

up that joint. This is where growth of long bones occurs. The proximal head of the femur is a common site for problems at the pressure epiphysis, such as *Legg-Calvé-Perthes disease* and *slipped femoral capital epiphysis*. A **traction epiphysis** is located where tendons attach to bones and are subjected to a pulling, or traction, force. Examples would be the greater and lesser trochanters of the femur and tibial tuberosity. Overuse can cause irritation and inflammation at this epiphysis. A common condition at the traction epiphysis of the tibial tuberosity in children whose bones are still growing is called *Osgood-Schlatter disease*. Problems at these pressure and traction epiphyses usually exist only during the bone-growing years and not once the epiphyses have fused and bone growth stops.

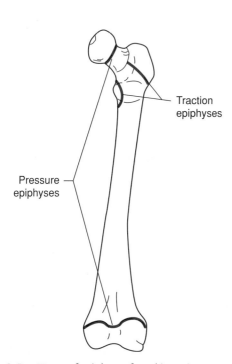

Traction
epiphyses

Pressure
epiphyses

Figure 2-5.   Types of epiphyses found in an immature bone.

Types of Bones

Long bones are so named because their length is greater than their width (Fig. 2-6A). They are the largest bones in the body and make up most of the appendicular skeleton. Long bones are basically tubular shaped with a shaft (diaphysis) and two bulbous ends (epiphysis). The wide part of the shaft nearest the epiphysis is called the metaphysis (see Fig. 2-3). The diaphysis consists of compact bone surrounding the marrow cavity. The metaphysis and epiphysis consist of cancellous bone covered by a thin layer of compact bone. Over the articular surfaces of the epiphysis is a thin layer of hyaline cartilage. Bone growth occurs at the epiphysis.

Short bones tend to have more equal dimensions of height, length, and width, giving them a cubical shape (Fig. 2-6B). They have a great deal of articular surface and, unlike long bones, usually articulate with more than one bone. Their composition is similar to long bones: they have a thin layer of compact bone covering cancellous bone, which has a marrow cavity in

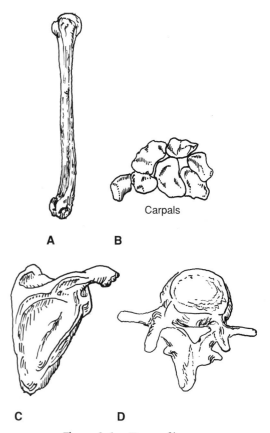

Carpals

A   **B**

C   **D**

Figure 2-6.   Types of bones.

Table 2-2	Types of Bones		
	Appendicular Skeleton		
Type	**Upper Extremity**	**Lower Extremity**	**Axial Skeleton**
Long bones	Clavicle	Femur	None
	Humerus	Fibula	
	Radius	Tibia	
	Ulna	Metatarsals	
	Metacarpals	Phalanges	
	Phalanges		
Short bones	Carpals	Tarsals	None
Flat bones	Scapula	Hip	Cranial bones (frontal, parietal)
		Patella	Ribs
			Sternum
Irregular bones	None	None	Vertebrae
			Cranial bones (sphenoid, ethmoid)
			Sacrum
			Coccyx
			Mandible, facial bones

the middle. Examples of short bones include the bones of the wrist (carpals) and ankle (tarsals).

Flat bones have a very broad surface but are not very thick. They tend to have a curved surface rather than a flat one (Fig. 2-6C). They are made up of two layers of compact bone with cancellous bone and marrow in between. The ilium and scapula are good examples of flat bones.

Irregular bones have a variety of mixed shapes, as their name implies (Fig. 2-6D). Examples are bones such as the vertebrae and sacrum that do not fit into the other categories. They are also composed of cancellous bone and marrow encased in a thin layer of compact bone.

Sesamoid bones, which resemble the shape of sesame seeds, are small bones located where tendons cross the ends of long bones in the extremities. They develop within the tendon and protect it from excessive wear. For example, the tendon of the flexor hallucis longus spans the bottom (plantar surface) of the foot and attaches on the great toe. If this tendon were not protected in some way at the ball of the foot, it would constantly be stepped on. Mother Nature is too clever to allow this to happen. Sesamoid bones are located on either side of the tendon near the head of the first metatarsal, providing a protective "groove"

for the tendon to pass through this weight-bearing area.

Sesamoid bones also change the angle of attachment of a tendon. The patella can be considered a sesamoid bone because it is encased in the quadriceps tendon and improves the mechanical advantage of the quadriceps muscle. As previously mentioned, sesamoid bones are also found in the flexor tendons that pass posteriorly into the foot on either side of the ankle. In the upper extremity they are found in the flexor tendons of the thumb near the metacarpophalangeal and interphalangeal joints. Occasionally, a sesamoid bone is located near the metacarpophalangeal joint of the index and little fingers.

Table 2-2 summarizes the types of bones of the axial and appendicular skeletons. It should be noted that there are no long or short bones in the axial skeleton, and there are no irregular bones in the appendicular skeleton. Sesamoid bones are not included in Table 2-2 because they are considered accessory bones and their shape and number vary greatly.

When looking at various bones, you will see holes, depressions, ridges, bumps, grooves, and various other kinds of markings. Each of these markings serves different purposes. Table 2-3 describes the different kinds of bone markings and their purposes.

Table 2-3   Bone Markings

Depressions and Openings

Marking	Description	Examples
1. Foramen	Hole through which blood vessels, nerves, and ligaments pass	Vertebral foramen of cervical vertebra *Foramen magnum*
2. Fossa	Hollow or depression	Glenoid fossa of scapula
3. Groove	Ditchlike groove containing a tendon or blood vessel	Bicipital (intercondylar) groove of humerus
4. Meatus	Canal or tubelike opening in a bone	External auditory meatus
5. Sinus	Air-filled cavity within a bone	Frontal sinus in frontal bone

Projections or Processes That Fit into Joints

Marking	Description	Examples
1. Condyle	Rounded knuckle-like projection	Medial condyle of femur, *Lateral condyle humerus*
2. Eminence	Projecting, prominent part of bone	Intercondylar eminence, tibia
3. Facet	Flat or shallow articular surface	Articular facet of rib, *Superior facet of the 12th thoracic vertebra*
4. Head	Rounded articular projection beyond a narrow necklike portion of bone	Femoral head, *Fibular Head*

Projections/Processes That Attach Tendons, Ligaments, and Other Connective Tissue

Marking	Description	Examples
1. Crest	Sharp ridge or border	Iliac crest of hip
2. Epicondyle	Prominence above or on a condyle	Medial epicondyle of humerus, *Lateral epicondyle of the femur*
3. Line	Less prominent ridge	Linea aspera of femur
4. Spine	Long, thin projection (spinous process)	Scapular spine
5. Tubercle	Small, rounded projection	Greater tubercle of humerus
6. Tuberosity	Large, rounded projection	Ischial tuberosity, *tuberosity of the 5th metatarsal*
7. Trochanter	Very large prominence for muscle attachment	Greater trochanter of femur

Review Questions

1. What are the differences between the axial and appendicular skeletons?

2. Give an example of compact bone and one of cancellous bone.

3. Which is heavier, compact bone or cancellous bone? Why?

4. What type of bone is mainly involved in an individual's growth in height? In what portion of the bone does this growth occur?

5. What is the purpose of sesamoid bone?

6. Name the bone markings that can be classified as:
   a. Depressions and openings
   b. Projections or processes that fit into joints
   c. Projections or processes that attach connective tissue

Classify the following bone markings:

7. Bicipital groove

8. Humeral head

9. Acetabulum

10. Scapular spine

11. Supraspinous fossa

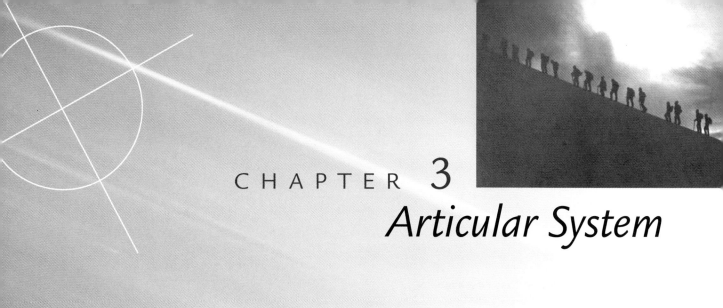

CHAPTER 3

Articular System

Types of Joints

Joint Structure

Common Pathological Terms

Planes and Axes

Degrees of Freedom

Review Questions

A joint is a connection between two bones. Although joints have several functions, perhaps the most important is to allow motion. Joints also help to bear the weight of the body and to provide stability. This stability may be mostly due to the shape of the bones making up the joint, as with the hip joint, or due to soft-tissue features, as seen in the shoulder and knee. Joints also contain synovial fluid, which lubricates the joint and nourishes the cartilage.

Types of Joints

A joint may allow a great deal of motion, as in the shoulder, or very little motion, as in the sternoclavicular joint. As with all differences, there are trade-offs. A joint that allows a great deal of motion will provide very little stability. Conversely, a joint that is quite stable tends to have little motion. There is often more than one term that can be used to describe the same joint. These terms tend to describe either the structure or amount of motion allowed.

A **fibrous joint** has a thin layer of fibrous periosteum between the two bones, as in the sutures of the skull. There are three types of fibrous joints: synarthrosis, syndesmosis, and gomphosis. A **synarthrosis,** or suture joint, has a thin layer of fibrous periosteum between the two bones, as in the sutures of the skull. The ends of the bones are shaped to allow them to interlock (Fig. 3-1A). With this type of joint there is essentially no motion between the bones. The purpose of this type of joint is to provide shape and strength. Another type of fibrous joint is a **syndesmosis,** or ligamentous joint. There is a great deal of fibrous tissue, such as ligaments and interosseous membranes, holding the joint together (Fig. 3-1B). A small amount of twisting or stretching

A. Synarthrosis (suture type)

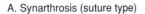

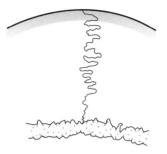

B. Syndesmosis (ligamentous type)

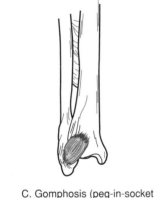

C. Gomphosis (peg-in-socket)

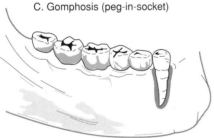

Figure 3-1.   Fibrous joints.

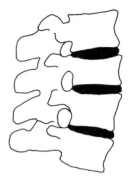

Figure 3-2.   Cartilaginous joint.

A **synovial joint** (Fig. 3-3) has no direct union between the bone ends. Instead, there is a cavity filled with synovial fluid contained within a sleevelike capsule. The outer layer of the capsule is made up of a strong fibrous tissue that holds the joint together. The inner layer is lined with a synovial membrane that secretes the synovial fluid. The articular surface is very smooth and covered with cartilage called *hyaline* or *articular cartilage.* The synovial joint is also called a **diarthrodial joint** because it allows free motion. It is not as stable as the other types of joints but does allow a great deal more motion. Table 3-1 provides a summary of the types of joints. The number of axes, the shape of the joint, and the type of motion allowed by the joint (Table 3-2) could further classify synovial, or diarthrodial, joints.

In a **nonaxial joint,** movement tends to be linear instead of angular (Fig. 3-4). The joint surfaces are relatively flat and glide over one another instead of one moving around the other. The motion that occurs between the carpal bones is an example of this type of motion.

movement can occur in this type of joint. The distal tibiofibular joint at the ankle and the distal radioulnar joint are examples. The third type of fibrous joint is called a **gomphosis,** which is Greek for "bolting together." This joint occurs between a tooth and the wall of its dental socket in the mandible and maxilla (Fig. 3-1C).

A **cartilaginous joint** (Fig. 3-2) has either hyaline cartilage or fibrocartilage between the two bones. The vertebral joints are examples of joints in which fibrocartilage (disks) are directly connecting the bones. The first sternocostal joint is an example of the direct connection made by hyaline cartilage. Cartilaginous joints are also called **amphiarthrodial joints** because they allow a small amount of motion, such as bending or twisting, and some compression. At the same time, these joints provide a great deal of stability.

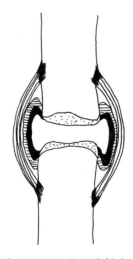

Figure 3-3.   Synovial joint.

Table 3-1	Joint Classification			
Type	**Motion**	**Structure**	**Example**	
Synarthrosis	None	Fibrous—suture	Bones in the skull	
Syndesmosis	Slight	Fibrous—ligamentous	Distal tibiofibular	
Gomphosis	None	Fibrous—peg-in-socket	Teeth in mandible and maxilla	
Amphiarthrosis	Little	Cartilaginous	Symphysis pubis, intervertebral disks	
Diarthrosis	Free	Synovial	Hip, elbow, knee	

Unlike most other types of diarthrodial joint motion, nonaxial motion occurs secondarily to other motion. For example, you can flex and extend your elbow without moving other joints; however, you cannot move your carpal bones by themselves. Motion of the carpals occurs when the wrist joint moves in either flexion and extension or abduction and adduction.

A **uniaxial joint** has angular motion occurring in one plane around one axis, much like a hinge. The elbow, or humeroulnar joint, is a good example of the convex shape of the humerus fitting into the concave-shaped ulna. The only motions possible are flexion and extension, which occur in the sagittal plane around the frontal axis. There are no other motions possible at this joint. The interphalangeal joints of the hand and foot also have this hinge motion (Fig. 3-5). The knee is a hinge joint, but this example must be clarified. During the last few degrees of extension, the femur rotates medially on the tibia. This rotation is not an active motion but the result of certain mechanical features present. Therefore, the knee is best classified as a uniaxial joint because it has *active* motion only around one axis.

Also at the elbow is the radioulnar joint, which demonstrates another type of uniaxial motion. The head of the radius pivots around the stationary ulna during pronation and supination of the forearm (Fig. 3-6). This pivot motion is in the transverse plane around the longitudinal axis. The motion of the atlantoaxial joint of C1 and C2 is also pivot motion. The first cervical vertebra *(atlas),* on which the head rests, rotates around the odontoid process of the second cervical vertebra *(axis).* This allows the head to rotate.

Biaxial joint motion, such as that found at the wrist, occurs in two different directions (Fig. 3-7). Flexion and extension occur around the frontal axis, and radial and ulnar deviation occur around the sagittal axis. This bidirectional motion also occurs at the metaphalangeal (MP) joints, where they are referred to as **condyloid** or *ellipsoidal* joints because of their shape.

The carpometacarpal (CMC) joint of the thumb is biaxial but differs somewhat from the condyloid joint. In this joint, the articular surface of each bone is concave in one direction and convex in the other. The bones fit together like a horseback rider in a saddle,

Table 3-2	Classification of Diarthroidal Joints			
Number of Axes	**Shape of Joint**	**Joint Motion**	**Example**	
Nonaxial	Irregular (plane)	Gliding	Intercarpals	
Uniaxial	Hinge	Flexion/extension	Elbow and knee	
	Pivot	Rotation	Atlas/axis, radius/ulna	
Biaxial	Condyloid	Flexion/extension, abduction/adduction	Wrist, MPs	
	Saddle	Flexion/extension, abduction/adduction, rotation (accessory)	Thumb, CMC	
Triaxial (multiaxial)	Ball and socket	Flexion/extension, abduction/adduction, rotation	Shoulder, hip	

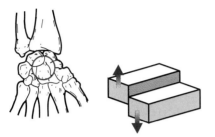

Figure 3-4.   Plane joint.

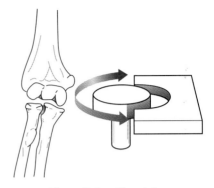

Figure 3-6.   Pivot joint.

which is why this joint is also descriptively called a **saddle joint** (Fig. 3-8).

The CMC joint is unlike the condyloid joint in that it allows a slight amount of rotation. Like the motion within the carpal bones, this rotation motion cannot occur by itself. If you try to rotate your thumb without also flexing and abducting, you find that you cannot do it. Yet, rotation does occur. Look at the direction to which the pad of your thumb is pointing when it is adducted. Abduct and flex your thumb and notice that the direction to which the pad is pointing has changed by approximately 90 degrees. This rotation has not occurred actively; rotation has occurred because of the shape of the joint. Therefore, although the CMC joint of the thumb is not a true biaxial joint because of the rotation allowed, it fits into this category best because the *active* motion allowed is around two axes.

With a **triaxial joint,** sometimes referred to as a *multiaxial joint,* motion occurs actively in all three axes (Fig. 3-9). The hip and shoulder allow motion in the frontal axis (flexion and extension), in the sagittal axis (abduction and adduction), and in the vertical axis (rotation). Obviously, triaxial joints allow more motion than any other type of joint. The triaxial joint is also referred to as a **ball-and-socket joint** because in the hip, for example, the ball-shaped femoral head fits into the concave socket of the acetabulum.

Joint Structure

There are many other structures associated with synovial joints (Fig. 3-10). First, there are **bones,** usually two, that articulate with each other. The amount of motion allowed at each joint and the direction of that motion are dictated by the shape of the bone ends and by the articular surface of each bone. For example, the shoulder joint has a smooth articular surface over most of the humeral head as well as over the glenoid fossa (shoulder socket). As a result, there is a great deal of shoulder motion, and that motion occurs in all directions. The knee, on the other hand, has a great deal of motion but in a specific direction. In examining the distal end of the femur, you will note that there are two ridges much like the rocker surfaces of a rocking chair. The proximal end of the tibia has two articular surfaces with a high area (intercondylar eminence) in between them. These articular surfaces allow a great deal of motion but, like the rocking chair, in only one direction.

The two bones of a joint are held together and supported by **ligaments,** which are bands of fibrous connective tissue. Ligaments also provide attachment for

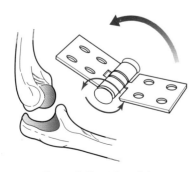

Figure 3-5.   Hinge joint.

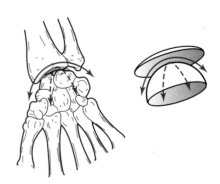

Figure 3-7.   Condyloid joint.

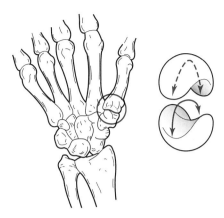

Figure 3-8. Saddle joint.

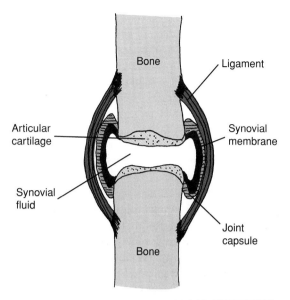

Figure 3-10. Synovial joint, longitudinal cross section.

cartilage, fascia, or, in some cases, muscle. Ligaments are flexible but not elastic. This flexibility is needed to allow joint motion, but the nonelasticity is needed to keep the bones in close approximation to each other and to provide some protection to the joint. In other words, ligaments prevent excessive joint movement. When ligaments surround a joint, they are called *capsular ligaments*.

In every synovial joint there is a joint **capsule** that surrounds and encases the joint and protects the articular surfaces of the bones (Fig. 3-11). In the shoulder joint, the capsule completely encases the joint, forming a partial vacuum that helps hold the head of the humerus against the glenoid fossa. In other joints, the capsule may not be as complete.

There are two layers to the capsule. There is the outer layer, which is made up of fibrous tissue and provides support and protection to the joint. This fibrous layer is

usually reinforced by ligaments. The inner layer is lined with a **synovial membrane,** which is a thick, vascular connective tissue that secretes synovial fluid. **Synovial fluid** is a thick, clear fluid, much like the white of an egg that lubricates the articular cartilage. This substance reduces friction and helps to keep the joint moving freely. It provides some shock absorption and is the major source of nutrition for articular cartilage.

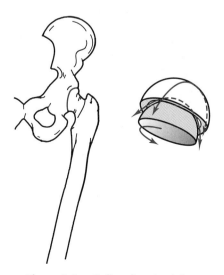

Figure 3-9. Ball-and-socket joint.

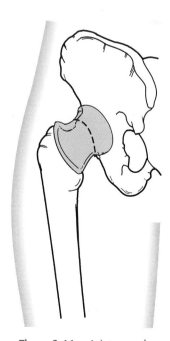

Figure 3-11. Joint capsule.

Cartilage is a dense fibrous connective tissue capable of withstanding a great amount of pressure and tension. There are basically three types of cartilage in the body: hyaline, fibrocartilage, and elastic. **Hyaline cartilage,** also called **articular cartilage,** covers the ends of opposing bones. With the help of synovial fluid, it provides a smooth articulating surface in all synovial joints. Hyaline cartilage has no blood or nerve supply of its own and must get its nutrition from the synovial fluid. Therefore, when it is damaged it is unable to repair itself.

Fibrocartilage acts as a shock absorber. This is especially important in weight-bearing joints such as the knee and vertebrae. At the knee, the semilunar-shaped cartilage called **menisci** build up the sides of the relatively flat articular surface of the tibia. Between the vertebral bones are the intervertebral **disks** (see Fig. 3-2). Because of their very dense structure, these disks are capable of absorbing an amazing amount of shock that is transmitted upward from weight-bearing forces.

In the upper extremity there is a fibrocartilaginous disk located between the clavicle and sternum. It is important for absorbing the shock transmitted along the clavicle to the sternum should you fall on your outstretched hand. This disk helps prevent dislocation of the sternoclavicular joint. It is also important in allowing motion. The disk, which is attached to the sternum at one end and the clavicle at the other, is much like a swinging door hinge that allows motion in both directions. This double-hung hinge allows the clavicle to move on the sternum as the acromial end is elevated and depressed. In effect, the fibrocartilage divides the joint into two cavities, allowing two sets of motion.

There are other functions of fibrocartilage in joints. The shoulder fibrocartilage, called **labrum,** deepens the shallow glenoid fossa, making it more of a socket to hold the humeral head (Fig. 3-12). Fibrocartilage also fills the gap between two bones. If you examine the wrist, you will notice that the ulna does not extend all the way to the carpal bones as does the radius. In this gap there is located a small triangular disk that acts as a space filler and allows force to be exerted on the ulna and carpals without causing damage.

The third type of cartilage, **elastic cartilage,** is designed to help maintain the shape of a structure. It is found in the external ear and eustachian (auditory) tube. It is also found in the larynx, where its motion is important to speech.

Muscles provide the contractile force that causes joints to move. They must, therefore, span the joint to have an effect on that joint. Muscles are soft and cannot attach directly to the bone. A **tendon** must connect

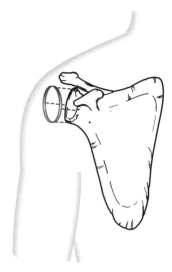

Figure 3-12.   Labrum.

them to bone. The tendon may be a cylindrical cord, like the long head of the biceps tendon, or a flattened band, like the rotator cuff. In certain locations tendons are encased in **tendon sheaths.** These fibrous sleeves surround the tendon when it is subject to pressure or friction, such as when it passes between muscles and bones or through a tunnel between bones. The tendons passing over the wrist all have tendon sheaths. These sheaths are lubricated by fluid secreted from their lining. An **aponeurosis** is a broad, flat tendinous sheet. Aponeuroses are found in several places where muscles attach to bones. The large, powerful latissimus dorsi muscle is attached at one end over a large area to several bones by means of an aponeurosis. In the anterior abdominal wall aponeuroses provide a base of muscular attachment where no bone is present but where great strength is needed. As the abdominal muscles approach the midline from both sides, they attach to an aponeurosis called the **linea alba.**

Found around most joints are small padlike sacs called **bursae.** Bursae are located in areas of excessive friction, such as under tendons and over bony prominences (Fig. 3-13). These sacs are lined with synovial

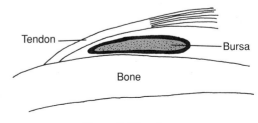

Figure 3-13.   Bursa.

membrane and filled with a clear fluid. Their purpose is to reduce friction between moving parts. For example, in the shoulder the deltoid muscle passes directly over the acromion process. Repeated motion would cause excessive wearing of the muscle tissue. However, the subdeltoid bursa, located between the muscle and acromion process, prevents excessive friction and reduces the likelihood of damage. The same arrangement occurs in the elbow where the triceps tendon attaches to the olecranon process. Some joints, such as the knee, have many bursae.

There are two types of bursa: natural bursa, which has just been discussed, and acquired bursa. It is possible to develop a bursa in an area that normally does not have excessive friction if, for some reason, this area has become the site of excessive friction. These *acquired bursae* tend to occur in places other than joints. For example, a person may develop a bursa on the lateral side of the third finger of the writing hand. This is often called the "student's bursa" because students often do a lot of writing and note taking. These bursae disappear when the activity is stopped or greatly reduced.

Common Pathological Terms

A **fracture** and a broken bone are synonymous. It is a break in the continuity of the bony cortex caused by direct, or indirect, force or pathology. Fractures in children tend to be incomplete ("greenstick") or epiphyseal. Fractures in the elderly tend to be of the hip (proximal femur) caused by a fall, or of the upper extremity as a result of a fall on the outstretched hand. Fractures are often described by type (i.e., closed), direction of fracture line (i.e., transverse), or position of bone parts (i.e., overriding).

Dislocation refers to the complete separation of the two articular surfaces of a joint. A portion of the joint capsule surrounding the joint will be torn. **Subluxation** is a partial dislocation of a joint and usually occurs over a period of time. A common example is a shoulder subluxation that develops after a person has had a stroke. Muscle paralysis and the weight of the arm slowly subluxes the shoulder joint.

A **sprain** is a partial or complete tearing of fibers of a ligament. A *mild* sprain involves the tearing of a few fibers with no loss of function. With a *moderate* sprain, there is partial tearing of the ligament with some loss of function. In a *severe* sprain, the ligament is completely torn (ruptured) and no longer functions. A **strain** refers to the overstretching of muscle fibers. As with sprains, strains are graded depending on severity.

Tendonitis is an inflammation of a tendon. **Tenosynovitis** refers to an inflammation of the tendon sheath. It is often caused by repetitive use. The tendon of the long head of the biceps and flexor tendons of the hand are common sites. **Synovitis** is an inflammation of the synovial membrane. **Bursitis** is an inflammation of the bursa. **Capsulitis** is an inflammation of the joint capsule.

Planes and Axes

Planes of action are fixed lines of reference along which the body is divided. There are three planes, and each plane is at right angles, or perpendicular, to the other two planes (Fig. 3-14).

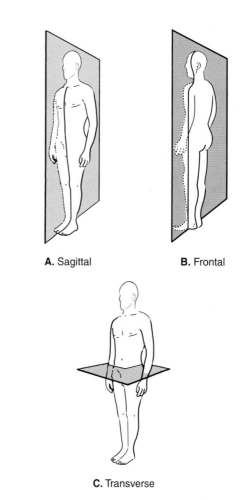

A. Sagittal   **B.** Frontal

C. Transverse

Figure 3-14. The planes of the body. *(A)* Sagittal plane. *(B)* Frontal plane. *(C)* Transverse plane.

The **sagittal plane** passes through the body from front to back and divides the body into right and left parts. Think of it as a vertical wall that the extremity moves along. Motions occurring in this plane are flexion and extension.

The **frontal plane** passes through the body from side to side and divides the body into front and back parts. It is also called the *coronal plane*. Motions occurring in this plane are abduction and adduction.

The **transverse plane** passes through the body horizontally and divides the body into top and bottom parts. It is also called the *horizontal plane*. Rotation occurs in this plane.

Whenever a plane passes through the midline of a part, whether it is the sagittal, frontal, or transverse plane, it is referred to as a cardinal plane because it divides the body into equal parts. The point where the three cardinal planes intersect each other is the **center of gravity.** In the human body that point is in the midline at about the level of, though slightly anterior to, the second sacral vertebra (Fig. 3-15).

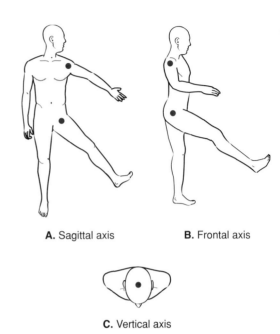

A. Sagittal axis   **B.** Frontal axis

C. Vertical axis

Figure 3-16.   The axes of the body. *(A)* Sagittal axis. *(B)* Frontal axis. *(C)* Vertical axis.

Axes are points that run through the center of a joint around which a part rotates (Fig. 3-16). The **sagittal axis** is a point that runs through a joint from front to back. The **frontal axis** runs through a joint from side to side. The **vertical axis,** also called the *longitudinal axis,* runs through a joint from top to bottom.

Joint movement occurs around an axis that is always perpendicular to its plane. Another way of stating this is that joint movement occurs *in a plane* and *around an axis*. A particular motion will always occur in the same plane and around the same axis. For example, flexion/extension will always occur in the sagittal plane around the frontal axis. Abduction/adduction will always occur in the frontal plane around the sagittal axis. Similar motions, such as radial and ulnar deviation of the wrist, will also occur in the frontal plane around the sagittal axis. The thumb is the exception because flexion/extension and abduction/adduction do not occur in these traditional planes. These motions, and their planes and axes, will be discussed in Chapter 12. Table 3-3 summarizes joint motion in relation to planes and axes.

Degrees of Freedom

Joints can also be described by the degrees of freedom, or number of planes, in which they can move. For example, a uniaxial joint has motion around one axis

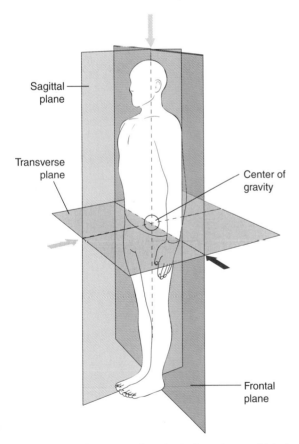

Sagittal plane

Transverse plane

Center of gravity

Frontal plane

Figure 3-15.   The center of gravity is the point at which the three cardinal planes intersect.

Table 3-3	Joint Motions	
Plane	**Axis**	**Joint Motion**
Sagittal	Frontal	Flexion/extension
Frontal	Sagittal	Abduction/adduction
		Radial/ulnar deviation
		Eversion/inversion
Transverse	Vertical	Medial/lateral rotation
		Supination/pronation
		Right/left rotation
		Horizontal abduction/ adduction

and in one plane. Therefore, it has one degree of freedom. A biaxial joint would have two degrees of freedom, and a triaxial joint would have three, which is the maximum number of degrees of freedom that an individual joint can have.

This concept becomes significant when dealing with one or more distal joints. For example, the shoulder has three degrees of freedom, the elbow and radioulnar joints each have one, and together they have five degrees of freedom. The entire limb from the finger to the shoulder would have 11 degrees of freedom.

Review Questions

1. There are three types of a joint that allows no motion. They are:

2. The two terms for a joint that allows a great deal of motion are:

3. Diarthrodial joints can be described in terms of three features.
   They are:
   a. _____
   b. _____
   c. _____

4. What type of joint structure connects bone to muscle?

5. What type of joint structure pads and protects *areas* of great friction?

6. How does hyaline cartilage differ from fibrocartilage? Give an example of each type of cartilage.

7. When the anterior surface of the forearm moves toward the anterior surface of the humerus, what joint motion is involved? In what plane is the motion occurring? Around what axis?

8. What joint motions are involved in turning the palm of the hand? In what plane and around what axis does that joint motion occur?

9. What joint motion is involved in returning the fingers to anatomical position from the fully spread position? In what plane and around what axis does the joint motion occur?

10. Identify the 11 degrees of freedom of the upper extremity.

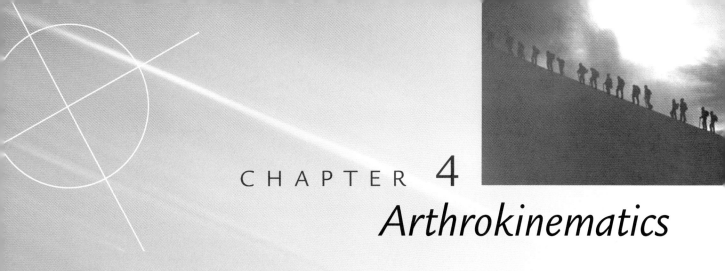

Osteokinematic Motion

   End Feel

Arthrokinematic Motion

   Accessory Motion Terminology

   Joint Surface Shape

   Types of Arthrokinematic Motion

   Convex-Concave Law

   Joint Surface Positions (Joint Congruency)

   Accessory Motion Forces

Points to Remember

Review Questions

Osteokinematic Motion

Joint movement is commonly thought of as one bone moving on another causing such motions as flexion, extension, abduction, or rotation. These movements, which are done under voluntary control, are often referred to as **classical, physiological,** or **osteokinematic motion.** This type of motion can be done in the form of isometric, isotonic, or even isokinetic exercises. When performed actively, muscles move joints through ranges of motion (ROMs). As we move our joints throughout the day, we are actively performing osteokinematic movements. These movements were described in Chapter 3. When a person moves a joint passively through its range of motion, it is usually done to assist in maintaining full motion or to determine the nature of the resistance at the end of the range. The latter is called the end feel of a joint.

End Feel

End feel is a subjective assessment of the *quality* of the feel when slight pressure is applied at the end of the joint's passive range of motion. It was first described by Cyriax (1983). He stressed the importance of how the end feel felt to the examiner's hands during passive motion.

   The three major types of end feel are bony, capsular, and empty end feel. **Bony end feel** is characterized by a hard and abrupt limit to joint motion. This occurs when bone contacts bone at the end of the ROM. This is sometimes called *hard end feel*. An example would be normal terminal elbow extension. **Capsular end feel** is characterized by a hard, leatherlike limitation of motion that has a slight give. This occurs in full normal joint motion of the shoulder and is related to capsular restriction. An **empty end feel** is characterized by a lack of mechanical limitation of joint range of motion. This occurs when motion is limited by pain and there is complete disruption of soft-tissue constraints. Empty end feel is not good.

Three additional characteristics can be used to quantify the limitation of joint motion. A rebound movement felt at the end of the ROM characterizes **springy block.** This occurs with internal derangement of a joint, such as torn cartilage. Asymptomatic limited ROM characterizes **soft tissue approximation.** This occurs when the soft tissue of body segments prevents further motion (e.g., at normal terminal elbow flexion). **Muscle guarding** is a reflex muscle spasm during motion. It is a protective response seen with acute injury. Palpation of the muscle will reveal the muscle in spasm. The ability to palpate normal end feel and to distinguish changes from normal end feel is important in protecting joints during ROM exercises.

Arthrokinematic Motion

Another way of looking at joint movement is to look at what is taking place within the joint at the joint surfaces. Called **arthrokinematic motion,** it is defined as the manner in which adjoining joint surfaces move on each other during osteokinematic joint movement. Therefore, osteokinematic motion is referred to as joint motion, and arthrokinematic motion is joint surface motion.

Accessory Motion Terminology

Terminology can be somewhat confusing because various experts use the same terminology somewhat differently. Paris describes **accessory movement** as motions that accompany (are accessory to) the classical movement and are essential to normal full range and painless function (Paris and Patla, 1986). He further divides this motion into (1) **joint play movements,** which are not under voluntary control and occur only in response to an external force, and (2) **component movements,** which take place within a joint to facilitate a particular active motion. An example of joint play exists at the end of all active ROMs. A component movement is the associated anterior glide of the tibia as the knee goes into extension. Kisner, on the other hand, refers to component movements as motions that accompany active motion, but are not under voluntary control (Kisner and Colby, 2002). An example would be shoulder girdle upward rotation. The motion, which cannot be done alone, must accompany shoulder flexion. Kisner

describes joint play as motions occurring within the joint that are necessary for normal joint function. They can be done passively by applying an external force but cannot be done actively by the individual. This describes such terms as glide, spin, and roll.

Regardless of how these accessory movements are defined, it is generally agreed that these accessory movements are necessary for joint mobilization. **Joint mobilization** is generally described as a passive oscillatory motion or sustained stretch that is applied at a slow enough speed by an external force that the individual can stop the motion. Gould describes joint mobilization as the attempt to improve joint mobility or decrease pain originating in joint structures by the use of selected grades of accessory movements. Further discussion of joint mobilization is beyond the scope of this book. These terms and related concepts are introduced to provide a basic understanding of joint movement. Another term, **manipulation,** is defined as a passive movement applied with a very forceful thrust within a short range that cannot be stopped. It is also applied under anesthesia. This maneuver is well beyond the scope of this text.

Joint Surface Shape

To understand arthrokinematics, one must recognize that the type of motion occurring at a joint depends on the shape of the articulating surfaces of the bones. Most joints have one concave bone end and one convex bone end (Fig. 4-1). A convex surface is rounded outward much like a mound. A concave surface is "caved" in much like a cave.

All joint surfaces are either ovoid or sellar. An **ovoid joint** has two bones forming a convex-concave relationship. For example, in the metacarpophalangeal joint, one surface is concave (proximal phalanx) and the other is convex (metacarpal) (see Fig. 4-1). Most synovial joints are ovoid. Usually in an ovoid joint, one bone end is larger than its adjacent bone end. This

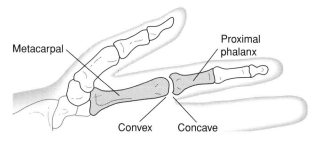

Figure 4-1.   Shape of bone surfaces of an ovoid joint—MCP joint of finger.

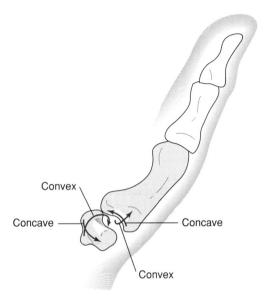

Figure 4-2. Shape of bone surfaces of a sellar joint—CMP joint of thumb.

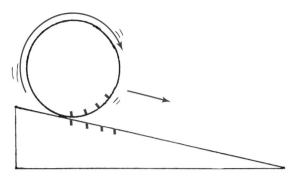

Figure 4-3. Roll—movement of one joint surface on another. New points on each surface make contact.

permits a greater ROM on a less articular surface, which reduces the size of the joint.

In a **sellar** or **saddle-shaped joint,** each joint surface is concave in one direction and convex in another. The carpometacarpal (CMP) joint of the thumb is perhaps the best example of a sellar joint (Fig. 4-2). If you look at the carpal bone (trapezium), it is concave in a front-to-back direction and convex in a side-to-side direction. The first metacarpal bone that articulates with the carpal bone has just the opposite shape. It is convex in a front-to-back direction and concave in a side-to-side direction.

Types of Arthrokinematic Motion

The types of arthrokinematic motion are roll, glide, and spin. Most joint movement involves a combination of all three of these motions. **Roll** is the rolling of one joint surface on another. New points on each surface come into contact throughout the motion (Fig. 4-3). Examples include the surface of your shoe on the floor during walking, or a ball rolling across the ground. **Glide,** or **slide,** is linear movement of a joint surface parallel to the plane of the adjoining joint surface (Fig. 4-4). In other words, one point on a joint surface contacts new points on the adjacent surface. An ice skater's skate blade (one point) sliding across the ice surface (many points) demonstrates the glide motion. **Spin** is the rotation of the movable joint surface on the fixed adjacent surface (Fig. 4-5). Essentially the same point on each surface

remains in contact with each other. Examples of this type of movement would be a top spinning on a table. If the top remains perfectly upright, the top spins in one place. Examples in the body would be any pure (relatively speaking) rotational movement such as the humerus rotating medially and laterally in the glenoid fossa, or the head of the radius spinning on the capitulum of the humerus.

As will be discussed in Chapter 18, the knee joint motion demonstrates clearly that all three types of arthrokinematic motion are necessary to obtain full knee flexion and extension. In this motion during weight-bearing, the femoral condyles roll on the tibial condyles. Because of the large range of flexion and extension permitted at the knee, the femur would roll off the tibia if the femoral condyles did not also glide posteriorly on the tibia. Because the medial and lateral femoral condyles are different sizes, and the medial and lateral aspects of the knee joint move at different speeds, there must be spin (medial rotation) of the femur on the tibia during the last 15 degrees of knee extension. In a non–weight-bearing activity, the same

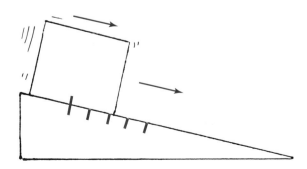

Figure 4-4. Glide—linear movement of one joint surface parallel to the other joint surface. One point on one surface contacts new points on other surface.

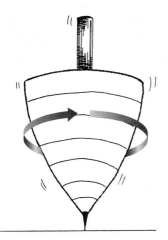

Figure 4-5. Spin—rotation of one joint surface on another. Same point on each surface remains in contact.

motions are occurring except that the tibia is moving on the femur, and the spin motion is lateral rotation of the tibia on the femur (see Fig. 18-3B).

Convex-Concave Rule

Knowing that a joint surface is concave or convex is important because shape determines motion. The **concave-convex rule** describes how the differences in shapes of bone ends require joint surfaces move in a specific way during joint movement. The law is described as follows:

A concave joint surface will move on a fixed convex surface in the same direction as the body segment is moving. For example, the proximal portion of the proximal phalanx is concave and the distal portion of the metacarpal is convex (Fig. 4-6). During finger extension (from finger flexion) the proximal phalanx

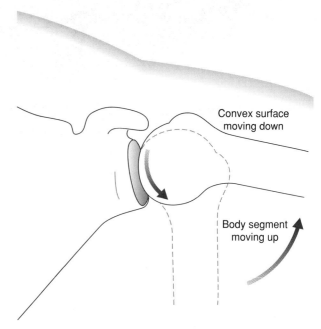

Figure 4-7. The convex surface moving in the opposite direction from the direction in which the body segment is moving.

moves in the same direction as the phalanx itself while moving on the convex metacarpal joint surface. To summarize, the **concave joint surface** moves in the **same direction** as the body segment's motion.

A convex joint surface will move on a fixed concave surface in the opposite direction as the moving body segment. For example, the head of the humerus is convex whereas the glenoid fossa of the scapula, in which it articulates, is concave (Fig. 4-7). During shoulder flexion, the convex surface of the humeral head moves

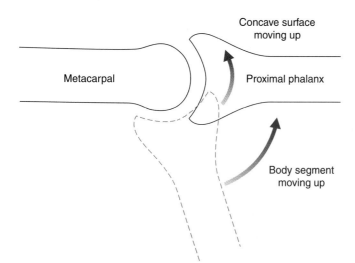

Figure 4-6. The concave surface moving in the same direction that the body segment is moving.

in the opposite direction (downward) from the rest of the humerus, which is moving upward. Thus, the **convex joint surface** moves in the **opposite direction** of body segment's movement.

There is an easy visual way to remember this rule. To represent a joint, make a fist with your left hand and place it inside your cupped right hand. Your left fist represents a convex joint surface of one bone. The left forearm represents the bone. Your cupped right hand represents a concave surface of the other bone. Keeping your hands at the same level, your wrist straight, and your left fist rotating inside the cupped hand, raise your left elbow. Notice that as your forearm (body segment) moves up, your fist (joint surface) rotates down. In other words, the convex surface moves in the opposite direction as the body segment's motion. Repeat the action, with the cupped hand moving on the fist. The concave surface (cupped hand) is moving in the same direction as the body segment's motion.

Joint Surface Positions (Joint Congruency)

The joint surfaces of an ovoid joint or sellar joint are congruent in one position and incongruent in all other positions. When a joint is **congruent,** the joint surfaces have maximum contact with each other, are tightly compressed, and difficult to distract (separate). The ligaments and capsule holding the joint together are taut. This is known as the **close-packed or closed-pack position.** It usually occurs at one extreme of the ROM. For example, if you place your knee in the fully extended position you can manually move the patella slightly from side to side and up and down. However, if you flex your knee, such patellar movement is *not* possible. Therefore, the close-packed position of the patellofemoral joint is knee flexion. Other close-packed positions are ankle dorsiflexion, metacarpophalangeal flexion, and extension of the elbow, wrist, hip, knee, and interphalanges. Table 4-1 gives a more detailed listing of the close-packed positions of joints. When ligaments and capsular structures are tested for stability and integrity, the joint is usually placed in the close-packed position. By the nature of the characteristics of a close-packed position, a joint usually is injured when in this position. For example, a knee joint that sustains a lateral force when it is extended (closed-packed position) is much more likely to be injured than when it is in a flexed or semiflexed position (loose-packed position). When a joint is swollen, it cannot be moved into the close-packed position.

In all other positions the joint surfaces are incongruent. The position of maximum incongruency is called

Table 4-1	Close-Packed Positions of Joints
Joint(s)	**Position**
Facet (spine)	Extension
Temporomandibular	Clenched teeth
Glenohumeral	Abduction and lateral rotation
Acromioclavicular	Arm abducted to 30°
Sternoclavicular	Maximum shoulder elevation
Ulnohumeral (elbow)	Extension
Radiohumeral	Elbow flexed 90°, forearm supinated 5°
Proximal radioulnar	5° supination
Distal radioulnar	5° supination
Radiocarpal (wrist)	Extension with ulnar deviation
Metacarpophalangeal (fingers)	Full flexion
Metacarpophalangeal (thumb)	Full opposition
Interphalangeal	Full extension
Hip	Full extension and medial rotation*
Knee	Full extension and lateral rotation of tibia
Talocrural (ankle)	Maximum dorsiflexion
Subtalar	Supination
Midtarsal	Supination
Tarsometatarsal	Supination
Metatarsophalangeal	Full extension
Interphalangeal	Full extension

Source: From Magee, DJ: Orthopedic Physical Assessment, ed 4. WB Saunders, Philadelphia, 2002, p 50, with permission.
*Some authors include abduction.

the **open-packed** or **loose-packed position.** It is also referred to as the **resting position.** Parts of the capsule and supporting ligaments are lax. There is minimal congruency between the articular surfaces. Further passive separation of the joint surfaces can occur in this position. Because the ligaments and capsular structures tend to be more relaxed, joint mobilization techniques are best applied in the open-packed position. It is these open-packed positions that allow for the roll, spin, and glide, necessary for normal joint motion. Table 4-2 gives a more detailed listing of the loose-packed positions of joints.

Also, in these open-packed positions a certain amount of **accessory motions,** or **joint play,** can be demonstrated. This is the passive movement of one articular surface

Table 4-2	Loose-Packed Positions of Joints
Joint(s)	**Position**
Facet (spine)	Midway between flexion and extension
Temporomandibular	Mouth slightly open (freeway space)
Glenohumeral	55° abduction, 30° horizontal adduction
Acromioclavicular	Arm resting by side in normal physiological position
Sternoclavicular	Arm resting by side in normal physiological position
Ulnohumeral (elbow)	70° flexion, 10° supination
Radiohumeral	Full extension and full supination
Proximal radioulnar	70° flexion, 35° supination
Distal radioulnar	10° supination
Radiocarpal (wrist)	Neutral with slight ulnar deviation
Carpometacarpal	Midway between abduction/ adduction and flexion/ extension
Metacarpophalangeal	Slight flexion
Interphalangeal	Slight flexion
Hip	30° flexion, 30° abduction and slight lateral rotation
Knee	25° flexion
Talocrural (ankle)	10° plantar flexion, midway between maximum inversion and eversion
Subtalar	Midway between extremes of range of movement
Midtarsal	Midway between extremes of range of movement
Tarsometatarsal	Midway between extremes of range of movement
Metatarsophalangeal	Neutral
Interphalangeal	Slight flexion

Source: From Magee, DJ: Orthopedic Physical Assessment, ed 4. WB Saunders, Philadelphia, 2002, p 50, with permission.

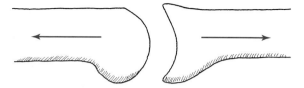

Figure 4-8.   Traction force causes bone ends to move apart from each other.

and shearing. Bending and rotary forces are the result of a combination of forces.

Traction, also called **distraction** or **tension,** occurs when external force is exerted on a joint causing the joint surfaces to be pulled apart (Fig. 4-8). Carrying a heavy suitcase or hanging from an overhead bar causes traction to the shoulder, elbow, and wrist joints. You can demonstrate this on another person by grasping their index finger at the proximal end of the middle phalanx with one thumb and index finger. Next, grasp the distal end of the proximal phalanx with your other thumb and index finger. Move the PIP joint into a slightly flexed position (loose-packed position), and pull gently in opposite directions. This description, and others to follow, is meant to describe the various forces, and is not a description of therapeutic technique. Extreme care must be exercised when performing these motions.

Approximation, also called **compression,** occurs when an external force is exerted on a joint causing the joint surfaces to be pushed closer together (Fig. 4-9). Doing a chair or floor push-up causes the joint surfaces of the shoulder, elbow, and wrist to be approximated. As a general rule, traction can assist the mobility of a joint, and approximation can assist the stability of a joint.

Shear forces occur parallel to the surface (Fig. 4-10). Shear force results in a glide motion at the joint. Using the positions described with distraction, place your thumbs on the dorsal surfaces and your index fingers on the palmar surfaces of the person's finger. With the PIP joint slightly flexed, gently move your two hands in an up-and-down motion. This motion describes anterior/posterior glide of the PIP joint.

over another. Because joint play is not a voluntary movement, it requires relaxed muscles and the external force of a trained practitioner to correctly demonstrate it.

Accessory Motion Forces

When applying joint mobilization, three main types of forces are used. Those forces are traction, compression,

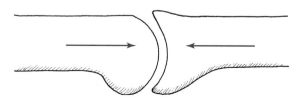

Figure 4-9.   Compression force causes bone ends to move toward each other.

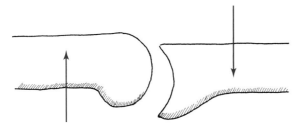

Figure 4-10.   Shear force causes bone ends to move parallel to and in opposite direction from each other.

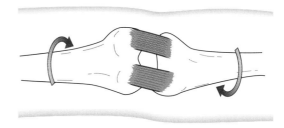

Figure 4-12.   Rotary force is a twisting motion.

Bending and rotary forces are actually a combination of forces. **Bending** occurs when an other-than-vertical force is applied, resulting in compression on the concave side and distraction on the convex side (Fig. 4-11). **Rotary** forces involve twisting, resulting in a combination of compression and shear (Fig. 4-12).

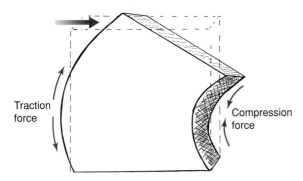

Traction
force

Compression
force

Figure 4-11.   Bending force causes compression on one side and traction on other side.

Points to Remember

- End feel can be described as bony, capsular, empty, springy block, soft-tissue approximation, or muscle guarding.
- Joint surface shape can be ovoid or sellar.
- Types of arthrokinematic motion are roll, glide, or spin.
- According to the concave-convex law, concave joint surfaces move in the same direction as the joint or body segment's motion while convex surfaces move in the opposite direction as the joint motion.
- When a joint is congruent, it is in the close-packed position. When the joint is incongruent, it is in the open-packed position.
- When mobilizing a joint, traction, compression, shear, bending, or rotary forces may be used.

Review Questions

1. a. Is shoulder flexion and extension an arthrokinematic or osteokinematic type of motion?
    b. Is shoulder distraction an arthrokinematic or osteokinematic type of motion?
2. You would feel what type of end feel when bending your knee to the end of the range?
3. Flex the shoulder from an extended position.
    a. Is the humerus moving on the scapula or is the scapula moving on the humerus?
    b. Is the proximal end of the humerus a concave or convex joint surface?
    c. Does the glenoid fossa of the scapula have a concave or convex joint surface?
    d. Is the concave surface moving on a fixed convex surface or is a convex surface moving on a fixed concave surface?
    e. Is the joint surface moving in the same or opposite direction as the joint motion?
4. Identify the accessory motion force(s) occurring in the following activities:
    a. Leaning on a table with your elbows extended.
    b. Transferring from a wheelchair to the car using a sliding board.
    c. Picking up one end of a table.

5. Is the close-packed position of the TMJ (jaw) when the teeth are clenched or mouth slightly open?

6. In terms of joint congruency, describe how a stack of Pringles potato chips fits together (see Fig. 12-2). Place a stack of two chips in front of you with the long end pointing toward you in an anterior-posterior position.

   Consider the joint surfaces of each chip in contact with the other

   a. Is the anterior/posterior shape of the bottom surface of the top chip concave or convex?

   b. Is the anterior/posterior shape the top surface of the bottom chip concave or convex?

   c. Is the medial/lateral shape of the bottom surface of the top chip concave or convex?

   d. Is the medial/lateral shape of the top surface of the bottom chip concave or convex?

   e. If these chips were a joint, would the shape of the joint be ovoid or sellar?

7. Rotating a quarter on its edge across the table demonstrates what type of arthrokinematics motion?

8. Lay the quarter flat on the table and hit it with your finger, send it across the table. This would be what type of arthrokinematics motion?

9. In comparing the size of a quarter and a nickel, note that the quarter is larger. Place a pencil mark on the quarter at the 6 and 12 o'clock positions. Lay a nickel flat on the table. Roll the quarter across the flat surface of the nickel, starting with the quarter at the 6 o'clock position at the edge of the nickel.

   a. Will the quarter reach the edge of the nickel before reaching the 12 o'clock position?

   b. Which arthrokinematic motion will you have to use on the quarter in addition to roll, so that the 12 o'clock mark can reach the opposite side of the nickel?

10. Hold a pencil vertically with the lead end on the table. Holding the eraser end between your thumb and index finger, roll the pencil between your fingers, keeping the lead end in contact with the table. This is demonstrating which type of arthrokinematic motion?

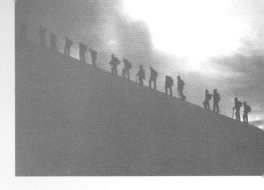

CHAPTER 5

Muscular System

Muscle Attachments

Muscle Names

Muscle Fiber Arrangement

Functional Characteristics of Muscle Tissue

Length-Tension Relationship in Muscle Tissue

Active and Passive Insufficiency

Types of Muscle Contraction

Roles of Muscles

Angle of Pull

Kinetic Chains

Points to Remember

Review Questions

Muscle Attachments

When a muscle contracts, it knows no direction; it simply shortens. If a muscle were unattached at both ends and stimulated, the two ends would move toward the middle. However, muscles are attached to bones and cross at least one joint, so when a muscle contracts, one end of the joint moves toward the other. The more movable bone, often referred to as the **insertion,** moves toward the more stable bone, the **origin.** For example, when the biceps brachii muscle contracts, the forearm moves toward the humerus, as when bringing a glass toward your mouth (Fig. 5-1A). The humerus is more stable because it is attached to the axial skeleton at the shoulder joint. The forearm is more movable because it is attached to the hand, which is quite movable. Therefore, the insertion is moving toward the origin, or explained another way, the more movable end is moving toward the more stable end. Another point that can be made about muscle attachments is that origins tend to be closer to the trunk and insertions tend to be more toward the distal end.

This arrangement can be reversed if the more movable end becomes less movable. For example, what would happen if the hand were holding onto a chinning bar when the biceps contracted? The biceps would still flex the elbow, but now the humerus would move toward the forearm. In other words, the origin would move toward the insertion (Fig. 5-1B). Some sources refer to this as **reversal of muscle action.** However, you should realize that the same joint motion is occurring (in this case, elbow flexion). What has changed is that instead of the insertion moving toward the origin, the origin is now moving toward the insertion. The proximal bone, which is usually more stable, has become more movable.

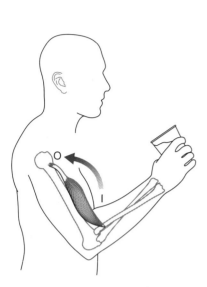

Insertion moves toward origin

A

Origin moves toward Insertion

B

Figure 5-1. Direction of movement of biceps muscle attachments.

Consider another example in a very simplistic form. Lying on your back, bring your knees up toward your chest. Using your hip flexors to flex your hip, you are moving the femur (more movable) toward your chest (more stable), or insertion toward origin. If someone holds your feet down, your femur would become the more stable end and your trunk, the more movable end. When your hip flexors contract, the origin would move toward the insertion. Closed kinetic chain exercises are based on the distal segment being fixed, and the proximal end being moved. This is another way of applying reversal of muscle action. Open and closed kinetic chains will be discussed later in this chapter.

Muscle Names

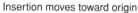

The name of a muscle can often tell you a great deal about that muscle. Muscle names tend to fall into one or more of the following categories:

1. Location
2. Shape
3. Action
4. Number of heads or divisions
5. Attachments = origin/insertion
6. Direction of the fibers
7. Size of the muscle

The tibialis anterior, as its name indicates, is located on the anterior surface of the tibia. The rectus (straight) abdominis muscle is a vertical muscle located on the abdomen. The trapezius muscle has a trapezoid shape, and the serratus anterior muscle (Fig. 5-2) has a serrated or jagged-shaped attachment anteriorly. The name of the extensor carpi ulnaris muscle tells you that its action is to extend the wrist (carpi) on the ulnar side. The triceps brachii muscle is a three-headed

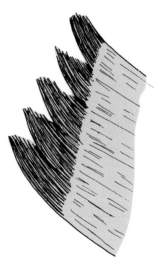

Figure 5-2. The serratus anterior muscle has a saw-toothed shape.

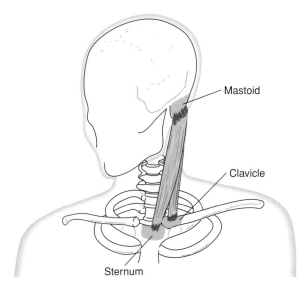

Figure 5-3. The sternocleidomastoid muscle is named for its attachments on the sternum, clavicle, and mastoid bone.

muscle on the arm, and the biceps femoris muscle is a two-headed muscle on the thigh. The sternocleidomastoid muscle (Fig. 5-3) attaches on the sternum, clavicle, and mastoid bones. The names of the external and internal oblique muscles describe the direction of the fibers and their location to one another. In the same way, the names pectoralis major and pectoralis minor indicate that although both of these muscles are in the same area, one is larger than the other.

Muscle Fiber Arrangement

Muscle fibers are arranged within the muscle in a direction that is either parallel or oblique to the long axis of the muscle (Fig. 5-4). **Parallel muscle** fibers tend to be longer, thus having a greater range of motion potential. **Oblique muscle** fibers tend to be shorter but are more numerous per given area than parallel fibers, which means that oblique-fibered muscles tend to have a greater strength potential but a smaller range-of-motion potential than parallel-fibered muscles. There are many types of each muscle fiber arrangement in the body.

Parallel-fibered muscles can be strap, fusiform, rhomboidal (rectangular), or triangular in shape. **Strap muscles** are muscles that are long and thin with fibers running the entire length of the muscle. The sartorius muscle in the lower extremity, the rectus abdominis in the trunk, and the sternocleidomastoid in the neck are examples of strap muscles.

A **fusiform muscle** has a shape similar to that of a spindle. It is wider in the middle and tapers at both ends where it attaches to tendons. Most, but not all, fibers run the length of the muscle. The muscle may be any length or size, from long to short or large to small. Examples of fusiform muscles can be found in the elbow flexors; that is, the biceps, brachialis, and brachioradialis muscles.

A **rhomboidal muscle** is four-sided, usually flat, with broad attachments at each end. Examples of this muscle shape are the pronator quadratus in the forearm, the rhomboids in the shoulder girdle, and the gluteus maximus in the hip region.

Triangular muscles are flat and fan shaped with fibers radiating from a narrow attachment at one end to a broad attachment at the other. An example of this type of muscle is the pectoralis major in the chest.

Oblique-fibered muscles have a feather arrangement in which a muscle attaches at an oblique angle to its tendon, much like feather tendrils attach to the quill. The different types of oblique-fibered muscles are unipennate, bipennate, and multipennate.

Unipennate muscles look like one side of a feather. There are a series of short fibers attaching diagonally along the length of a central tendon. Examples are the

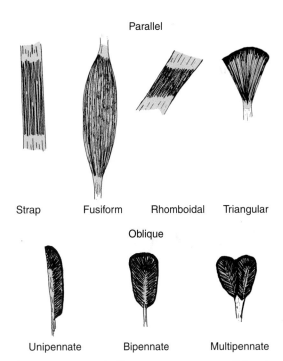

Figure 5-4. Muscle fiber arrangements, parallel and oblique.

tibialis posterior muscle of the ankle, semimembranosus of the hip and knee, and the flexor pollicis longus muscle of the hand.

The **bipennate muscle** pattern looks like that of a common feather. Its fibers are obliquely attached to both sides of a central tendon. The rectus femoris muscle of the hip and the interossei muscles of the hand are examples of this pattern.

Multipennate muscles have many tendons with oblique fibers in between. The deltoid and subscapularis muscles at the shoulder demonstrate this pattern.

Functional Characteristics of Muscle Tissue

Muscle tissue has the properties of irritability, contractility, extensibility, and elasticity. No other tissue in the body has all of these characteristics. To better understand these properties, you might find it helpful to know that muscles have a **normal resting length.** This is defined as the length of a muscle when it is unstimulated, that is, when there are no forces or stresses placed upon it. **Irritability** is the ability to respond to a stimulus. A muscle contracts when stimulated. This can be a natural stimulus from a motor nerve or an artificial stimulus such as an electrical current. **Contractility** is the ability to shorten or contract when it receives adequate stimulation. This may result in the muscle shortening, staying the same, or lengthening. **Extensibility** is the ability of a muscle to stretch or lengthen when a force is applied. **Elasticity** is the ability to recoil or return to normal resting length when the stretching or shortening force is removed. Saltwater taffy has extensibility, but not elasticity. You can stretch it, but once the force is removed the taffy will remain stretched. A wire spring has both extensibility and elasticity. Stretch the wire, and it will lengthen. Remove the stretch, and the wire spring will return to its original length. The same can be said of a muscle. However, unlike the taffy or wire spring, a muscle is able to shorten beyond its normal resting length.

The properties of a muscle are summarized as follows: Stretch a muscle, and it will lengthen (extensibility). Remove the stretch, and it will return to its normal resting position (elasticity). Stimulate a muscle, and it will respond (irritability) by shortening (contractility); then remove the stimulus and it will return to its normal resting position (elasticity).

Length-Tension Relationship in Muscle Tissue

Tension refers to the force built up within a muscle. Stretching a muscle builds up *passive tension,* much like stretching a rubber band. It involves the noncontractile units of a muscle. *Active tension* comes from the contractile units, and can be compared to releasing one end of a stretched rubber band. The total tension of a muscle is a combination of passive and active tension. **Tone** is the slight tension that is present in a muscle at all times, even when the muscle is resting. It is a state of readiness that allows the muscle to act more easily and quickly when needed.

Although there is variation between muscles, it can generally be said that a muscle is capable of being shortened to approximately one half of its normal resting length. For example, a muscle that is approximately 6 inches long can shorten to approximately 3 inches. Also, a muscle can be stretched about twice as far as it can be shortened. Therefore, this same muscle can be stretched 3 inches beyond its resting length to an overall length of 9 inches. The **excursion** of a muscle is that distance from maximum elongation to maximum shortening. In this example, the excursion would be 6 inches (Fig. 5-5).

Usually a muscle has sufficient excursion to allow the joint to move through the joint's entire range. This is certainly true of muscles that span only one joint. However, a muscle spanning two or more joints may not have sufficient excursion to allow the joint to move through the combined range of all the joints it crosses.

One of the factors determining the amount of tension in a muscle is its length. It has been demonstrated

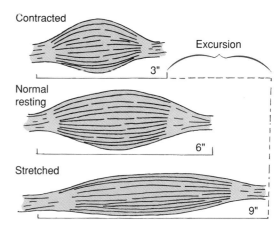

Figure 5-5.   Excursion of a muscle.

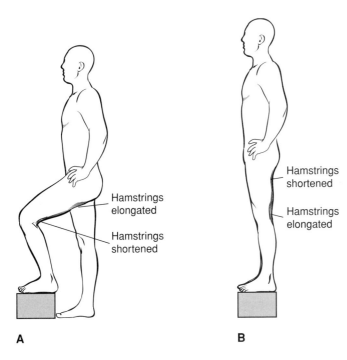

A   B

Figure 5-6. Optimal length-tension relationship of hamstrings when going up stairs. *(A)* When the foot is placed on the step, the hamstrings are being stretched over the hip while shortened over the knee. *(B)* Stepping up requires the hip to extend (hamstrings are contracting = shortening) and the knee to extend (hamstrings are being stretched).

that a muscle is strongest if put on a stretch prior to contracting. Many examples of this concept can be cited. Think of what you do when kicking a ball. First you hyperextend your hip and then forcefully flex it. In other words, you put the hip flexors on a stretch before contracting them. This is similar to pulling back on a rubber band before snapping it.

There is an optimum range of a muscle within which it contracts most effectively. As with a rubber band, a muscle contraction is strongest when it is on a stretch, and loses power quickly as it shortens. Therefore, two-joint muscles have the advantage over one-joint muscles of maintaining greater contractile force through a wider range. They do so by contracting over one joint while being elongated over another. Consider your hamstring muscles when climbing stairs. Hamstring function is to extend the hip and flex the knee. When you go up stairs, you start by flexing the hip and knee (Fig. 5-6A). This elongates the hamstrings over the hip and shortens them over the knee. Next, your hip goes into extension (shortening the muscle), while your knee also goes into extension (elongating the muscle) (Fig. 5-6B). In other words, the hamstring muscles are being shortened over the hip while they are being elongated over the knee. Therefore, they are able to maintain an optimal length-tension relationship throughout the range.

Active and Passive Insufficiency

In a one-joint muscle, the excursion of the muscle will be greater than the range of motion allowed by the joint. However, with a two-joint or multijoint muscle, the muscle's excursion is less than the combined range allowed by the joints. The tension within the muscle becomes insufficient at both extremes. It can neither be elongated nor shortened any farther. Brunnstrom uses the terms "active" and "passive insufficiency" to describe these conditions.

When a muscle reaches a point where it cannot shorten any farther, it is called **active insufficiency.** Active insufficiency occurs to the agonist (the muscle that is contracting). Consider the hamstrings as an example. The hamstring muscles are two-joint muscles located on the posterior thigh. They extend the hip and flex the knee. There is sufficient tension to perform either hip extension or knee flexion, but not both simultaneously. Notice that if you flex your knee while your hip is extended, you cannot complete the full knee range. The muscles have "insufficient power" to contract (shorten) over both joints at the same time (Fig. 5-7A). They have become actively insufficient. The fact that more range of motion exists can be shown by grabbing your ankle and pulling the knee into more flexion (Fig. 5-7B). Be careful when trying this exercise that you do not get a muscle cramp. In other words, in this

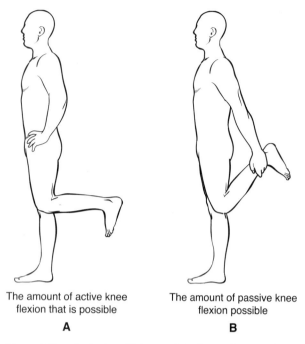

The amount of active knee
flexion that is possible

A

The amount of passive knee
flexion possible

B

Figure 5-7.   Active insufficiency of the hamstring muscle.

two-joint muscle that is contracting over both joints at the same time, the muscle (hamstring) will run out of the contractility before the joints (hip and knee) run out of range of motion.

Passive insufficiency occurs when a muscle cannot be elongated any farther without damage to its fibers. Passive insufficiency occurs to the antagonist (the muscle that is relaxed and is on the opposite side of the joint from the agonist). Agonist and antagonists are terms described in more detail later in this chapter.

Consider the hamstring muscle as an example of passive insufficiency. The hamstring is long enough to be stretched over each joint individually (hip flexion or knee extension), but not both. If you flex your hip with your knee flexed, you can complete the range. As you can see in Figure 5-8A, the individual can touch the toes by flexing the hip and the knee. The hamstrings are being stretched over only one joint (the hip). You can also extend your knee fully when the hip is extended (see Fig. 5-6B) because the hamstrings are being stretched over only the knee. However, if you try to flex your hips to touch your toes with your knee extended (Fig. 5-8B), you will experience pain in the posterior thigh well before you reach full hip flexion. Your hamstring muscles are telling you to stop. They are being stretched over both joints at the same time and have become passively insufficient. They cannot be stretched any farther.

Stretching

Generally speaking, an agonist usually becomes actively insufficient (cannot contract any farther) before the antagonist becomes passively insufficient (cannot be stretched farther). We can use this concept to good advantage when we purposely stretch a muscle to either maintain or regain its normal resting length. Some activities require a great deal of flexibility, so stretching is done to lengthen the resting length of a muscle. In all of these situations, stretching should be performed on relaxed muscles. A person is put in a position that will stretch a muscle, usually a two-joint muscle, over all joints simultaneously within the pain limits of that muscle. If you wanted to stretch your hamstring muscles, you would put the knee in extension and slowly flex the hip to the point where you feel discomfort but not beyond to the point of extreme pain. To stretch a one-joint muscle, it is necessary to put any two-joint muscles on a slack over the joint not crossed by the one joint-muscle. In other words, to stretch the soleus muscle, which crosses the ankle only, the gastrocnemius muscle, which crosses the ankle and knee, must be put on a slack over the knee. This can be accomplished by flexing the knee while dorsiflexing the ankle. Otherwise, if you attempt to dorsiflex the ankle when the knee is extended, you may be stretching the gastrocnemius more than the soleus.

There are various methods of stretching used for different situations and sometimes for different results. These different methods are important, but beyond the scope of this discussion.

Tendon Action of a Muscle (Tenodesis)

Some degree of opening and closing the hand can be accomplished by using the principle of passive

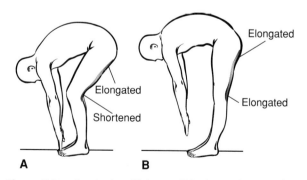

A   **B**

Figure 5-8.   Passive insufficiency of the hamstring muscle. *(A)* The hamstring being stretched (elongated) over only one joint allows more joint range of motion. *(B)* Stretching the muscle over both joints (the hip and knee) allows less individual joint range of motion.

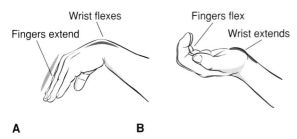

A   **B**

Figure 5-9. Tenodesis, the functional use of passive insufficiency, demonstrated on the finger flexor and extensor muscles. Each group cannot be stretched over the wrist, MP, PIP, and DIP joints at the same time. (A) Passive insufficiency of the finger extensors occurs when the wrist is flexed, causing the fingers to extend. (B) Passive insufficiency of the finger flexors occurs when the wrist is extended, causing the fingers to flex.

insufficiency. The finger flexors and extensors are multijoint muscles. They cross the wrist, the metaphalangeal (MP) joints, the proximal (PIP), and sometimes the distal (DIP) interphalangeal joints. We have already noticed that a two-joint or multijoint muscle does not have sufficient length to be stretched over all joints simultaneously. Something has to give. If you rest your flexed elbow on the table in a pronated position, relax, and let your wrist drop into flexion, you will notice that your fingers have a tendency to extend passively (Fig. 5-9A). Conversely, if you supinate your forearm and relax your wrist into extension, your fingers will have a tendency to close (Fig. 5-9B). If these tendons were a little tight, this opening and closing

would be more pronounced. This is called **tenodesis** or **tendon action of a muscle.** A person who is quadriplegic and has no voluntary ability to open and close the fingers can use this principle to grasp and release light objects. By supinating the forearm, the weight of the hand and gravity causes the wrist to fall into hyperextension. This closes the fingers creating a slight grasp. Pronating the forearm causes the wrist to fall into flexion, thus opening the fingers and releasing an object.

Types of Muscle Contraction

There are three basic types of muscle contraction: isometric, isotonic, and isokinetic. An **isometric contraction** occurs when a muscle contracts, producing force without changing the length of muscle (Fig. 5-10A). The term isometric originates from the Greek meaning "same length." To demonstrate this action, in the sitting position place your right hand under your thigh and place your left hand on your right biceps muscle. Now, pull up with your right hand or, in other words, attempt to flex your right elbow. Note that there was no real motion at the elbow joint, but you did feel the muscle contract. This is an isometric contraction of your right biceps muscle. The muscle contracted, but no joint motion occurred.

Next, hold a weight in your hand while flexing your elbow to bring the weight up toward your shoulder (Fig. 5-10B). You will feel the biceps muscle contract, but this time there is joint motion. This is an **isotonic**

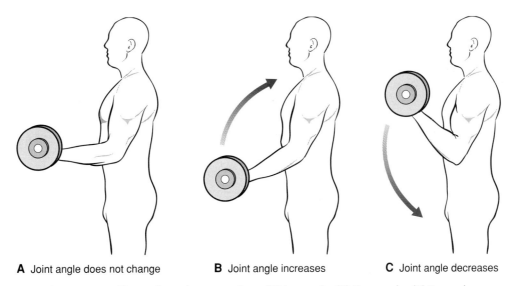

A Joint angle does not change   **B** Joint angle increases   **C** Joint angle decreases

Figure 5-10. Types of muscle contractions: (A) Isometric, (B) Concentric, (C) Eccentric.

contraction. An isotonic contraction occurs when a muscle contracts, the muscle length changes, and the joint angle changes.

Occasionally you will read a text that describes an isometric contraction as a *static,* or *tonic, contraction* and an isotonic contraction as *phasic.* Although these terms mean essentially the same thing, they have fallen into disuse, and specific differences between these terms no longer seem relevant.

The term isotonic originates from the Greek meaning "same tone or tension." Use of this term is not without its critics because it is felt that tension created within a muscle does not remain constant throughout its range. Therefore, this term is not as significant as its two types. An isotonic contraction can be subdivided into concentric and eccentric contractions. A **concentric contraction** occurs when there is joint movement, the muscles shorten, and the muscle attachments (O and I) move toward each other (Fig. 5-10B). It is sometimes referred to as a *shortening contraction.* Picking up the weight, as described earlier, is an example of a concentric contraction of the biceps muscle.

If you continue to palpate the biceps muscle while setting the weight back down on the table, you will feel that the biceps muscle (not the triceps muscle) continues to contract, even though the joint motion is elbow extension. What is occurring is an eccentric contraction of the biceps muscle.

An **eccentric contraction** occurs when there is joint motion but the muscle appears to lengthen; that is, the muscle attachments separate (Fig. 5-10C). After bringing the weight up to shoulder level, realize that if you relaxed your biceps muscle, the pull of gravity on your hand, forearm, and the weight would cause them to drop to the table. If you used your triceps muscle to extend the elbow (concentrically), your hand and weight would fall onto the tabletop with great force and speed. However, what you did by slowly returning the weight to the tabletop was to slow down the pull of gravity. You did this by eccentrically contracting the biceps (elbow flexor).

Eccentric contractions are sometimes referred to as *lengthening contractions.* This is somewhat misleading because, although the muscle is lengthening at a gross level, it is shortening microscopically. What the muscle is actually doing is returning to its normal resting position from a shortened position. An eccentric contraction can produce much greater forces than a concentric contraction can.

Frequently, different types of muscle contractions are used in various exercises. Quadriceps "setting" exercises are isometric contractions of the quadriceps

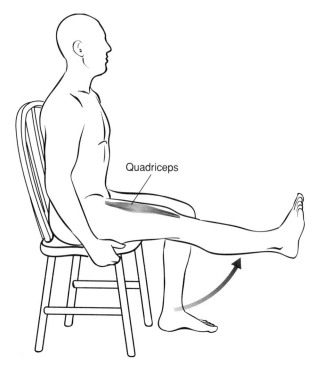

Figure 5-11.   Concentric contraction of quadriceps muscle.

muscle. Flexing and extending the knee are isotonic contractions. Sitting on a chair and extending the knee is a concentric contraction of the quadriceps muscle (Fig. 5-11), whereas flexing the knee and returning it to the starting position would be an eccentric contraction of the quadriceps muscle. If you were lying on the floor in a prone position and flexed your knee to 90 degrees, you would be doing a concentric contraction of the hamstring muscles. Straightening your knee would be an eccentric contraction of the same muscles. What is happening? Straightening the knee while sitting and bending the knee while prone involve moving the lower leg *against gravity.* Bending the knee while sitting and straightening the knee while prone involve moving the part *with gravity* and actually slowing down gravity. Generally speaking, eccentric contractions are used in deceleration activities and concentric contractions are used in acceleration activities.

Therefore, it can be summarized that the two types of isotonic contractions have the following features.

Concentric Contractions
1. Muscle attachments move closer together.
2. Movement is usually occurring against gravity (a "raising" motion).
3. It is an acceleration activity.

Eccentric Contractions

1. Muscle attachments move farther apart.
2. Movement usually occurs with gravity (a "lowering" motion).
3. The contraction is used with a deceleration activity.

However, it should be noted that not all concentric and eccentric contractions demonstrate all of the above listed features every time. Of course, there are exceptions. Here is an example. In the sitting position, have someone give resistance while you flex your knee. What type of contraction is it, and what muscle group is contracting? The answer is a concentric contraction of the hamstring muscles (knee flexors). In this case, your lower leg is moving down (with gravity), but gravity is not being slowed down. This is because a force (the other person's resistance) greater than the pull of gravity is being overcome.

Consider another example. If you hold on to the handle of an overhead pulley and pull it down into shoulder extension, you are doing a concentric contraction of the shoulder extensors. While your arm is moving in the same direction as gravity, you are overcoming a force greater than gravity (i.e., the overhead pulley weight). To prove this, keep holding the pulley handle but relax your shoulder muscles. Notice that your arm does not fall toward the ground. Why? The pulley weight is greater than the gravity weight (force of gravity).

Next, if you return the pulley handle to the starting position (shoulder flexion) slowly, and under control, you are doing an eccentric contraction of the shoulder extensors. Why? You are moving against gravity (a "raising" motion). However, in this case, you are decelerating the external force (the pulley weights).

Elastic tubing is a common method of providing resistance while exercising. While it can be used effectively with concentric contractions, it has greater limitations with eccentric contractions. If you attached elastic tubing over the top of a door and pulled down, you would be duplicating the action of the overhead pulley. Pulling down would be a concentric contraction of the shoulder extensors. However, returning to the starting position using elastic tubing is not as effective as an eccentric contraction with the pulleys. The initial motion is a strong eccentric contraction, but the elasticity quickly loses its tension. Therefore, using tubing for eccentric contraction must be done only in the early part of the motion, and not be considered effective throughout the entire range. It is possible to have effective eccentric contraction through smaller ranges using elastic tubing, such as forearm pronation and supination, but not with wide ranges, such as elbow flexion and extension.

Another, though less common, type of muscle contraction is an **isokinetic contraction.** It can be done only with special equipment. The *Cybex* and *Orthotron* were the first machines to produce such contractions. With an isokinetic contraction, resistance to the part varies, but the velocity, or speed, stays the same. This differs from an isotonic contraction in which the resistance remains constant but the velocity varies.

Consider the example of the person with the 5-pound weight attached to the leg. While the person straightens and flexes the knee (isotonic contraction), the amount of resistance stays the same. That 5-pound weight remained 5 pounds throughout the range. Because of other factors, such as angle of pull, it is easier to move the leg in the middle and at the end of the range than at the beginning. In other words, the speed at which the person is able to move the leg varies throughout the range.

In an isokinetic contraction, the speed is preset and will stay the same no matter how hard a person pushes. However, the resistance will vary. If the person pushes harder, the machine will give more resistance, and if the person does not push as hard, there will be less resistance.

Why are isokinetic muscle contractions significant? A complete discussion of the merits of isokinetic exercise in comparison with other forms of exercise is best covered in a more detailed discussion of therapeutic exercise, which is beyond the scope of this book. However, there are two significant advantages. Isokinetic exercises can alter or adjust the amount of resistance given through the range of motion, whereas an isotonic contraction cannot. This is important because a muscle is not as strong at the beginning or end of its range as it is in the middle. Because the muscle is strongest in the midrange, more resistance should be given there, and less resistance at the beginning and end. An isotonic contraction cannot do this; therefore, there may be too much resistance in the weaker parts of the range and not enough resistance in the stronger parts.

Accommodating resistance is also important because of the pain factor. If pain suddenly develops during the exercise, the person's response is to stop exercising, or not to work as hard. With an isotonic contraction, this response cannot happen quickly or even safely. With an isokinetic exercise, if the person stops working, the machine also stops. If the person does not contract as hard, the machine does not give as much resistance.

Table 5-1	Types of Muscle Contraction		
Type	**Speed**	**Resistance**	**Joint Motion**
Isometric	Fixed	Fixed (0 degrees/sec)	No
Isotonic	Variable	Fixed	Yes
Isokinetic	Fixed	Variable (accommodating)	Yes

Hopefully, this will give you some idea of the value of isokinetic exercise. There are, however, some drawbacks. For example, isokinetic exercise requires special equipment, and that equipment is expensive. There is a time and place for all of these types of muscle contractions. It is important that you recognize the differences among them. Table 5-1 summarizes the major differences among these three types of muscle contractions.

Roles of Muscles

Muscles assume different roles during joint motion, depending on such variables as the motion being performed, the direction of the motion, and the amount of resistance the muscle must overcome. If any of these variables change, the muscle's role may also change. The roles a muscle can assume are those of an agonist, antagonist, stabilizer, or neutralizer. An **agonist** is a muscle or muscle group that causes the motion. It is sometimes referred to as the **prime mover.** A muscle that is not as effective but does assist in providing that motion is called an **assisting mover.** Factors that determine whether a muscle is a prime mover or an assisting mover include size, angle of pull, leverage, and contractile potential. During elbow flexion, the biceps muscle is an agonist, and because of its size and angle of pull, the pronator teres muscle is an assisting mover.

An **antagonist** is a muscle that performs the opposite motion of the agonist. In the case of elbow flexion, the antagonist is the triceps muscle. Keep in mind that the role of a muscle is specific to a particular joint action. In the case of elbow extension, the triceps muscle is the agonist and the biceps muscle is the antagonist. However, in elbow flexion, the biceps muscle is the agonist and the triceps muscle is the antagonist.

The antagonist has the potential to oppose the agonist, but it is usually relaxed while the agonist is working. When the antagonist contracts at the same time as the agonist, a **cocontraction** results. A cocontraction occurs when there is a need for accuracy. Some experts feel that cocontractions are common when a person learns a task, especially a difficult one; thus, as the task is learned, cocontraction activity tends to disappear.

A **stabilizer** is a muscle or muscle group that supports, or makes firm, a part and allows the agonist to work more efficiently. For example, when you do a push-up, the agonists are the elbow extensor muscles. The abdominal muscles (trunk flexor muscles) act as stabilizers to keep the trunk straight, while the arms move the trunk up and down. A stabilizer is sometimes referred to as a fixator.

Remember, a muscle knows no direction when it contracts. If a muscle can do two (or more) actions, but only one is wanted, a **neutralizer** contracts to prevent the unwanted motion. For example, the biceps muscle can flex the elbow and supinate the forearm. If only elbow flexion is wanted, the supination component must be ruled out. Therefore, the pronator teres muscle, which pronates the forearm, would contract to counteract the supination component of the biceps muscle, and only elbow flexion would occur. A neutralizer may also allow a muscle to perform more than one role. Wrist ulnar deviation is such an example. The flexor carpi ulnaris muscle causes flexion and ulnar deviation of the wrist. The extensor carpi ulnaris muscle causes extension and ulnar deviation. In ulnar deviation, these muscles contract and accomplish two things. They neutralize each other's flexion/extension component while acting as agonists in wrist ulnar deviation.

A **synergist** is a muscle that works with one or more other muscles to enhance a particular motion. It is a term used by some authors to encompass the role of agonists, assisting movers, stabilizers, and neutralizers. The disadvantage of this term is that although it indicates that the muscle is working, it does not indicate how.

Angle of Pull

Several factors determine the role that a muscle will play in a particular joint motion. Determining whether a muscle has a major role (prime mover), a minor role (assisting mover), or no role at all will depend on such factors as its size, angle of pull, the joint motions possible, and the location of the muscle in relation to the

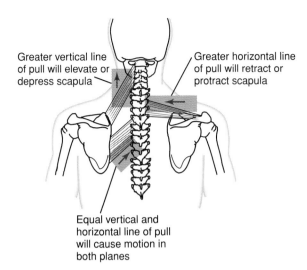

Greater vertical line of pull will elevate or depress scapula

Greater horizontal line of pull will retract or protract scapula

Equal vertical and horizontal line of pull will cause motion in both planes

Figure 5-12. Angle of pull as a determinant of muscle action.

joint axis. Visualizing the muscle, particularly in relation to other muscles performing the same action, will give you an idea about size as a factor. For example, compare the size of the triceps with that of the anconeus (see Figs. 10-17 and 10-18). It is easy to see that the anconeus will have little effect on joint motion compared to the triceps. Next, you know the motions that a particular joint allows. In the case of the elbow, the motions possible are flexion and extension. The triceps and anconeus cross the joint posterior to the joint axis. Because the triceps is much larger than the anconeus, it crosses the elbow posteriorly, and extensors must cross the elbow posteriorly, it is logical that the triceps is a prime mover in elbow extension.

Not all muscles are so obvious in their action. Angle of pull is usually a major factor. Most muscles pull at a diagonal. As will be discussed in Chapter 7 regarding torque, most muscles have a diagonal line of pull. That diagonal line of pull is the resultant force of a vertical force and a horizontal force. In the case of the shoulder girdle, muscles with a greater vertical angle of pull will be effective in pulling the scapula up or down (elevating or depressing the scapula). Muscles with a greater horizontal pull will be more effective in pulling the scapula in or out (protracting or retracting). Muscles with a more equal horizontal and vertical pull will have a role in both motions. Figure 5-12 gives an example of each. The levator scapula has a stronger vertical component, the middle trapezius has a stronger horizontal component, and the rhomboids have a more equal pull in both directions. As you will see when these muscles are described later in Chapter 8, the levator scapula is a

prime mover in scapular elevation and the middle trapezius is a prime mover in retraction, whereas the rhomboids are prime movers in both elevation and retraction.

Kinetic Chains

The concept of open versus closed kinetic chain exercises has evolved into movement and exercise. In engineering terms, a kinetic chain consists of a series of rigid links connected in such a way as to allow motion. Because these links are connected, movement of one link causes motion at other links in a predictable way. Applying this to the human body, a **closed kinetic chain** requires that the distal segment is fixed (closed) and the proximal segment(s) moves (Fig. 5-13). For example, when you rise from a sitting position, your knees extend, causing your hips and ankles to move as well. With your foot fixed on the ground, there is no way you can move your knee without causing movement at the hip and knee.

However, if you were to remain seated and extend your knee, your hip and ankle would not move. This is an **open kinetic chain** activity. The distal segment is

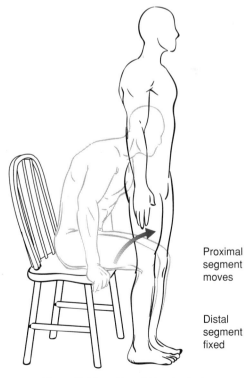

Proximal segment moves

Distal segment fixed

Figure 5-13. Closed kinetic chain.

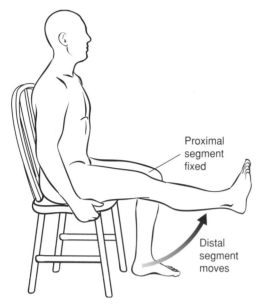

Figure 5-14.   Open kinetic chain.

free to move while the proximal segment(s) can remain stationary (Fig. 5-14). With open-chain activities, the limb segments are free to move in many directions. For example, if you are lying on a bed with your arm in the air, you can move your shoulder, elbow, wrist, and hand in many directions, either together or individually. This is open-chain activity. The distal segment is not fixed but is free to move.

However, if you took hold of an overhead trapeze, your hand, the distal segment, would be fixed or closed. As you flexed your elbow, your shoulder would have to go into some extension. As your elbow extended, your shoulder would have to go into some flexion. With closed-chain activities, the limb segments move in limited and predictable directions. Other examples of upper extremity closed-chain activities occur during crutch walking and pushing a wheelchair. The crutch tip (distal segment) is fixed on the ground and the body (proximal segment) moves. The hands on the wheelchair rims are the distal segments and joints proximal to the hands move in a connected fashion, i.e., the elbows extend and the shoulders flex.

Closed-chain exercise equipment includes such things as the bench press, rowing machine, stationary bicycle, and StairMaster. Examples of open-chain exercise equipment would be the Cybex and free weights.

Manual muscle testing is all open-chain movement. The treadmill is a combination of open- and closed-chain exercise. The weight-bearing portion would be closed-chain, and the non–weight-bearing portion would be open-chain movement.

The following listing illustrates the interrelationships of the concepts discussed in this chapter. Keep in mind that these are general statements and not absolute ones.

Exercise Terminology

Concentric	**Eccentric**
Usually open chain	Can be open or closed chain
Usually non–weight-bearing	Can be weight-bearing or non–weight-bearing
Open Chain	**Closed Chain**
Can be concentric or eccentric	Can be concentric or eccentric
Usually non–weight-bearing	Usually weight-bearing
Non–Weight-Bearing	**Weight-Bearing**
Can be concentric or eccentric	Usually eccentric
Usually open chain	Usually closed chain

Points to Remember

- The two ends of a muscle are referred to as the origin or insertion.

- Usually the insertion moves toward the origin.

- When the origin moves toward the insertion, it is referred to as reversal of muscle action.

- Active insufficiency is when a muscle cannot contract any further.

- Passive insufficiency is when a muscle cannot be elongated any further.

- Muscle contractions are of three basic types: isometric, concentric, or eccentric.

- A muscle can assume the role of agonist, antagonist, stabilizer, or neutralizer depending upon a particular situation.

- Kinetic chain movement depends upon whether the distal segment is fixed (closed) or free to move (open).

Review Questions

1. Usually, when a muscle contracts, the distal attachment moves toward the proximal attachment.
   a. What is another name to describe the distal attachment?
   b. What is another name for the proximal attachment?

2. What is the term for describing a muscle contraction in which the proximal end moves toward the distal end?

3. The flexor carpi radialis performs wrist flexion and radial deviation. The flexor carpi ulnaris performs wrist flexion and ulnar deviation.
   a. In what wrist action do the two muscles act as agonists?
   b. In what wrist action do they act as antagonists?

4. The following chart identifies the hip motions of three muscles. Hip extension is the desired motion.

Muscle	Extension	Lateral Rotation	Medial Rotation
Gluteus maximus	X	X	
Hamstrings	X		
Gluteus minimus			X

   a. Which of these muscles are acting as agonists in hip extension?
   b. What motion must be neutralized so the agonists can do only hip extension?
   c. What muscle must act as a neutralizer to rule out the undesired motion?

5. What is the term for the situation in which a muscle contracts until it can contract no farther even though more joint range of motion is possible?

6. Is walking downhill a concentric or eccentric contraction of your quadriceps muscle?

7. Sitting with a weight in your hand, forearm pronated, elbow extended, and shoulder medially rotated, slowly raise your hand out to the side and upward.
   a. What is the joint motion at the shoulder?
   b. Is an isometric, concentric, or eccentric muscle contraction occurring at the shoulder?
   c. What type of muscle contraction is occurring at the elbow?

8. Lying supine with your arm at your side and with a weight in your hand, raise the weight up and over your shoulder. (Hint: Think about gravity's effect throughout the range.)
   a. What is the joint motion at the shoulder?
   b. Is the muscle action during the first 90 degrees of the motion concentric or eccentric?
   c. Are the shoulder flexors or extensors responsible for this action?
   d. Is the muscle action during the second 90 degrees of the motion concentric or eccentric?
   e. Are the shoulder flexors or extensors responsible for this action?

9. Identify the following in terms of open or closed kinetic chain activities:
   a. Wheelchair push-ups
   b. Exercises with weight cuffs
   c. Overhead wall pulleys

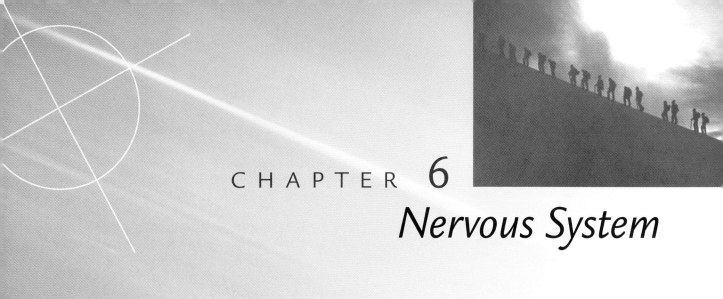

CHAPTER 6

Nervous System

Nervous Tissue (Neurons)

The Central Nervous System

 Brain

 Spinal Cord

The Peripheral Nervous System

 Cranial Nerves

 Spinal Nerves

 Functional Significance of Spinal Cord Level

 Plexus Formation

 Common Peripheral Nerve Pathologies

Review Questions

The nervous system is the highly complex mechanism in our bodies that controls, stimulates, and coordinates all other body systems. As outlined in Figure 6-1, it can be anatomically divided into the central nervous system (CNS), the peripheral nervous system (PNS), and the autonomic nervous system (ANS). The CNS includes the brain and spinal cord, and the PNS includes nerves outside the spinal cord. The ANS controls mostly visceral structures. The subdivisions of the ANS are the sympathetic nervous system and the parasympathetic nervous system. These operate as a check-and-balance system for each other. The sympathetic system deals with stress and stimulation whereas the parasympathetic system deals with conserving energy.

Specific description of the various parts of each system and their functions is beyond the scope of this text. A fairly brief anatomical and functional description of the CNS and PNS as they affect muscle movement will be given. This description will be focused at the gross, not the cellular, level.

Nervous Tissue (Neurons)

The fundamental unit of nervous tissue is the neuron (Fig. 6-2). It contains a **cell body** with fiber branches coming into and going away from it. The term "nerve cell" is synonymous with *neuron,* and includes all of its processes (dendrites and axons).

Dendrites are fiber branches that receive impulses from other parts of the nervous system and bring those impulses toward the cell body. **Axons** transmit impulses away from the cell body, are located on the side opposite the dendrites, and usually consist of a single branch. The inner part of the axon is often surrounded by a fatty sheath called **myelin,** which in turn is surrounded by a

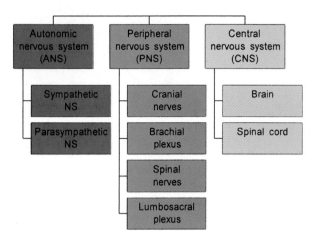

Figure 6-1. The nervous system.

transparent **neurilemma.** The myelin is interrupted approximately every half-millimeter. This break in the myelin is referred to as the **node of Ranvier.**

Myelin is a white, fatty substance found in the CNS and PNS. One of its functions is to increase the speed of impulse conduction in the myelinated fiber. Myelin does not cover cell bodies or certain nerve fibers. Areas that contain mostly unmyelinated fibers are referred to as **gray matter,** whereas areas that contain mostly myelinated fibers are called **white matter** (Fig. 6-3). Areas of gray matter include the cerebral cortex and the central portion of the spinal cord. White matter includes the major tracts within the spinal cord and fiber systems, such as the internal capsule within the brain.

A **nerve fiber** is the conductor of impulses from the neuron. Transmission of impulses from one neuron to another occurs at a **synapse,** which is a small gap between neurons involving very complex physiological actions.

A **tract** is a group of myelinated nerve fibers within the CNS that carries a specific type of information from one area to another. Depending on its location within the CNS, the group of fibers may be referred to as a *fasciculus, peduncle, brachium, column,* or *lemniscus.* A group of fibers within the PNS may be called a *spinal nerve, nerve root, plexus,* or *peripheral nerve,* depending on location. An example of the pathway of a tract can be seen in Figure 6-17.

Motor and sensory neurons are the two major types of nerve fibers in peripheral nerves. A **motor (efferent) neuron** has a large, multipolar cell body with multi-branched dendrites and a long axon (Fig. 6-2B). The cell body and dendrites are located within the anterior horn of the spinal cord (Fig. 6-3). Depending upon an author's use of terms, ventral and anterior are synonymous, as are dorsal and posterior. The axon leaves the

anterior horn through the white matter and is organized with other similar axons in the **anterior (ventral) root,** which is located just outside the spinal cord in the area of the intervertebral foramen. The axon continues down the peripheral nerve to its termination in a **motor endplate (axon terminal)** of a muscle fiber. A motor neuron conducts **efferent** impulses from the spinal cord to the periphery (Figs. 6-3 and 6-4).

The **sensory afferent neuron** has a dendrite, which arises in the skin and runs all the way to its cell body in the dorsal root ganglion (see Fig. 6-2A), located in the intervertebral foramen. The axon travels through the posterior (dorsal) root of the spinal nerve and into the spinal cord through the posterior horn. The axon may end at this point, or it may enter the white matter and ascend to a different level of the spinal cord or to the brainstem. A sensory neuron sends **afferent** impulses from the periphery to the spinal cord (Figs. 6-3 and 6-4).

Both sensory and motor impulses travel along nerve fibers located outside the spinal cord, but within peripheral nerves. Motor impulses travel from the CNS to the periphery. Sensory impulses travel from the periphery to the CNS (Fig. 6-4).

A third type of neuron is an **interneuron** (Fig. 6-3). It is found within the CNS. Its function is to transmit or integrate sensory or motor impulses.

The Central Nervous System

The main components of the CNS are the brain and the spinal cord. The brain is made up of the cerebrum, brainstem, and cerebellum. (Trivia fans will note that the brain weighs about 3 pounds.)

Brain

Cerebrum

The **cerebrum** is the largest and main portion of the brain (Fig. 6-5), and it is responsible for the highest mental functions. It occupies the anterior and superior area of the cranium above the brainstem and cerebellum. The cerebrum is made up of right and left **cerebral hemispheres** joined in the center by the **corpus callosum.**

Each cerebral hemisphere has a **cortex,** or outer coating, that is many cell layers deep, and each hemisphere is divided into four **lobes** (Fig. 6-6). The **frontal lobe** occupies the anterior portion of the skull, and the **occipital lobe** takes up the posterior portion. The **parietal lobe** lies between the frontal and occipital lobe, and the **temporal lobe** lies under the frontal and parietal lobes just above the ear.

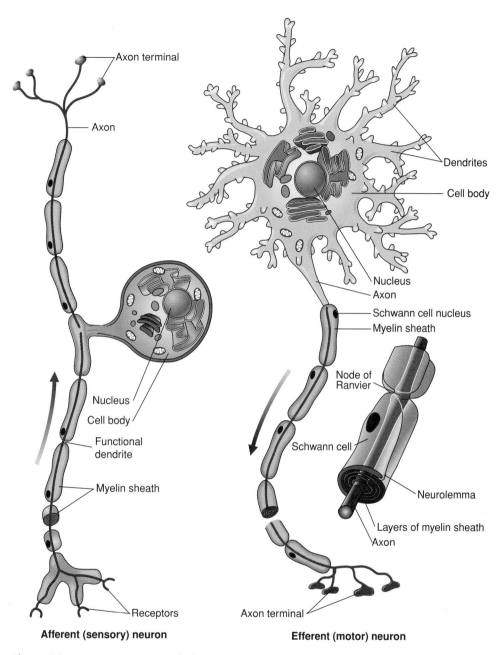

Figure 6-2. Neuron structure including *(A)* typical sensory and *(B)* motor neurons. (From Scanlon, VC, and Sanders, T: Essentials of Anatomy and Physiology, ed 4. FA Davis, Philadelphia 2003, p 157, with permission.)

Each lobe has many known functions. Specific locations of some functions have yet to be discovered. The area of brain activity that has to do with personality is located in the frontal lobe. The frontal lobe also controls motor movement and expressive speech. The occipital lobe is responsible for vision and recognition of size, shape, and color. The parietal lobe controls gross sensation, such as touch and pressure. It also controls fine sensation, such as the determination of texture, weight, size, and shape. Brain activity associated with reading skills is also located in the parietal lobe. The temporal lobes are the centers for behavior, hearing, and language reception and understanding. The interested student can find detailed maps of the brain functions in most anatomy and neurology texts.

Deep within the cerebral hemispheres, beneath the cortex, is the **thalamus** (see Fig. 6-5). This mass of nerve cells serves as a relay station for body sensations;

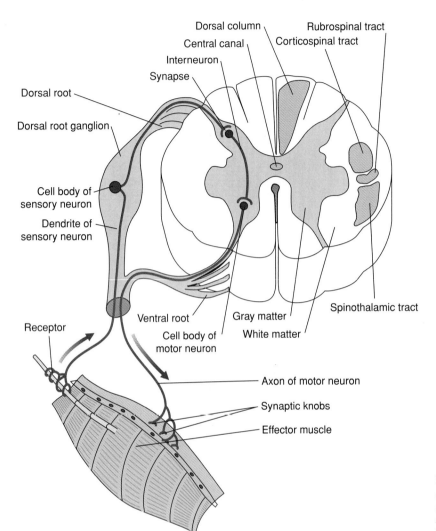

Dorsal column
Central canal
Interneuron
Synapse
Dorsal root
Dorsal root ganglion
Rubrospinal tract
Corticospinal tract
Cell body of sensory neuron
Dendrite of sensory neuron
Receptor
Ventral root
Cell body of motor neuron
Gray matter
White matter
Spinothalamic tract
Axon of motor neuron
Synaptic knobs
Effector muscle

Figure 6-3. Cross section of spinal cord and the three types of neurons. (From Scanlon, VC, and Sanders, T: Essentials of Anatomy and Physiology, ed 4. FA Davis, Philadelphia 2003, p 160, with permission.)

it is here where pain is perceived. Also deep inside the brain is the **hypothalamus,** which is important to hormone function and behavior. The **basal ganglia,** also in this area, are important in coordination of motor movement.

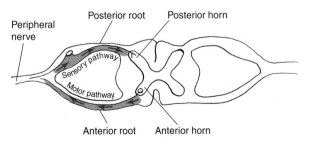

Peripheral nerve
Posterior root
Posterior horn
Sensory pathway
Motor pathway
Anterior root
Anterior horn

Figure 6-4. Sensory and motor pathways within the spinal cord.

Brainstem

Lying below the cerebrum is the brainstem, which can be divided into three parts: the midbrain, pons, and medulla (see Fig. 6-5). The upper portion of the brainstem is the midbrain, located somewhat below the cerebrum. The **midbrain** is the center for visual reflexes. Pons is Latin for "bridge," and is located between the midbrain and medulla. The **medulla oblongata** is the most caudal or inferior portion of the brainstem. It is usually referred to simply as the *medulla,* meaning "middle" or "inner." The medulla is continuous with the spinal cord, with the transition being at the base of the skull where it passes through the foramen magnum. The medulla is the center for automatic control of respiration and heart rate.

Most of the cranial nerves come from the brainstem area, and all fiber tracts from the spinal cord and peripheral nerves to and from higher centers of the brain go through this area.

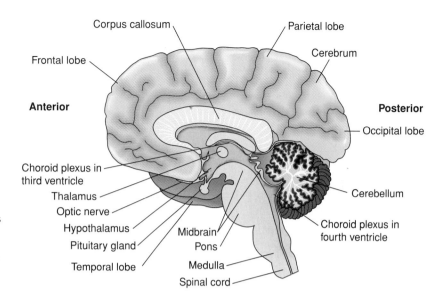

Figure 6-5. The brain. Note that this illustration identifies only a few of the major structures of the brain.
(From Scanlon, VC, and Sanders, T: Essentials of Anatomy and Physiology, ed 4. FA Davis, Philadelphia 2003, p 167, with permission.)

Cerebellum

In Latin, **cerebellum** means "little brain." It is located in the posterior portion of the cranium behind the pons and medulla (see Fig. 6-5). It is covered superiorly by the posterior portion of the cerebrum. The main functions of the cerebellum are control of muscle coordination, tone, and posture.

Brain Protection

The brain has basically three levels of protection: bony, membranous, and fluid. Surrounding the brain is the **skull,** made up of several bones with joints fused together for greater strength (Fig. 6-7).

Within the skull are three layers of membrane, called *meninges* (Figs. 6-8 and 6-12), that cover the brain and provide support and protection. The thickest, most fibrous, tough outer layer is called the **dura mater,** which means "hard mother" in Latin. The middle, thinner layer is called **arachnoid** or, less commonly, *arachnoid mater.* (*Arachnoid,* from Greek for "spider," means "spider-like.") The inner, delicate layer is called the **pia mater** (Latin for "tender mother"), which carries blood vessels to the brain. These cranial meninges are continuous with the spinal meninges that surround the spinal cord.

Between the layers of the arachnoid and pia mater is the **subarachnoid space** through which circulates **cerebrospinal fluid** (Fig. 6-8). This fluid surrounds

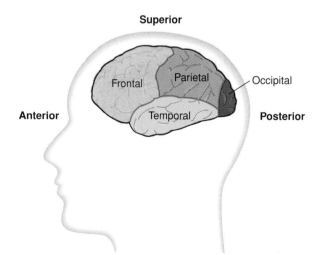

Figure 6-6. Each cerebral hemisphere has four lobes.

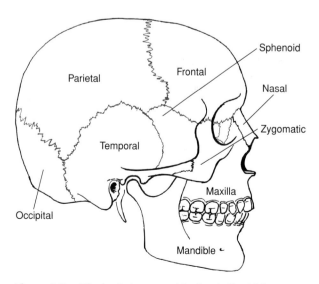

Figure 6-7. The brain is encased in the skull, which consists of nine bones. The fibrous, immovable joints between these bones offer maximum protection.

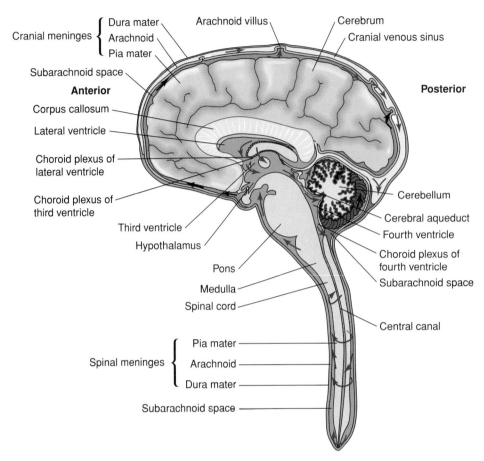

Figure 6-8.   Circulation of cerebrospinal fluid. The arrows indicate flow. (From Scanlon, VC, and Sanders, T: Essentials of Anatomy and Physiology, ed 4. FA Davis, Philadelphia 2003, p 176, with permission.)

the brain and fills the four **ventricles** within the brain. The ventricles are four small cavities containing a capillary network (choroid plexus) that produces cerebrospinal fluid. There are two lateral ventricles, a third ventricle, and a fourth ventricle. The main function of the cerebrospinal fluid is shock absorption.

Brain Blood Supply

The blood supply to the brain comes from branches of the internal carotid and vertebral arteries (Fig. 6-9). The right and left common carotid arteries arise from the aortic arch and run the length of the neck in an anterior lateral position. At about the level of the jaw, each divides into the external and internal carotid arteries. The **external carotid arteries** supply the scalp, dura, and skull. The **internal carotid arteries** enter the middle cranial fossa through the carotid canal in the temporal bone to supply primarily the anterior portion of the brain. Immediately upon entering the cranial cavity, the internal carotid artery branches into the middle and anterior cerebral arteries (Fig. 6-10A). The middle cerebral artery

is actually a continuation of the internal carotid and supplies the lateral cerebral hemispheres. The anterior cerebral arteries supply the medial surface of the brain.

The right and left vertebral arteries also branch off the aortic arch (see Fig. 6-9). They ascend the neck through the transverse foramens of the cervical vertebrae and enter the base of the brain through the foramen magnum to supply primarily the posterior portion of the brain. The vertebral arteries give off branches to the medulla and cerebellum and join together to form the **basilar artery** (see Fig. 6-10A), which also supplies parts of the cerebellum, as well as the pons and midbrain. The basilar artery branches to form the **posterior cerebral arteries,** which supply the occipital lobes and part of the temporal lobes.

The anterior and posterior cerebral arteries are connected at the base of the brain and form a cerebral arterial circle, often referred to as the **circle of Willis** (see Fig. 6-10B) after the English physician, Thomas Willis, who first described this interconnection. The anterior and posterior cerebral arteries are joined by the **posterior**

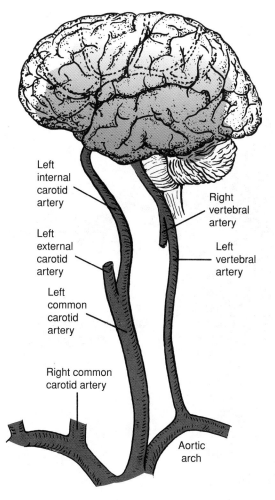

Figure 6-9. The four major arteries to the brain. (From Curtis, BA: Neurosciences: The Basics. Lea & Febiger, Malvern, PA, 1990, p 92, with permission.)

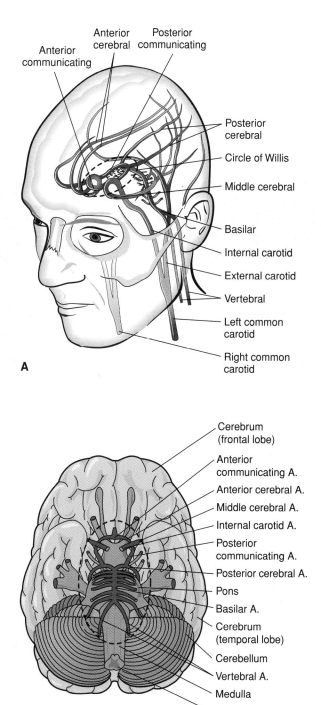

A

B

Figure 6-10. Circle of Willis. (From Scanlon, VC, and Sanders, T: Essentials of Anatomy and Physiology, ed 4. FA Davis, Philadelphia 2003, p 289, with permission.)

communicating artery. The right and left anterior cerebral arteries are joined by the **anterior communicating artery.** The significance of this circle is that failure of one of these major arteries usually does not seriously decrease blood flow to the region supplied by that artery.

Spinal Cord

A continuation of the medulla, the spinal cord runs within the vertebral canal from the foramen magnum to the cone-shaped **conus medullaris** at approximately the level of the second lumbar vertebra (Fig. 6-11). Below this level is a collection of nerve roots running down from the spinal cord much like a horse's tail, hence the name **cauda equina.** The cauda equina is made up of the nerve roots for L2 through S5. A threadlike, nonneural filament running from the conus medullaris is the **filum terminale.**

The spinal cord is approximately 17 inches in length. It is enclosed in the same three protective layers as the brain: the outer dura mater, the arachnoid membrane, and the inner pia mater (Fig. 6-12). As with the brain, cerebrospinal fluid flows in the space between the arachnoid layer and pia mater.

The **vertebral foramen** is the passageway for the spinal cord and is surrounded and protected by the bony structures of each individual vertebra (Fig. 6-13). Each vertebra is made up of a **body,** the anterior weight-bearing portion, and the posterior **neural arch** consisting of pedicles, transverse processes, lamina, and a spinous process (Fig. 6-14). The opening formed between these

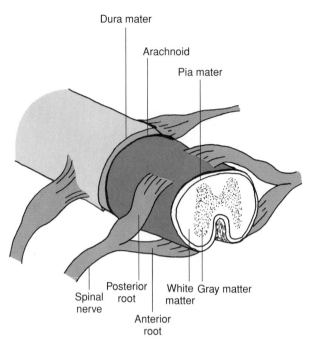

Figure 6-12. The three layers of the meninges surround the spinal cord and the brain.

two parts is the vertebral foramen. This opening is not to be confused with the **intervertebral foramen** located on the sides of the vertebral column. The intervertebral foramen is the opening formed by the superior vertebral notch of the vertebra below and the inferior vertebral notch of the vertebra above (Fig. 6-15). Through this opening, the spinal nerve root exits the vertebral canal.

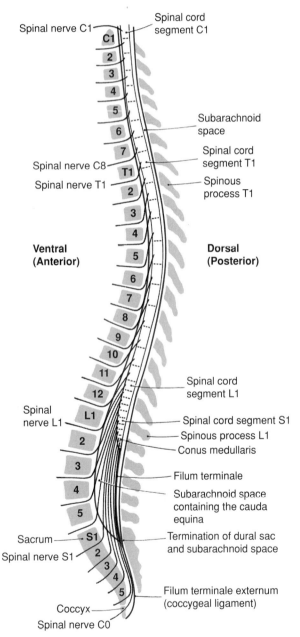

Figure 6-11. The spine and spinal cord. (From Gilman, S, and Newman, SW: Manter and Gatz's Essentials of Clinical Neuroanatomy and Neurophysiology, ed 10. FA Davis, Philadelphia, 2003, p 8, with permission.)

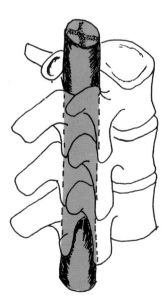

Figure 6-13. The spinal cord runs through the vertebral foramen.

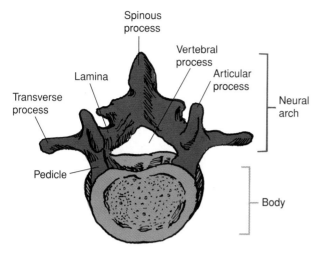

Figure 6-14.   The vertebra provides bony protection for the spinal cord.

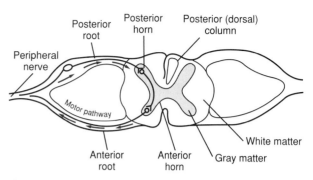

Figure 6-16.   Cross section of spinal cord showing gray and white matter.

A cross-sectional view of the spinal cord reveals peripheral white matter and central gray matter. The **gray matter** is in the middle of the cord in an **H** or "butterfly" shape (Fig. 6-16). It contains neuronal cell bodies and synapses. The top portion of the **H** is the **posterior horn,** which transmits sensory impulses. The lower portion, the anterior horn, transmits motor impulses.

The **posterior columns,** also called the *dorsal columns,* are located in the posterior medial portions of the spinal cord. These columns transmit the sensations of proprioception, pressure, and vibration (Fig. 6-16).

White matter contains ascending (sensory) and descending (motor) fiber pathways. Each pathway carries a particular type of impulse, such as touch, from and to a specific area. These various pathways cross over from one side of the body to the other at different levels. It is this crossover phenomenon that results in a stroke on the left side of the brain affecting the right side of the body.

The pathway of particular significance to muscle control is the **corticospinal tract** (Fig. 6-17). It is located lateral to the posterior column and posterior horn.

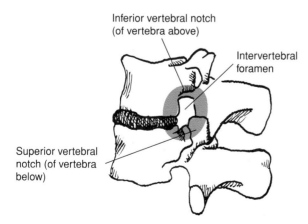

Figure 6-15.   Two vertebrae combine to form an opening (intervertebral foramen) on each side through which passes a spinal nerve root.

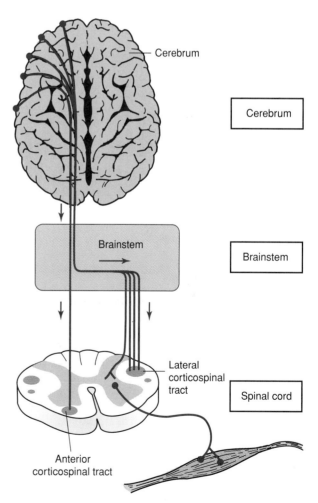

Figure 6-17.   Pathway of corticospinal tract from the brain's motor cortex to the spinal cord.

Table 6-1	Clinical Differences Between Upper and Lower Motor Neuron Lesions	
Sign	Upper Motor Neuron Lesion	Lower Motor Neuron Lesion
Paralysis	Spasticity present	Flaccid
Muscle atrophy	Not significant	Marked
Fasciculations and fibrillations	Not present	Present
Reflexes	Hyperreflexia	Hyporeflexia
Babinski reflex	Present	Not present
Clonus	Present	Not present

As its name implies, it runs from the motor area of the cerebral cortex to the spinal cord crossing over at about the level of the lower part of the brainstem. Corticospinal pathways synapse in the anterior horn just prior to leaving the spinal cord.

Motor neurons that synapse above this level are called **upper motor neurons.** Those that synapse at or below the anterior horn are called **lower motor neurons.** Injury to these two types of neurons results in quite different clinical signs. In other words, if a lesion occurs between the brain and the spinal cord proximal to the anterior horn, it will be considered an upper motor neuron lesion. If the lesion occurs between the anterior horn of the spinal cord and the periphery, it will be a lower motor neuron lesion. Paralysis will usually result in either case; however, clinical signs differ greatly (these are contrasted in Table 6-1).

Examples of diagnoses involving upper motor neuron lesions include spinal cord injuries, multiple sclerosis, parkinsonism, cerebral vascular accident, and various types of head injuries. Examples of diagnoses involving lower motor neuron lesions are muscular dystrophy, poliomyelitis, myasthenia gravis, and peripheral nerve injuries.

To summarize, motor impulses travel from the brain down the spinal cord through the anterior horn and out to the periphery via peripheral nerves. Sensory impulses from the periphery travel up the peripheral nerves into the spinal cord via the posterior, or dorsal, horn, then up the spinal cord to the brain.

The Peripheral Nervous System

The PNS is, for the most part, made up of all the nervous tissue outside the vertebral canal. It actually begins at the anterior horn of the spinal cord, sending motor impulses out to the muscles and receiving sensory impulses from the skin.

Cranial Nerves

There are 12 pairs of cranial nerves that are both numbered and named. They have their origins in the brain and can best be seen at their origins on the inferior surface of the brain (Fig. 6-18). They are sensory nerves, motor nerves, or mixed (a combination of both). Their functions are summarized in Table 6-2.

Table 6-2	Cranial Nerves		
Number	Name	Type	Function
I	Olfactory	Sensory	Smell
II	Optic	Sensory	Vision
III	Oculomotor	Motor	Muscles of eye
IV	Trochlear	Motor	Muscles of eye
V	Trigeminal	Mixed	Sensory: Face area Motor: Chewing muscles
VI	Abducens	Motor	Muscles of eye
VII	Facial	Mixed	Sensory: Tongue area Motor: Muscles of face
VIII	Vestibulocochlear (auditory)	Sensory	Hearing
IX	Glossopharyngeal	Mixed	Sensory: Tongue, pharynx, middle ear Motor: Muscles of pharynx
X	Vagus	Mixed	Sensory: Heart, lungs, GI tract, ear Motor: Heart, lungs, GI tract
XI	Spinal accessory	Motor	Sternocleidomastoid and trapezius muscles
XII	Hypoglossal	Motor	Muscles of tongue

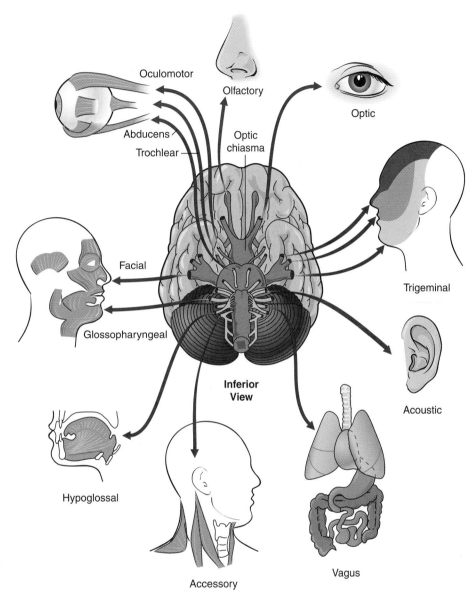

Oculomotor

Olfactory

Optic

Optic chiasma

Abducens

Trochlear

Optic

Facial

Trigeminal

Glossopharyngeal

Inferior
View

Acoustic

Hypoglossal

Vagus

Accessory

Figure 6-18.   Cranial nerves and their distributions. (From Scanlon, VC, and Sanders, T: Essentials of Anatomy and Physiology, ed 4. FA Davis, Philadelphia, 2003, p 178, with permission.)

Of the 12 cranial nerves, the trigeminal (V), facial (VII), and spinal accessory (XI) (often shortened to accessory) nerves are the ones most significant in terms of their control over certain muscles. In the following chapters, innervation of muscles will be given along with the summary description of each muscle.

Spinal Nerves

There are 31 pairs of spinal nerves. The spinal nerves are made up of 8 cervical, 12 thoracic, 5 lumbar, 5 sacral, and 1 coccygeal nerves (Fig. 6-19). The first seven cervical nerves (C1 to C7) exit the vertebral column above the corresponding vertebra. For example, C3 nerve exits over the C3 vertebra. Because there is one more cervical nerve than vertebra, this arrangement changes with the eighth cervical nerve (C8). It exits under the C7 vertebra and over the T1 vertebra. The T1 nerve exits *under* the T1 vertebra, and so on down the vertebral column.

Branches of Spinal Nerves

Once outside the spinal cord the anterior (motor) and posterior (sensory) roots join together to form the spinal nerve (Fig. 6-20), which passes through the bony intervertebral foramen. Almost immediately, the nerve sends a branch called the **posterior (dorsal) ramus.** This

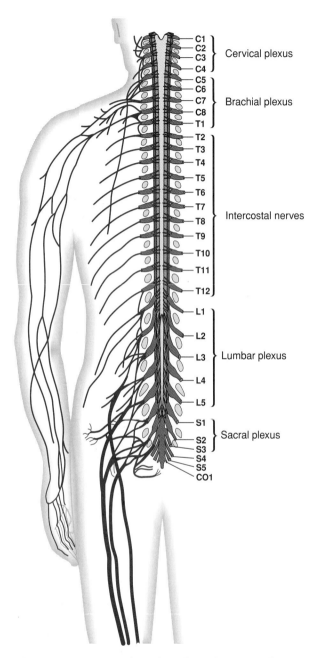

Figure 6-19. Anterior branches of spinal nerves in thoracic region give rise to intercostal nerves. Spinal nerves in other regions combine to form complex networks called plexuses. (From Scanlon, VC, and Sanders, T: Essentials of Anatomy and Physiology, ed 4. FA Davis, Philadelphia, 2003, p 163, with permission.)

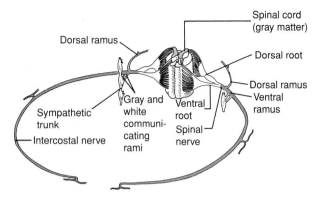

Figure 6-20. Anterior lateral view of a thoracic spinal cord segment and the two branches of its spinal nerves. (From Pratt, NE: Clinical Musculoskeletal Anatomy. JB Lippincott, Philadelphia, 1991, p 44, with permission.)

Located just peripheral to the posterior ramus is a branch to the autonomic nervous system. It is involved with such functions as blood pressure regulation. Although these functions are vital, they will not be discussed here. Instead, emphasis will be on the motor functions that occur mostly via the anterior ramus.

Dermatomes

The area of skin supplied with the **sensory fibers** of a spinal nerve is called the **dermatome** (Fig. 6-21). There is often overlap of contiguous dermatomes. Complete anesthesia of the area will not occur unless more than two spinal nerves have lost function. If an injury involves only one spinal nerve, sensation will be decreased or altered, but it will not be absent.

Thoracic Nerves

There are 12 pairs of thoracic nerves. With the exception of T1, which is part of the brachial plexus, they maintain their segmental relationship and do not join with the other nerves. Each nerve branches into a posterior and anterior ramus (see Fig. 6-19). The posterior rami innervate the muscles of the back and the overlying skin. The anterior rami become **intercostal nerves,** innervating the anterior trunk and intercostal muscles as well as the skin of the anterior and lateral trunk.

Functional Significance of Spinal Cord Level

As illustrated in Figure 6-22, it should be remembered that the spinal nerves in the cervical region exit the spinal cord above the vertebra. The C8 spinal nerve

branch on all spinal nerves innervates the deep muscles of the back as well as the skin covering these muscles. The spinal nerve continues as the **anterior (ventral) ramus.** These rami (plural of ramus) innervate all muscles and skin areas not innervated by the posterior rami.

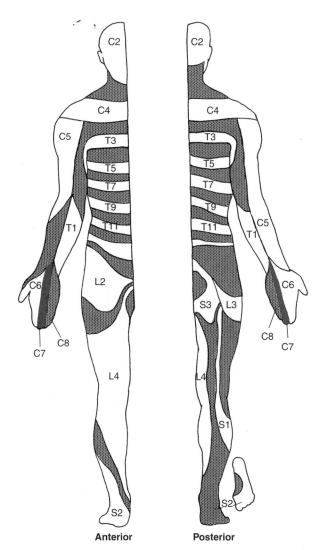

Anterior   **Posterior**

Figure 6-21.   Dermatomes: segmental areas of innervation of the skin. (Modified from Gilman, S, and Newman, SW: Manter and Gatz's Essentials of Clinical Neuroanatomy and Neurophysiology, ed 10. FA Davis, Philadelphia, 2003, p 44.)

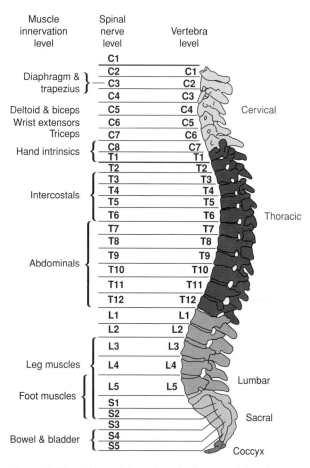

Figure 6-22.   The position of a spinal nerve exiting the vertebral column and its corresponding vertebral level. Also shown is a comparison of spinal cord level and muscle innervation. Cross-sectional view.

comes out below the C7 vertebra because there is one more cervical nerve than vertebrae. Starting with the T1 spinal nerve, all spinal nerves below T1 come out below the same numbered vertebra.

In this same illustration, one can gain an appreciation for the general innervation level of major muscles (Fig. 6-22). It should be noted that most muscles take innervation from more than one spinal level. Therefore, an injury at one spinal level may weaken a muscle, but some function will remain. For example, the elbow flexors receive innervation from the C5 and C6 spinal level. An injury at the C5 vertebral level will weaken elbow flexion but function will not be completely

absent. This is because the C5 spinal nerve exits the spinal cord above the C5 vertebra while the C6 spinal nerve exits below the C5 vertebra. Therefore, the C5 spinal nerve may not be injured, allowing the elbow flexors to continue to receive partial innervation.

Although there is slight variation among individuals, some general statements can be made about the level of function at various levels of the spinal cord. A person with a spinal cord injury at C3 or above would not have the function of the diaphragm and would be unable to breathe without assistance. Below that level, although breathing would be compromised, a person would probably be able to breathe without assistance. With C5 spinal cord involvement, innervation of the shoulder abductors and elbow flexors remains intact allowing increased function of the upper extremities. The wrist extensors receive innervation from C6 to C8 whereas the triceps are innervated at C7 to C8. The intrinsic muscles of the hand are the last to be innervated in the upper extremity at C8 to T1.

In the thoracic level, muscles receive innervation at each spinal level. Because the intercostals and erector spinae muscles receive innervation throughout the thoracic region, the lower the level of injury, the more muscles remain intact. The abdominal muscles receive innervation from the lower thoracic levels.

The lumbar and sacral regions are controlled by plexus innervation, so once again, the level of injury will be important in knowing which muscles are functioning. The hip flexors and knee extensors are innervated between L2 and L4. Next are the hip adductors at L2 to L3 and the hip abductors at L4 to L5. The hip extensors and knee flexors are innervated at L5 through S2. The ankle motions are innervated between L4 and S2. Last to receive innervation is bowel and bladder control at S4 to S5.

Sensation changes as one proceeds down the spinal cord. Figure 6-21 shows the sensory innervation (dermatomes) at various levels. A person with a C3 spinal cord injury will have sensation only from the top of the head to the neck. At T3, the entire upper extremity and chest, level with the axilla, are innervated. An injury at L3 would show innervation in an irregular pattern to approximately the midthigh level.

Autonomic dysreflexia, also know as **hyperreflexia,** is a serious and potentially life-threatening complication associated with spinal cord injuries at or above T10, although those with injuries at or above T6 are most susceptible. It is usually triggered by a noxious stimulus below the level of injury, such as a distended bladder. Symptoms include a severe headache, sudden hypertension, facial flush, sweating, and gooseflesh. Blood pressure may rise to dangerous levels, and if not treated, can lead to stroke or death.

Plexus Formation

Except for the thoracic nerves, the anterior rami of the spinal nerves will join together and/or branch out forming a network known as a **plexus.** There are three major plexuses (see Fig. 6-19):

1. The cervical plexus, made up of C1 through C4 spinal nerves, innervates the muscles of the neck.
2. The brachial plexus, made up of C5 through T1, innervates muscles of the upper limb.
3. The lumbosacral plexus, made up of L1 through S5, innervates muscles of the lower limb.
   a. Lumbar portion, L1 through L4, supplies mostly muscles of the thigh.
   b. Sacral portion, L5 through S3, supplies mostly muscles of the leg and foot.

Cervical Plexus

The anterior rami of the first four cervical nerves (C1 to C4) join together in various ways to form the **cervical plexus** (see Fig. 6-19). This plexus will not be described in detail because only a few muscles covered in this text receive their innervation from the cervical plexus.

There is a branch from C2 going to the sternocleidomastoid, and branches from C3 and C4 supply the trapezius. The levator scapulae receive innervation from C3 through C5. The anterior scalene gets some innervation from C4, and the middle scalene from C3 and C4. Perhaps one of the most significant nerves of the cervical plexus is the *phrenic nerve,* which is formed by branches of C3 through C5 and innervates the diaphragm.

Brachial Plexus

The **brachial plexus** is formed by the anterior rami of C5 through T1 spinal nerves. It splits and joins several times before ending in five main peripheral nerves. Its network arrangement consists of roots, trunks, divisions, cords, and finally peripheral (terminal) nerves, as shown in Figure 6-23.

There are five roots made up of the anterior rami of C5, C6, C7, C8, and T1. These roots join together forming three **trunks.** The three trunks, named for their position relative to each other, are:

1. The superior trunk coming from C5 and C6
2. The middle trunk coming from C7
3. The inferior trunk coming from C8 and T1

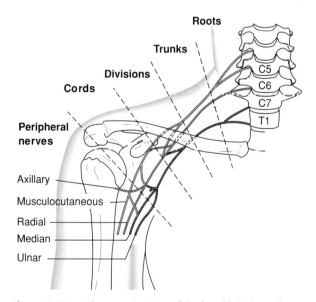

Figure 6-23. The organization of the brachial plexus from the nerve roots to the peripheral nerves. Some lesser motor and sensory nerves have been omitted.

Each trunk splits into an anterior and posterior **division,** named for their position relative to each other.

Next are the three **cords,** named according to their relationship to the axillary artery. They are formed by the joining of various trunk divisions. The lateral cord comes from the anterior division of the superior and middle trunks. The posterior cord arises from the posterior divisions of all three trunks, and the medial cord comes from the anterior division of the inferior trunk. The five **peripheral nerves,** which are branches of the cords, form the terminal nerves of the plexus as follows:

1. *Musculocutaneous nerve:* From the lateral cord
2. *Axillary nerve:* A branch of the posterior cord
3. *Radial nerve:* A branch of the posterior cord
4. *Median nerve:* From the lateral and medial cords
5. *Ulnar nerve:* From the medial cord

This network arrangement is not a plot to make learning more difficult; rather, it provides muscles with innervation from more than one level. In the event of trauma or disease, perhaps not all levels of innervation will be involved. Therefore, a muscle may be weakened but not completely paralyzed.

For the most part, these five peripheral nerves innervate the muscles of the upper limb; however, some muscles receive innervation from nerves that have branched off the plexus superior to the formation of the peripheral nerves. These branches are noted in Figure 6-23. The dorsal scapular nerve comes off the anterior ramus of C5 and innervates the rhomboids and levator scapulae muscles. The suprascapular nerve comes off the superior trunk and innervates the supraspinatus and infraspinatus muscles. The medial pectoral nerve comes off the medial cord and innervates the pectoralis major and minor muscles, while the lateral pectoral nerve comes off the lateral cord to provide additional innervation to the pectoralis major. The subscapular nerve comes off the posterior cord and innervates the subscapularis and teres major muscles. The thoracodorsal nerve also comes off the posterior cord to innervate the latissimus dorsi. All other muscles of the upper extremity receive innervation from the five terminal nerves described in the following.

Terminal Nerves of the Brachial Plexus

The five terminal nerves of the brachial plexus have been summarized according to:

1. The segment, or root, of the spinal cord from which they originate.
2. The major muscles they innervate.
3. The major sensory distribution.
4. The main motor impairments that would be seen following damage to the nerve.

Axillary Nerve (Fig. 6-24)

Spinal cord segment	C5, C6
Muscle innervation	Deltoid, teres minor
Sensory distribution	Lateral arm over lower portion of deltoid
Clinical motor features of paralysis	Loss of shoulder abduction Weakened shoulder lateral rotation

Musculocutaneous Nerve (Fig. 6-25)

Spinal cord segment	C5, C6
Muscle innervation	Coracobrachialis, biceps, brachialis
Sensory distribution	Anterior lateral surface of forearm
Clinical motor features of paralysis	Loss of elbow flexion Weakened supination

Radial Nerve (Fig. 6-26)

Spinal segment	C6, C7, C8, T1
Muscle innervation	Triceps, anconeus, brachioradialis, supinator, wrist, finger, and thumb extensors
Sensory distribution	Posterior arm, posterior forearm, and radial side of posterior hand
Clinical motor features of paralysis	Loss of elbow, wrist, finger and thumb extension: (commonly called "wrist drop")

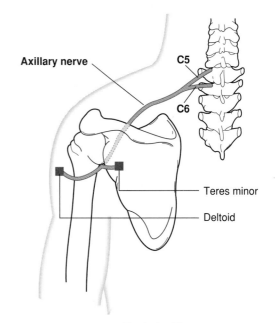

Posterior View

Figure 6-24. The axillary nerve.

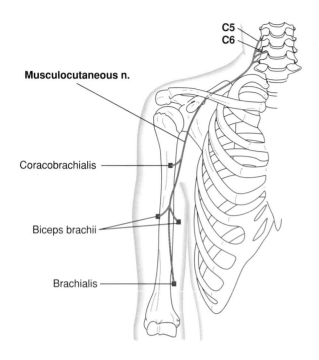

Anterior View

Figure 6-25.   The musculocutaneous nerve.

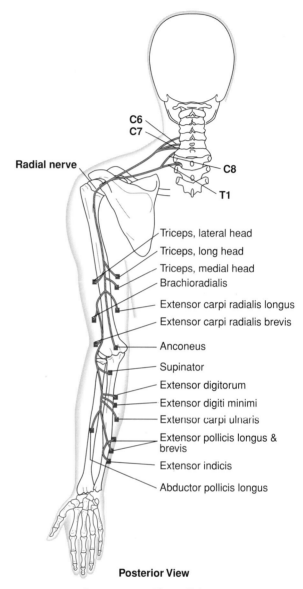

Posterior View

Figure 6-26.   The radial nerve.

Median Nerve (Fig. 6-27)

Spinal cord segment	C6, C7, C8, T1
Muscle innervation	Pronators
	Wrist and finger flexors on radial side
	Most thumb muscles
Sensory distribution	Palmar aspect of thumb, second, third, fourth (radial half) fingers
Clinical motor features of paralysis	Loss of forearm pronation
	Loss of thumb opposition, flexion, and abduction ("ape hand")

Ulnar Nerve (Fig. 6-28)

Spinal cord segment	C8, T1
Muscle innervation	Flexor carpi ulnaris
	Flexor digitorum profundus (medial half)
	Interossei
	Fourth and fifth lumbricales
Sensory distribution	Fourth finger (medial portion), fifth finger
Clinical motor features of paralysis	Loss of wrist ulnar deviation
	Weakened wrist, finger flexion
	Weakened fourth and fifth finger flexion ("pope's blessing")
	Loss of thumb adduction
	Loss of most intrinsics ("claw hand")

Lumbosacral Plexus

The lumbosacral plexus is formed by the anterior rami of L1 through S3 (Fig. 6-29). Some sources will sepa-

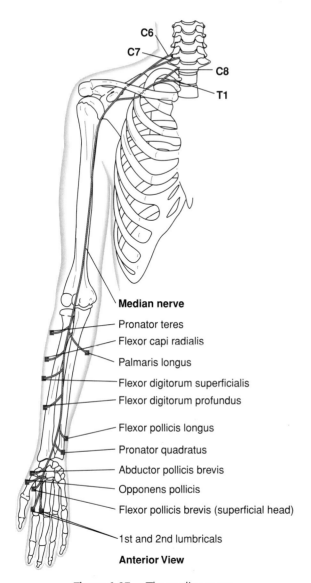

Median nerve
- Pronator teres
- Flexor capi radialis
- Palmaris longus
- Flexor digitorum superficialis
- Flexor digitorum profundus
- Flexor pollicis longus
- Pronator quadratus
- Abductor pollicis brevis
- Opponens pollicis
- Flexor pollicis brevis (superficial head)
- 1st and 2nd lumbricals

Anterior View

Figure 6-27. The median nerve.

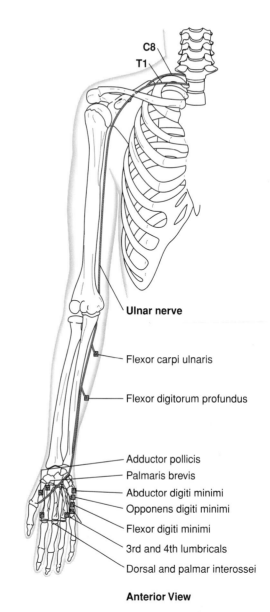

Ulnar nerve
- Flexor carpi ulnaris
- Flexor digitorum profundus
- Adductor pollicis
- Palmaris brevis
- Abductor digiti minimi
- Opponens digiti minimi
- Flexor digiti minimi
- 3rd and 4th lumbricals
- Dorsal and palmar interossei

Anterior View

Figure 6-28. The ulnar nerve.

rate this into a **lumbar plexus** (L1 through L4), which innervates most muscles of the thigh, and a **sacral plexus** (L5 through S3), which innervates mostly muscles of the leg and foot. Because there are several muscles of the lower limb that receive innervation from both plexuses, they will be discussed here as one plexus.

The lumbosacral plexus does not have as much dividing and joining of nerves as does the brachial plexus. It has eight roots that each divide into an upper and lower branch. L3 is the only root that does not divide. Most of these branches divide into an anterior and posterior division. These divisions join in various ways to form the six main peripheral nerves.

The upper branch of L1 divides into the iliohypogastric and ilioinguinal nerves. The lower branch of L1 and the upper branch of L2 form the genitofemoral nerve. These three nerves are primarily sensory in nature and will not be discussed in detail.

The anterior divisions of L2, L3, and L4 form the **obturator nerve.** Posterior divisions of the same roots form the **femoral nerve.** The posterior divisions of L4 through S1 form the **superior gluteal nerve,** and the posterior divisions of L5 through S2 make up the **inferior gluteal nerve.** The **sciatic nerve** is made up of branches from L4 through S3. It is actually the tibial and common peroneal nerves joined by a common

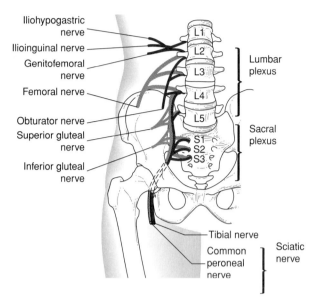

Figure 6-29. Anterior view of the lumbosacral plexus. (From Pratt, NE: Clinical Musculoskeletal Anatomy. JB Lippincott, Philadelphia, 1991, p 175, with permission.)

sheath, and it separates into the two nerves just above the knee. The **common peroneal nerve** comes from L4 through S2, while the **tibial nerve** is made up of anterior divisions of L4 through S3. If all of this is confusing, perhaps the illustrations in Figures 6-29 through 6-34 plus the summary that follows will provide some clarity. This summary is similar to the one provided for the brachial plexus.

Terminal Nerves of the Lumbosacral Plexus

Like the nerves of the upper extremity, the nerves of the lower extremity have been summarized according to:

1. The segment, or root, of the spinal cord from which they came.
2. The major muscles they innervate.
3. The major sensory distribution.
4. The main motor impairments that would be seen following severance of the nerve.

Femoral Nerve (Fig. 6-30)

Spinal cord segment	L2, L3, L4
Muscle innervation	Iliopsoas, sartorius, pectineus, quadriceps femoris
Sensory distribution	Anterior and medial thigh, medial leg, and foot

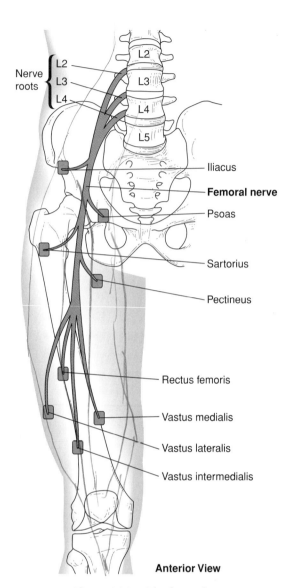

Figure 6-30. The femoral nerve.

Clinical motor features of paralysis	Weakened hip flexion Loss of knee extension

Obturator Nerve (Fig. 6-31)

Spinal cord segment	L2, L3, L4
Muscle innervation	Hip adductors Obturator externus
Sensory distribution	Middle part of medial thigh
Clinical motor features of paralysis	Loss of hip adduction Weakened hip lateral rotation

Sciatic Nerve (made up of tibial and common peroneal nerves) (Fig. 6-32)

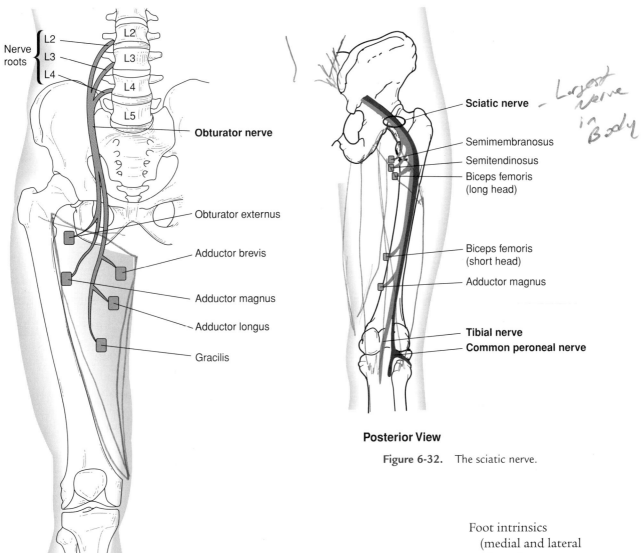

Obturator nerve

Nerve roots { L2 L3 L4 }

Obturator externus

Adductor brevis

Adductor magnus

Adductor longus

Gracilis

Anterior View

Figure 6-31. The obturator nerve.

Sciatic nerve — Largest nerve in Body

Semimembranosus

Semitendinosus

Biceps femoris (long head)

Biceps femoris (short head)

Adductor magnus

Tibial nerve

Common peroneal nerve

Posterior View

Figure 6-32. The sciatic nerve.

Spinal segment	L4, L5, S1, S2, S3
Muscle innervation	Hamstring muscles
Sensory distribution	None
Clinical motor features of paralysis	Weakened hip extension Loss of knee flexion

Tibial Nerve (divides into the medial and lateral plantar nerves) (Fig. 6-33)

Spinal cord segment	L4, L5, S1, S2, S3
Muscle innervation	Popliteus Ankle plantar flexors Tibialis posterior
	Foot intrinsics (medial and lateral plantar)
Sensory distribution	Posterior lateral leg, lateral foot
Clinical motor features of paralysis	Loss of ankle plantar flexion Weakened ankle inversion Loss of toe flexion

Common Peroneal Nerve (divides into superficial and deep peroneal nerves (Fig. 6-34)

Spinal segment	L4, L5, S1, S2
Muscle innervation	Peroneals (mostly superficial peroneal)
	Tibialis anterior (deep peroneal)
	Toe extensors (deep peroneal)

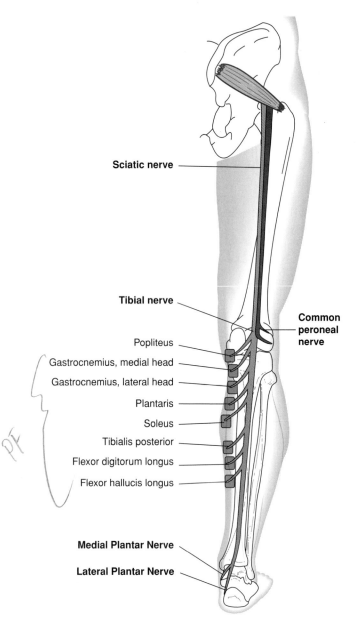

Figure 6-33. The tibial nerve. It divides into the medial and lateral plantar nerves.

Sensory distribution	Anterior lateral aspect of leg and foot
Clinical motor features of paralysis	Loss of ankle dorsiflexion ("foot drop")
	Loss of toe extension
	Loss of ankle eversion

Common Peripheral Nerve Pathologies

Typical muscle paralysis patterns can be seen depending upon the peripheral nerve involved and the level at

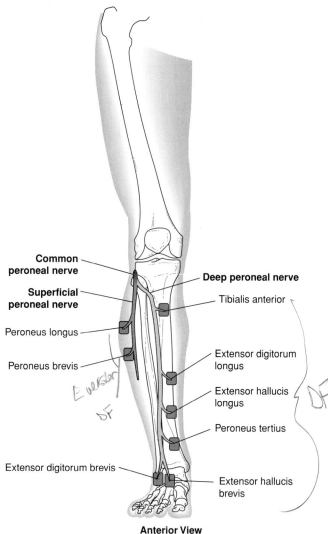

Figure 6-34. The peroneal nerves. The common peroneal nerve divides into the superficial and deep peroneal nerves.

which it is injured. In the upper extremity, **Erb's palsy** is a traction injury to the upper brachial plexus of the baby, most commonly occurring during a difficult childbirth. The affected arm hangs with the shoulder in extension and medial rotation with the elbow extended, forearm pronated, and wrist flexed. It is sometimes known as *"waiter's tip position."* **"Burner"** or **"stinger"** syndrome occurs when there is a stretch or compression injury to the brachial plexus from a blow to the head or shoulder. This is relatively common in football players and is also seen in wrestlers and gymnasts. It is usually short-lived and produces no residual effects. Symptoms include immediate burning pain, prickly paresthesia radiating from the neck, numbness, and even brief paralysis of the arm. These symptoms should resolve within minutes, although shoulder weakness and muscle tenderness of the neck may continue for a few days.

Scapular winging occurs when an injury to the *long thoracic nerve* weakens or paralyzes the serratus anterior muscle causing the medial border of the scapula to rise away from the rib cage. Injury to the *axillary nerve* will make it difficult to abduct the shoulder joint, whereas elbow flexion will be greatly weakened by a lesion of the *musculocutaneous nerve*. **Wrist drop** (loss of wrist extension) and a weakened ability to release objects (finger extension) will result from a high *radial nerve* injury, which is often a complication of a midhumeral fracture. A *median nerve injury* can weaken wrist flexion and thumb position. Loss of thumb opposition is referred to as **"ape hand,"** because apes are unable to oppose the thumb. Inability to flex the thumb, index, and middle finger gives the appearance of the **pope's blessing.** Carpal tunnel syndrome results from compression of the median nerve at the wrist as it passes through the carpal tunnel. **Claw hand** results from a loss of the intrinsic muscles due to ulnar nerve damage. The proximal phalanges are hyperextended and the middle and distal phalanges are in extreme flexion.

In the lower extremity, a lesion of the *femoral nerve* results in paralysis of the quadriceps muscle group. Sciatica refers to pressure on the *sciatic nerve* causing pain that runs down the posterior thigh and leg. A lesion of this nerve high in the thigh will result in paralysis of the hamstring muscle group and all muscles below the knee. Damage to the *common peroneal nerve* can result in **foot drop.** A common cause for this is cast pressure at the head of the fibula where this nerve is quite superficial as it lies over the bony fibular head.

Review Questions

1. The spinal cord extends to about what vertebral level?

2. What makes up gray matter? White matter?

3. Name the bony, membranous, and fluid features that protect the brain from trauma.

4. What is the circle of Willis? What is the functional significance of the circle of Willis?

5. What are the differences between upper and lower motor neurons?

6. How do thoracic nerves differ from cervical or lumbar nerves?

7. What is the difference between an afferent and an efferent nerve fiber?

8. In an individual who has lost the ability to oppose the thumb, what nerve is involved? What is a common term for this condition?

9. In an individual who has lost the ability to pick up the toes (ankle dorsiflexion), what nerve is involved? What is a common term for this condition?

10. Claw hand involves the loss of what muscle group? What nerve is primarily involved?

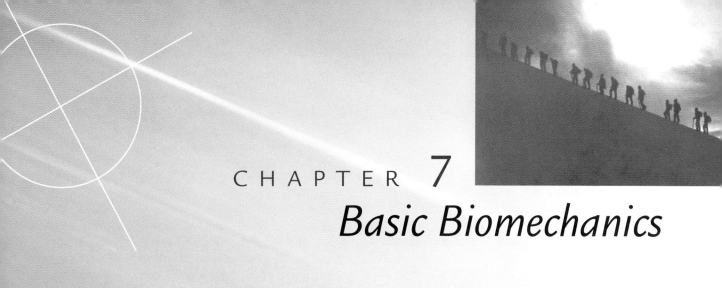

CHAPTER 7

Basic Biomechanics

Laws of Motion

Force

Torque

Stability

Simple Machines

   Levers

   Mechanical Advantages

   Pulleys

   Wheel and Axle

   Inclined Plane

Points to Remember

Review Questions

The human body, in many respects, can be referred to as a living machine. It is important when learning about how the body moves (kinesiology) to also learn about the forces placed on the body causing movement. As illustrated in Figure 7-1, **mechanics** is the branch of physics dealing with the study of forces and the motion produced by their actions. **Biomechanics** involves taking the principles and methods of mechanics and applying them to the structure and function of the human body. As mentioned in Chapter 1, mechanics can be divided into two main areas: statics and dynamics. **Statics** deals with factors associated with nonmoving, or nearly nonmoving systems. **Dynamics** involves factors associated with moving systems and can be divided into kinetics and kinematics. **Kinetics** deals with forces causing movement in a system, whereas kinematics involves the time, space, and mass aspects of a moving system. **Kinematics** can be divided into osteokinematics and arthrokinematics. **Osteokinematics** deals with the manner in which bones move in space without regard to the movement of joint surfaces, such as shoulder flexion/extension. **Arthrokinematics** deals with the manner in which adjoining joint surfaces move in relation to each other, that is, in the same or opposite direction.

Various mechanical terms must be defined before we begin a discussion of these topics. **Force** is a push or pull action. A **vector** is a quantity having both magnitude and direction. Force is a vector. For example, if you were to throw a ball, you would throw it in a certain direction and with a certain speed. A **scalar** quantity describes only magnitude. Common scalar terms are length, area, volume, and mass. Everyday examples would be such things as 5 feet, 2 acres, 12 fluid ounces, and 150 pounds. **Mass** refers to the amount of matter that a body contains. In this example, the amount of

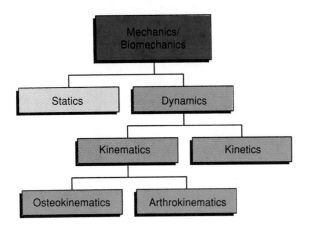

Figure 7-1. Mechanics/Biomechanics relationship flow chart.

matter within and making up the body is the mass. **Inertia** is the property of matter that causes it to resist any change of its motion in either speed or direction. Mass is a measure of inertia; that is, its resistance to a change in motion.

Kinetics is a description of motion with regard to what causes motion. **Torque** is the tendency of force to produce rotation about an axis. **Friction** is a force developed by two surfaces, which tends to prevent motion of one surface across another. For example, there is a great deal of friction between the bottom of a foot covered by a sock and the carpeted floor making sliding difficult. However, there is relatively little friction between the sock and a highly polished hardwood floor. **Velocity** is a vector that describes speed and is measured in units such as feet per second or miles per hour.

Laws of Motion

Motion is happening all around you—people walking, cars traveling on highways, airplanes flying in the air, water flowing in rivers, balls being thrown, and so on. Isaac Newton's three laws explain all types of motion. Newton's first law of motion states that an object at rest tends to stay at rest, and an object in motion tends to stay in motion. This is sometimes referred to as the **law of inertia,** because inertia is the tendency of an object to stay at rest or in motion. To demonstrate this law, consider riding in a car. If the car moves forward quickly from a starting position, your body pushes against the back of the seat and your neck probably hyperextends. Your body was at rest before the car

moved, and it tended to stay at rest as the car started to move. Once moving, if the car were to stop suddenly, your body would be thrown forward and your neck would go into extreme flexion because your body was in motion and tended to stay in motion when the car stopped. Many of the people with neck injuries from automobile accidents have, unfortunately, demonstrated this law.

A force is needed to overcome the inertia of an object and cause the object to move, stop, or change direction. The acceleration of the object depends on the strength of the force applied and the mass of the object. For example, kick a soccer ball and it will roll along the grass. If no forces act on it, the ball will roll forever. However, the force of friction acting on the ball causes the ball to stop. There is friction between any two surfaces. In this case, it is the friction of the grass on the surface of the ball that causes the ball to stop rolling.

A soccer ball can be used to demonstrate Newton's second law. First, mildly kick the ball and notice how far it travels. Next, kick the ball about twice as hard as the first kick. Notice that the ball will travel approximately twice as far. **Acceleration** is any change in the velocity of an object. The soccer ball is accelerating when it starts moving. If you were to kick the ball again even harder, it would travel proportionately farther. This is Newton's second law of motion, the **law of acceleration:** the amount of acceleration depends on the strength of the force applied to an object. Acceleration can also deal with a change in direction. Force is needed to change direction and, according to the law, the change in direction of an object depends on the force applied to it.

Another part of Newton's second law deals with the mass of an object. **Mass** is the amount of matter in an object. Acceleration is inversely proportional to the mass of an object. If you apply the same amount of force to two objects of differing mass, the object with greater mass will accelerate less than the object with less mass. You can demonstrate this by first rolling a soccer ball, then rolling a bowling ball with the same amount of force. The heavier bowling ball will not travel nearly as far.

Newton's third law of motion, the **law of action-reaction,** states that for every action there is an equal and opposite reaction. The strength of the reaction is always equal to the strength of the action, and it occurs in the opposite direction. This can be demonstrated by jumping on a trampoline. The action is you jumping down on the trampoline. The reaction is the trampoline pushing back with the same amount of force. This causes you to rebound up in the opposite direction that you jumped. The harder you jump, the higher you rebound.

As stated, no motion can occur without a force. There are basically two types of force that will cause the body to move. Forces can be internal, such as muscular contraction, ligamentous restraint, or bony support. Forces can also be external, which could be gravity or any externally applied resistance such as weight, friction, and so on.

Force

Force is one of those concepts that everyone understands, but is difficult to define. To create a force, one object must act on another. Force can either be a push, which creates compression, or pull, which creates tension. Movement occurs if one side pushes (or pulls) harder than the other.

Forces are vector quantities. A **vector** quantity describes both magnitude and direction. A person pulling a heavy load with a rope would be an example of a vector. The tension in the rope represents the magnitude of the vector, and the direction of the rope represents the direction of the vector.

A vector force can be shown graphically by a straight line of appropriate length and direction. Figure 7-2 shows two people (forces) pulling on a boat, but at right angles to each other. The characteristics of force include:

1. Magnitude (each person is pulling equally in this case)
2. Direction (shown by the arrow)
3. Point of application

Forces can be described by the effect they produce. A **linear force** results when two or more forces are acting along the same line. Figure 7-3A shows two people pulling a boat with the same rope in the same direction. Figure 7-3B shows two people pushing on opposite sides of the bed with equal force, but along the same line. Although this is an example of linear force because the two people are pushing along the same line, no motion occurs because they are pushing with equal force in opposite directions.

Parallel forces occur in the same plane and in the same or opposite direction. An example of this would be the three-point pressures of bracing (Fig. 7-4). Two forces, in this case the X and Y, are parallel to each other and pushing in the same direction, while a third parallel force, the back brace, is pushing

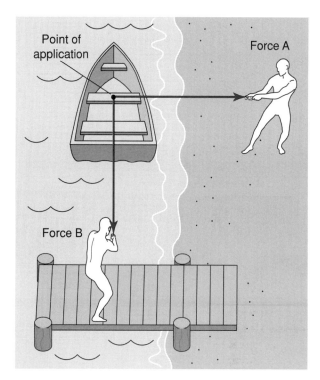

Figure 7-2.   Concurrent force system. Two people pulling at different angles to each other through a common point of application.

against them. This third force must always be located between the two parallel forces. To be effective, it must be of sufficient strength to counter the two forces.

Another example, as shown in Figure 7-5, is two children sitting on a seesaw. The forces are the two children, and the counterforce is the support bar in the middle. Because of this counterforce, a rotary movement occurs when one of the parallel forces is greater than the other.

To produce **concurrent forces,** two or more forces must act from a common point but pull in different (divergent) directions, such as the two people pulling on the boat in Figure 7-6. The net effect of these two divergent forces is called the **resultant force,** and lies somewhere in between.

Because forces are vectors, they can be shown graphically using what is called the **parallelogram method.** Using Figure 7-6 as an example, first draw in vectors for the two forces (solid lines). Secondly, complete the parallelogram using dotted lines. Lastly, draw in the diagonal of the parallelogram (middle line and arrow). This diagonal line represents the resultant force.

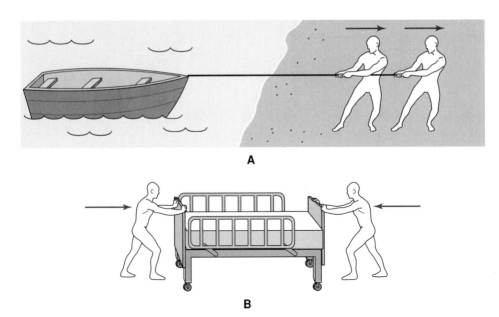

A

B

Figure 7-3.   Linear forces. *(A)* Two people pulling in same direction. *(B)* Two people pushing with same force in opposite directions.

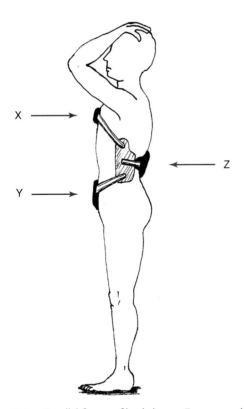

Figure 7-4.   Parallel forces of body brace. Forces *x* and *y* are parallel in the same direction while force *z* is parallel, but in the opposite direction. Force *z* must be in between forces *x* and *y* to provide stability. If force *z* were at either end, instead of the middle, motion would occur.

An example of resultant force in the body is the anterior and posterior parts of the deltoid muscle (Fig. 7-7). Both parts have a common attachment (the insertion) but they pull in different directions. When both parallel forces are equal, the resultant force causes the shoulder to abduct. If the pull of the two forces were not equal, that is, if the pull of the anterior deltoid were stronger than that of the posterior, the resultant force would show that the motion would be more in the direction of the anterior deltoid (Fig. 7-8). The shoulder would flex and abduct in a forward, diagonal direction.

A **force couple** occurs when two forces act in an equal but opposite direction resulting in a turning effect. An example would be the fingers (force *a*) and the thumb (force *b*) unscrewing a jar lid (Fig. 7-9). With the jar lid in the right hand, the fingers move to the left while the thumb moves to the right; together they move the jar lid counterclockwise, loosening or

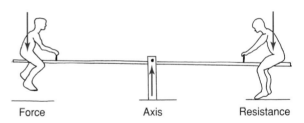

| Force | Axis | Resistance |

Figure 7-5.   Parallel forces of two children on seesaw with counterforce in the middle.

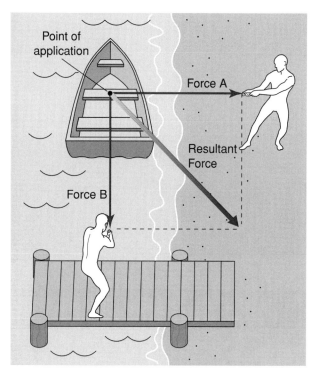

Figure 7-6. A parallelogram shows graphically the resultant force of two divergent forces pulling on the boat.

unscrewing it. Look at Figure 7-3B. What would happen if the person on the right moved toward the right side on the head of the bed and the person on the left moved toward the left side of the foot on the bed?

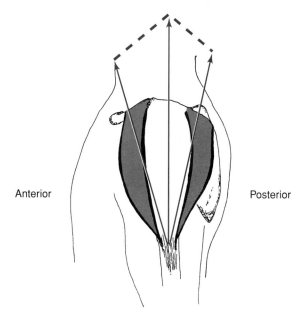

Figure 7-7. Resultant force of equal forces of anterior and posterior deltoid muscles.

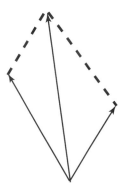

Figure 7-8. Resultant force of unequal forces moves toward the stronger force.

Assuming that they are pushing with equal force, a force couple would be created and the bed would rotate.

Torque

Torque, also known as **moment of force,** is the ability of force to produce rotation about an axis. It can be thought of as rotary force. The amount of torque a lever has depends on the amount of force exerted and the distance it is from the axis. Use of a wrench demonstrates torque. The twisting force (torque) exerted by the wrench can be increased either by:

1. Increasing the force applied to the handle
2. Increasing the length of the handle

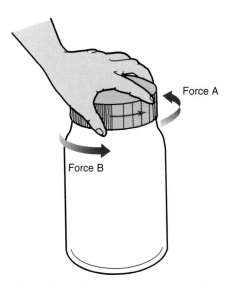

Figure 7-9. Force couple unscrewing lid.

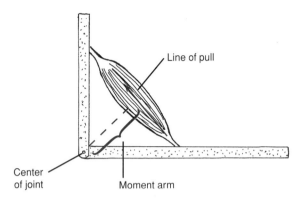

Figure 7-10. Moment arm of biceps is the perpendicular distance between the muscle's point of attachment and the center of the joint.

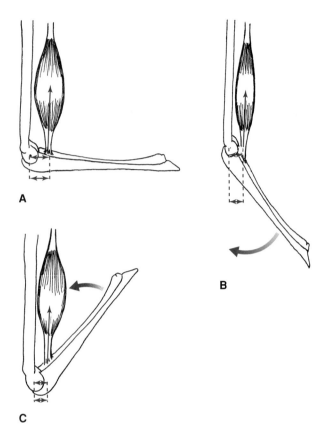

Figure 7-11. Effect of moment arm on torque. *(A)* Moment arm and angular force are greatest at 90 degrees. *(B)* Moment arm decreases as joint moves toward 0 degrees and stabilizing force increases. *(C)* Moment arm decreases as joint moves beyond 90 degrees toward 180 degrees and dislocating force increases. In both cases, when the stabilizing and dislocating forces are increasing, the angular force is decreasing. Stated another way, a muscle is most efficient at moving a joint or rotating when the joint is at 90 degrees. It becomes less efficient at moving or rotating when the joint angle is either increasing or decreasing.

Torque is also the amount of force needed by a muscle contraction to cause rotary joint motion.

Torque about any point (axis) equals the product of the force magnitude (how strong the force is) and its perpendicular distance from the line of action of the force to the axis of rotation. The perpendicular distance is called the **moment arm** or *torque arm* (Fig. 7-10). Therefore, the moment arm of a muscle is the perpendicular distance between the muscle's line of pull and the center of the joint (axis of rotation). Torque is greatest when the angle of pull is at 90 degrees (Fig 7-11A), and decreases as the angle of pull either decreases (Fig. 7-11B) or increases (Fig. 7-11C) from that perpendicular position.

No torque is produced if the force is directed exactly through the axis of rotation. Although this is not quite possible for a muscle, it comes very close. For example, if the biceps contracts when the elbow is nearly or completely extended, there is very little torque produced (Fig. 7-11B). The perpendicular distance between the joint axis and the line of pull is very small. Therefore, the force generated by the muscle is primarily a **stabilizing force,** in that nearly all of the force generated by the muscle is directed back into the joint, pulling the two bones together.

Contrary to that, when the angle of pull is at 90 degrees (Fig. 7-11A), the perpendicular distance between the joint axis and the line of pull is much larger. Therefore, the force generated by the muscle is primarily an **angular force** (or movement force), in that most of the force generated by the muscle is directed at rotating the joint and not stabilizing the joint.

As a muscle contracts through its range of motion (ROM), the amount of angular or stabilizing force changes. As the muscle increases its angular force, it decreases its stabilizing force and vice versa. At 90 degrees, or halfway through its range, the muscle has its greatest angular force. Past 90 degrees, the stabilizing force becomes a **dislocating force** because the force is directed away from the joint (Fig. 7-11C).

Some muscles have a much greater stabilizing force than angular force throughout the range, and therefore are more effective at stabilizing the joint than moving it. The coracobrachialis of the shoulder joint is a good example (see Fig. 9-17). Its line of pull is mostly vertical and quite close to the axis of the shoulder joint. Therefore, it has a very short moment arm, which makes this muscle more effective at stabilizing than at flexing the shoulder joint.

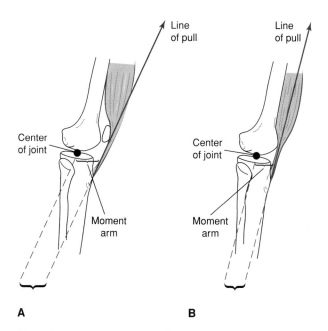

Figure 7-12. Moment arm of quadriceps muscle with a patella *(A)* and without a patella *(B)*.

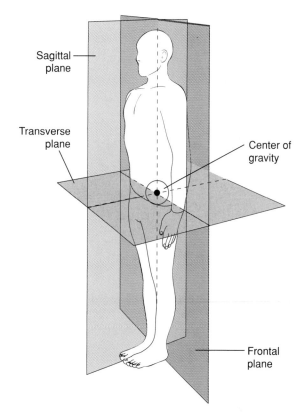

Figure 7-13. The center of gravity is the point at which the three cardinal planes intersect.

The angular force of the quadriceps muscle is increased by the presence of the patella. The patella, a sesamoid bone encapsulated in the tendon, increases the moment arm of the quadriceps muscle, allowing the muscle to have a greater angular force (Fig. 7-12A). Without a patella, the moment arm is smaller and much of the force of the quadriceps is directed back into the joint (Fig. 7-12B). Although this is good for stability, it is not effective for motion. To have effective knee motion, it is vital that the quadriceps provide a strong angular force.

In summary, if the moment arm is greater, then the angular force (torque) is greater. Moment arm is determined by measuring the perpendicular distance between the axis of rotation (joint axis) and the line of force (muscle's line of pull). Moment arm, size of the muscle, and contractile strength of the muscle all determine how effective a muscle is in causing joint motion.

Stability

When an object is balanced, all torques acting on it are even, and it is in a **state of equilibrium.** How secure or precarious this state of equilibrium is depends primarily on the relationship between the object's center of gravity and base of support. To understand the principles of stability, certain terms must be defined. **Gravity** is the mutual attraction between the earth and an object. **Gravitational force** is always directed vertically downward toward the center of the earth. Practically speaking, gravitational force is always directed toward the ground. **Center of gravity** (COG) is the balance point of an object at which torque on all sides is equal. It is also the point at which the planes of the body intersect, as shown in Figure 7-13.

In the human body, the COG is located in the midline at about the level of, though slightly anterior to, the second sacral vertebra of an adult. Because body proportions change with age, the COG of a child is higher than that of an adult. To demonstrate this, move your right arm up over your head and touch your left ear. Now, ask a 3-year-old child to do the same. You will notice that while you can easily touch your ear, the child's hand reaches only to about the top of the head (Fig. 7-14). The child's head is much larger in proportion to the arms and rest of the body.

As a point of interest: A body proportion made famous by the illustration of Leonardo deVinci is height-arm span. The length of an adult's outstretched arms is equal to his or her height (Fig. 7-15).

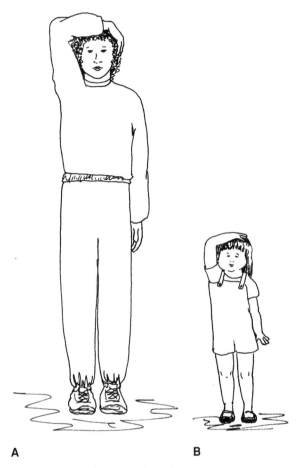

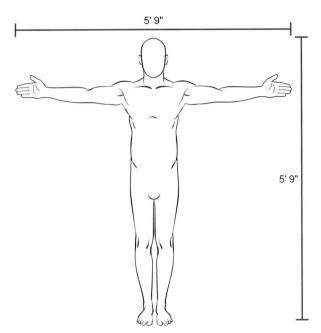

Figure 7-15. In an adult, arm span and body height are equal.

A **B**

Figure 7-14. Body proportions change as a person grows.

Base of support (BOS) is that part of a body that is in contact with the supporting surface. If you were to outline the surface of the body in contact with the ground, you would have identified the BOS. **Line of gravity (LOG)** is an imaginary vertical line passing through the COG toward the center of the earth. These are shown in Figure 7-16.

There are basically three states of equilibrium (Fig. 7-17). **Stable equilibrium** occurs when an object is in a position that to disturb it would require its COG to be raised. A simple example is that of a brick. When the widest part of the brick is in contact with the surface (BOS), it is quite stable (Fig. 7-17A). To disturb it, the brick would have to be tipped up in any direction, thus raising its COG. The same could be said of a person lying flat on the floor. **Unstable equilibrium** occurs when only a slight force is needed to disturb an object. Balancing a pencil on the pointed end is a good example. A similar example is that of a person standing on one leg. Once balanced, it takes very little force to knock the pencil over (Fig. 7-17B). **Neutral equilibrium**

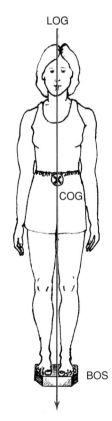

Figure 7-16. Center of gravity (COG), line of gravity (LOG), and base of support (BOS).

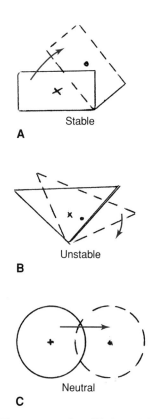

A Stable

B Unstable

C Neutral

Figure 7-17. Three states of equilibrium. *(A)* Stable. *(B)* Unstable. *(C)* Neutral.

exists when an object's COG is neither raised nor lowered when it is disturbed. A good example would be a ball. As the ball rolls across the floor, its COG remains the same (Fig. 7-17C).

The following principles demonstrate the relationships between balance, stability, and motion.

1. The lower the COG, the more stable the object. In Figure 7-18, both triangles have the same base of support. However, the triangle on the left is

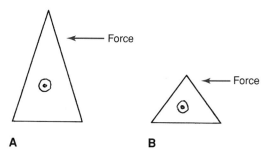

A   **B**

Force

Force

Figure 7-18. Relationship of height of center of gravity to stability. *(A)* is less stable because it has a higher COG. *(B)* Lower COG is more stable.

taller, has a higher COG, and thus is more unstable than the triangle on the right. It would take less force to disturb the taller triangle.

2. The COG and LOG must remain within the BOS for an object to remain stable. (Keep in mind that the LOG passes through the COG. Therefore what can be said of one can be said of the other. For the purpose of clarity, from this point forward, the term COG will be used.) The wider the BOS, the more stable the object. In the example in Figure 7-19, the book, resting entirely on its BOS (tabletop), is quite stable. As you push it off the edge, it becomes less stable. When its COG is no longer over its BOS, the book will fall.

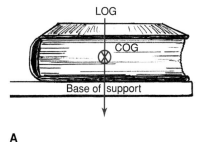

LOG

COG

Base of support

A

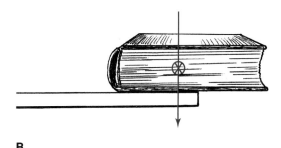

B

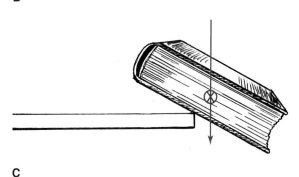

C

Figure 7-19. Relationship of COG to BOS. *(A)* The book is very stable because its COG is in the middle of its BOS. *(B)* The book is less stable because its COG is near the edge of its BOS. *(C)* The book is unstable and will fall because its COG is beyond its BOS.

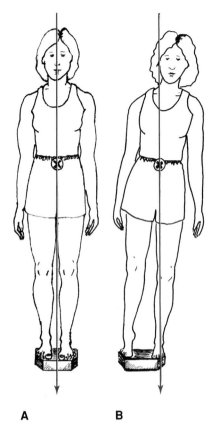

A   **B**

Figure 7-20. Relationship of COG to BOS. *(A)* She is stable—her COG is in the middle of her BOS. *(B)* She is less stable because her COG is near the edge of her BOS.

Another example would be a woman standing upright on both feet (Fig. 7-20). Her COG lies at or near the center of the base of support. As she leans to the side, her COG moves toward the border of her BOS. As soon as her COG passes beyond the BOS, she becomes unstable, and if her posture is not corrected or her BOS widened, she will fall. To lean further without losing her balance she could either extend her opposite arm or widen her stance. In either case, her COG would move back over her BOS.

3. Stability increases as the BOS is widened in the direction of the force. A person standing at a bus stop on a very windy day would be more stable when facing into the wind and placing one foot behind the other, thus widening the BOS in the direction of the wind (Fig. 7-21).

4. The greater the mass of an object, the greater its stability. This concept is observed by looking at the size of players on a football team. Linebackers are traditionally heavier, and thus harder to push over. Halfbacks, whose job is to run with the ball,

are much lighter. It can be said that what is gained in stability is lost in speed and vice versa.

5. The greater the friction between the supporting surface and the BOS, the more stable the body will be. Walking on an icy sidewalk is a slippery experience because there is essentially no friction between the ice and the shoe. Sanding the sidewalk increases the friction of the icy surface, thus improving traction. Having a surface with a great deal of friction is not always desirable. Pushing a wheelchair across a hardwood floor is much easier than pushing one across a carpeted floor. The carpet creates more friction, making it harder to push the wheelchair.

6. People have better balance while moving if they focus on a stationary object rather than on a moving object. Therefore, people learning to walk with crutches would be more stable by focusing on an object down the hall than by looking down at their moving feet or crutches.

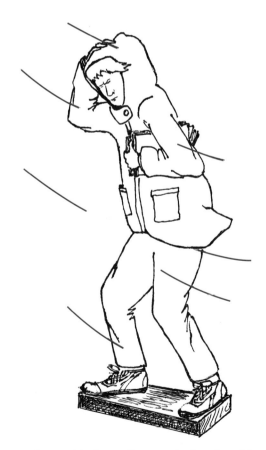

Figure 7-21. Wider base of support in direction of force increases stability.

Simple Machines

In engineering, various machines are used to change the magnitude or direction of a force. The four simple machines are the lever, the pulley, the wheel and axle, and the inclined plane. Examples of each of these machines, except for the inclined plane, can be found in the human body. The lever, the wheel and axle, and the inclined plane allow a person to exert a force greater than could be exerted by using muscle power alone; the pulley allows force to be applied more efficiently. This increase in force is usually at the expense of speed and can be expressed in terms of mechanical advantage, which will be described later.

Levers

There are three classes of levers, each with a different purpose and a different mechanical advantage. We use levers daily to help us accomplish various activities. The wheelbarrow, crowbar, manual can opener, scissors, golf club, tennis racket, and the playground seesaw are but a few examples. Different types of levers can also be found in the human body. To understand the structure and function of levers, you should be familiar with certain terms.

A **lever** is a rigid bar that can rotate about a fixed point when a force is applied to overcome resistance. The fixed point about which the lever rotates is the **axis (A),** sometimes referred to as the *fulcrum.* In the human body, the **force (F)** that causes the lever to move is usually, but not always, muscular. The **resistance (R)** that must be overcome for motion to occur can include the weight of the part being moved, gravity, or an external weight. The **force arm (FA)** is the perpendicular distance, or length, between the line of force and the axis while the **resistance arm (RA)** is the perpendicular distance, or length, between the line of resistance and the axis (Fig. 7-22). The arrangement of the axis *A* in relation to the force *F* and the resistance *R* determines the type of lever.

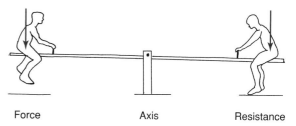

Figure 7-23. First-class lever. FAR (F = force; A = axis; R = resistance).

Classes of Levers

In **a first-class lever,** the axis is located between the force and the resistance:

$$\text{First-class lever} \quad F\text{———————}R$$
$$A$$

A good example of this would be a playground seesaw (Fig. 7-23). The seesaw (lever arm) rotates on a crossbar (axis), which is located somewhere between a child sitting on one end of the board and pushing down against the ground (force) and the weight of the child sitting at the other end (resistance).

A **second-class lever** has the axis at one end, the resistance in the middle, and the force at the other end:

$$\text{Second-class lever} \quad \frac{R \qquad F}{A}$$

The wheelbarrow is a second-class lever (Fig. 7-24). The wheel at the front end is the axis, the contents of the wheelbarrow are the resistance, and the person pushing the wheelbarrow is the force.

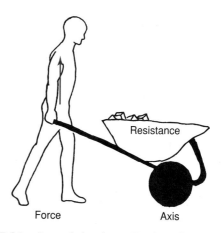

Figure 7-24. Second-class lever. FRA (F = force; R = resistance; A = axis).

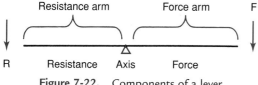

Figure 7-22. Components of a lever.

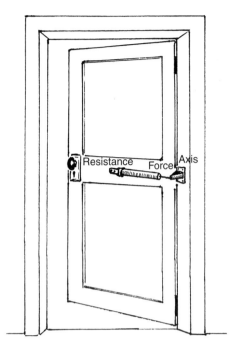

Figure 7-25.   Third-class lever.

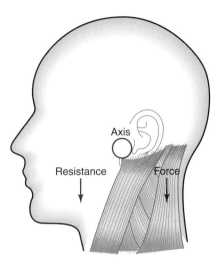

Figure 7-26.   First-class lever.

A **third-class lever** has the axis at one end with the force in the middle and resistance at the opposite end:

$$\text{Third-class lever} \quad \dfrac{\text{F} \quad \text{R}}{\text{A}}$$

An example of this type of lever would be a screen door that has a spring attachment (Fig. 7-25). The axis is the door hinges, the force is the spring that closes the door, and the resistance is the door itself.

As mentioned, each of these levers has a different purpose or mechanical advantage. The first-class lever is best designed for balance. An example in the human body would be the head sitting on the first cervical vertebra, moving up and down (Fig. 7-26). The vertebra would be the axis, the weight of one side of the head would be the resistance, and the muscles, pulling down on the opposite side of the head, would be the force. If, for example, you lowered your head to your chest, your head would rotate about the vertebra (axis). To return to the upright position, your posterior neck muscles (force) must contract to pull the weight of your head up against gravity (resistance). If you look up to the sky, your head would rock back, and you would need to use your anterior neck muscles to pull your head back to the upright position. Although force and resistance may change places, depending on the motion, the axis is always in the middle.

The second-class lever is best used for power, and there are surprisingly few, if any, examples in the body. Most authorities believe that there are no pure second-class levers in the body in which the force is a muscle contracting concentrically. Some will give the example of the action of the ankle plantar flexor muscles when a person stands on tiptoes (Fig. 7-27). In this case, the axis is the MP (metatarsophalangeal) joints in the foot, the resistance is the tibia and the rest of the body weight above it, and the force is provided by the ankle plantar flexors. As you can see, the plantar flexors do

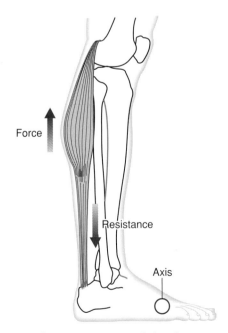

Figure 7-27.   Second-class lever.

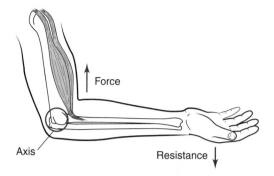

Figure 7-28. Third-class lever.

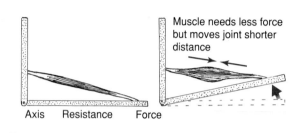

A

B

Figure 7-29. Third-class levers favor distance *(A)*, and second-class levers favor force *(B)*.

not have to move the joint very far, but they do have a great deal of weight or resistance to overcome.

The advantage of the third-class lever is ROM (also called speed and distance). This is, by far, the most common lever in the body. An example would be the biceps muscle during elbow flexion (Fig. 7-28). The axis is the elbow joint, the force is that exerted by the biceps muscle attached to the proximal radius, and the resistance is the weight of the forearm and hand. For the hand to be truly functional, it must be able to move through a wide ROM. The resistance will vary depending on what, if anything, is in the hand.

Why are there so many third-class levers, which favor ROM (speed and distance), and so few second-class levers, which favor power, in the body? Probably because the advantage gained from increased ROM is more important than the advantage gained from increased power. Examine the roles of the biceps and brachioradialis muscles in elbow flexion (Fig. 7-29). They both span the elbow but attach on the radius at very different places. The biceps muscle attaches to the proximal end of the radius, and the brachioradialis muscle attaches to the distal end. The biceps muscle acts as the force in a third-class lever because it attaches between the axis (elbow) and the resistance (forearm). The brachioradialis muscle is the force in a second-class lever because it attaches at the end of the lever arm, putting the resistance (forearm) in the middle. For example, say that each muscle is capable of contracting approximately 4 inches. Remember that a muscle is capable of being shortened to half of its resting length. Therefore, the brachioradialis muscle will be able to move the distal end of the forearm and, subsequently, the hand approximately 4 inches because its attachment is near the distal end. The biceps muscle, with its attachment at the proximal end, will move the proximal end of the forearm approximately 4 inches, which will move the hand at the distal end much far-

ther. Because the main function of the upper extremity is to allow the hand to move through a wide range, it makes sense that most of these muscles act as third-class levers.

Factors That Change Class

Under certain conditions a muscle may change from a second-class to a third-class lever, and vice versa. For example, the brachioradialis has been described as a second-class lever with the weight of the forearm being the main resistance. The weight of the forearm is located between the axis (elbow) and the force (distal muscle attachment) as shown in Figure 7-29B. However, if you put a weight in the hand, that weight now becomes the resistance and is located farther from the axis than the force (muscle) (Fig. 7-30). Therefore, the brachioradialis is now working as a third-class lever.

The direction of the movement in relation to gravity is another factor that will affect lever class. For example, the biceps illustrated in Figure 7-31A is a third-class lever because it contracts concentrically to flex the elbow. The muscle is the force and the forearm is the resistance. The force is between the axis and resistance; therefore, it is a third-class lever. If you put a weight in the hand, it would still be a third-class lever. However, if the muscle contracted eccentrically, it would become a second-class lever. What has changed?

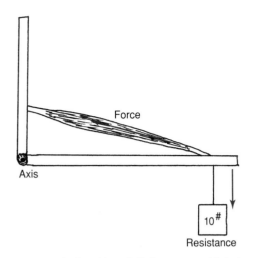

Figure 7-30. The brachioradialis becomes a third-class lever when a weight is placed in the hand.

Mechanical Advantage

Another important feature of levers and other machines is **mechanical advantage,** which is defined as the ratio between the force arm and the resistance arm. The mechanical advantage (MA) of a lever is deter-

mined by dividing the length of the force arm by the length of the resistance arm (MA = FA ÷ RA).

When the force arm (*FA*) is greater than the resistance arm (*RA*), as with a second-class lever, the mechanical advantage (*MA*) is greater than 1. For example, if a force arm were 2 feet and the resistance arm were 1 foot, the mechanical advantage would be:

$$MA = FA \div RA \qquad MA = 2 \div 1 \qquad MA = 2$$

This means that the force arm has twice the length as the resistance arm. Therefore, it has twice the torque (rotary force). If, however, the force arm were shorter (1 foot) and the resistance arm were longer (2 feet) as with a third-class lever, the mechanical advantage would be:

$$MA = FA \div RA \qquad MA = 1 \div 2 \qquad MA = 1/2$$

In other words, the force arm has half the length of the resistance arm. Therefore, it has half the torque (rotary force).

What is always true of simple machines is that what is gained in force is lost in distance, and vice versa. In other words, to move an object using less force (mechanical advantage greater than 1) will also require that the force arm move a greater distance. Conversely, by using more force (mechanical advantage less than 1), the force arm will need to move a shorter distance. If the mechanical advantage equaled 1, the force arm and resistance arm would be equal and the system would be balanced, as in a first-class lever.

An example in therapeutic exercise is the application of force to a patient's lower leg while the patient tries to keep the knee extended. It takes less force on your part if you place your hand distally versus proximally (Fig. 7-32). In this case the axis (*A*) is the knee

As the elbow extends, moving the same direction as the pull of gravity, the biceps must contract eccentrically to slow the pull of gravity. Gravity and its pull on the forearm becomes the force. The biceps becomes the resistance slowing elbow extension (Fig. 7-31B). With the resistance now in the middle between the force and the axis, the biceps becomes a second-class lever.

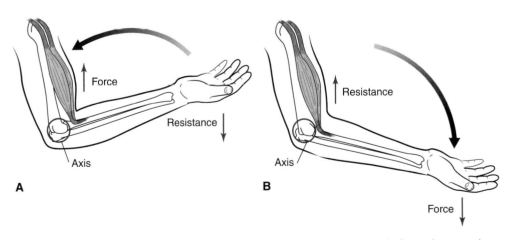

A   **B**

Figure 7-31. *(A)* The biceps is a third-class lever when contracting concentrically, and a second-class lever when contracting eccentrically.

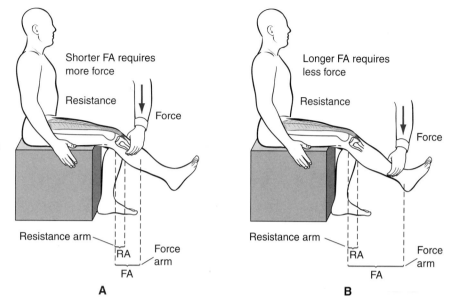

Figure 7-32. *(A)* Shorter force arm requires more force. *(B)* Longer force arm requires less force than does a shorter force arm. Strictly speaking, the RA and FA shown here are correct only if the line of force and line of resistance are both vertical. However, what is important here is the advantage of a longer force arm versus a shorter force arm.

joint, the resistance *(R)* is the insertion of the quadriceps muscle, and the force *(F)* is your hand on the lower leg. In Figure 7-32A, the resistance arm is 2 inches and the force arm is 4 inches. The mechanical advantage can be calculated as follows:

$$MA = FA \div RA \qquad MA = 4 \div 2 \qquad MA = 2$$

In Figure 7-32B, the *RA* remains at 2 inches and the *FA* is 10 inches. Its mechanical advantage is calculated as follows:

$$MA = FA \div RA \qquad MA = 10 \div 2 \qquad MA = 5$$

Simply stated, less force is needed to cause motion when the mechanical advantage is greater.

If the force arm and resistance arm are the same length, and the amount of force and resistance are equal, then the system is balanced and no motion will occur. Using the seesaw example, if child A and child B each weigh 40 pounds, and are both sitting 5 feet from the crossbar, the seesaw will be balanced. If child A moves one foot closer to the crossbar, the system is no longer balanced. Child A would go up, and child B would go down (Fig. 7-33). Child A needs to either add weight (more force) or move back (lengthen *FA*) to balance the seesaw again. Remember, with a longer force arm and a shorter resistance arm, less force is needed to cause motion.

Apply this concept to the wheelbarrow (Fig. 7-34). What is the difference between placing a load of bricks closer to the wheel axis (1 foot) or farther away (2 feet)? Although the force arm (where you place your hands on the handles) remains the same (3 feet), the length of

the resistance arm changes. It becomes longer if the bricks are placed farther from the wheel (Fig. 7-34A) and shorter as the bricks are placed closer to the wheel (Fig. 7-34B). When there is a longer resistance arm,

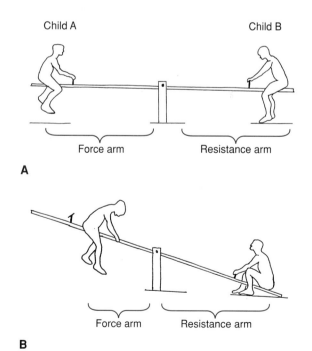

Figure 7-33. *(A)* When lever arms are equal, the system is balanced. *(B)* The force arm is shorter. To balance the system, the force arm needs to be lengthened or more weight (force) needs to be added to the force arm.

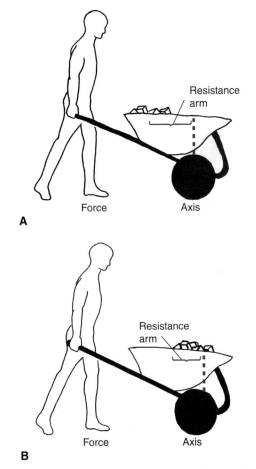

A

B

Figure 7-34. A shorter resistance arm requires less force. Loading bricks in front closer to axis *(B)* shortens the resistance arm.

more force is needed; conversely, when there is a shorter resistance arm, less force is needed.

Another example involves lifting or carrying (Fig. 7-35). Which is going to take less energy, holding a box 2

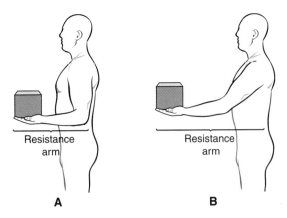

A   **B**

Figure 7-35. A shorter resistance arm *(A)* requires less force, which is done by carrying box closer to the body.

inches from your body or 10 inches from your body? The answer is 2 inches. When the box is held 10 inches away from your body, the resistance arm is longer; therefore, more force is required to overcome its resistance.

There are many applications of the mechanical advantage of levers in rehabilitation. The importance of levers can be seen in such things as saving energy or making tasks possible when strength is limited. To summarize, less force is required if you put the resistance as close to the axis as possible, and apply the force as far from the axis as possible.

Pulleys

A **pulley** consists of a grooved wheel that turns on an axle with a rope or cable riding in the groove (Fig. 7-36). Its purpose is to either change the direction of a force, or

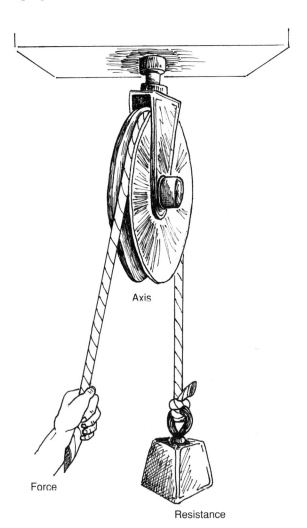

Figure 7-36. Pulley system.

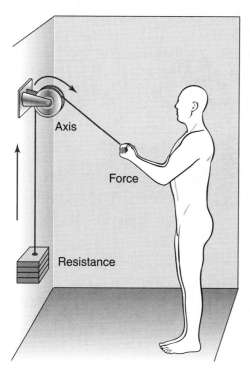

Figure 7-37.   Fixed pulley. Its purpose is to change direction.

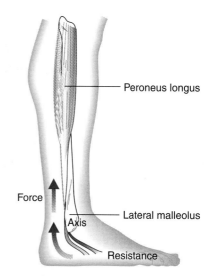

Figure 7-38.   The lateral malleolus acts as a pulley, allowing the peroneus longus to change its direction of pull.

to increase or decrease the magnitude of a force. A **fixed pulley** is a simple pulley attached to a beam. It acts as a first-class lever with F on one side of the pulley (axis) and R on the other. It is used only to change direction. Clinical examples of this can be found in both overhead and wall pulleys (Fig. 7-37) and home cervical traction units. In the body, the lateral malleolus of the fibula acts as a pulley for the tendon of the peroneus longus and changes its direction of pull (Fig. 7-38).

A **movable pulley** has one end of the rope attached to a beam then the rope runs through the pulley to the other end where the force is applied. The load (resistance) is suspended from the movable pulley (Fig. 7-39). The load is supported by both segments of the rope on either side of the pulley so it has a mechanical advantage of 2. It will require only half as much force to lift the load because the amount of force gained has doubled. Although only half of the force is needed to lift the load, the rope must be pulled twice as far. In other words, what is gained in force is lost in distance. Examples of a movable pulley are not found in the human body.

Wheel and Axle

The **wheel and axle** is another, though less common, type of simple machine found in the body. It is actually a lever in disguise. The wheel and axle consists of a

wheel, or crank, attached to and turning together with an axle. It is typically used to increase the force exerted. Turning about a large radius (wheel) requires less force, whereas turning about a small radius (axle) requires a greater force. An example of a wheel and axle would be a faucet handle (Fig. 7-40). The handle(s) is the wheel and the stem is the axle. Turning the faucet requires a certain amount of force. However, take off the handle and you are left with only the axle (see Fig. 7-41B). Try turning it

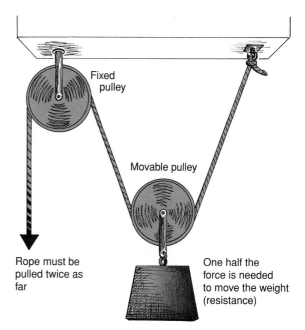

Figure 7-39.   A movable pulley has a mechanical advantage for force, at the expense of distance.

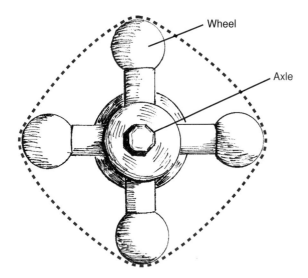

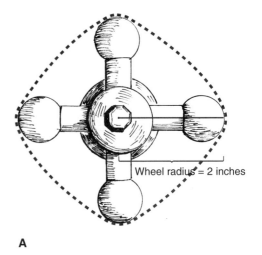

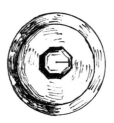

Figure 7-40. A faucet handle is a wheel and axle.

Axle radius = ¹⁄₈ inch

B

Figure 7-41. The radius of a wheel divided by the radius of the axle determines the mechanical advantage.

and you will realize that a great deal more strength is needed to turn it. Simply stated, the larger the wheel in relation to the axle, the easier it is to turn the object. This is referred to as mechanical advantage (MA).

Calculation of the mechanical advantage of a wheel and axle is essentially the same as for a lever, only some of the terms are different. Wheel-and-axle mechanical advantage is calculated by dividing the radius of the wheel by the radius of the axle (Fig. 7-41):

$$MA = \text{radius of wheel} \div \text{radius of axle}$$

Therefore, calculating the mechanical advantage between the faucet *with* the handle and the faucet *without* the handle would be as follows:

$$MA \text{ (with handle)} = \text{radius of wheel} \div \text{radius of axle}$$

$$MA = 2 \text{ inches} \div \tfrac{1}{8} \text{ inch} = 16$$

The MA (without handle) is when the radius of the wheel and axle are the same, so the calculation would be as follows:

$$MA = \tfrac{1}{8} \text{ inch} \div \tfrac{1}{8} \text{ inch} = 1$$

Hence, with the larger mechanical advantage, it is easier to turn the handle, but the further the handle must be turned. Assume that you are treating a person with severe arthritis in the hands who is unable to turn the faucet handles easily. If you replace the handle with a long, lever-type handle (Fig. 7-42), you still have a wheel and axle. Visualize the 3-inch handle as one spoke of the wheel with the rest of the wheel missing. Its mechanical advantage would be calculated as follows:

$$MA = 3 \text{ inches} \div \tfrac{1}{8} \text{ inch} = 24$$

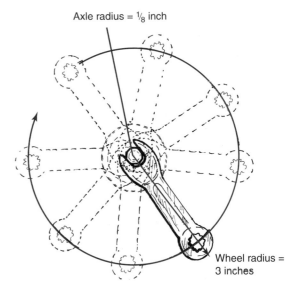

Figure 7-42. A longer radius requires less force to turn the wheel.

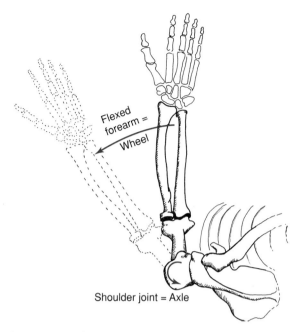

Figure 7-43.   The upper extremity acting as a wheel and axle.

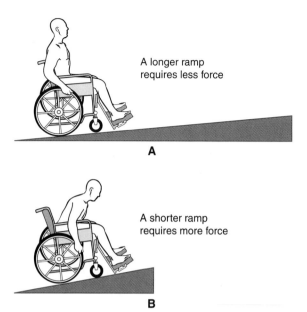

A longer ramp
requires less force

A

A shorter ramp
requires more force

B

Figure 7-44.   Inclined plane as a wheelchair ramp. A longer ramp (A) requires less force but greater distance to reach a certain height. A shorter ramp (B) requires more force but less distance to reach same height.

The faucet handle will be much easier to turn because of its greater mechanical advantage. The longer the handle of the faucet, the easier it is to turn. Keep in mind that although it is easier to turn the handle, the handle must be turned a greater distance.

To give an example of a wheel and axle in the human body, think of performing passive shoulder rotation on a patient. It can best be visualized by looking down on the shoulder from a superior view (Fig. 7-43). The shoulder joint serves as the axle and the forearm serves as the wheel. With the elbow flexed, the wheel is much longer than the axle, and thus, much easier to turn.

Inclined Plane

Although there are no examples of an inclined plane in the human body, the concept of wheelchair accessibility often depends on this type of simple machine. An **inclined plane** is a flat surface that slants. It exchanges increased distance for less effort. The longer the length of a wheelchair ramp, the greater distance the wheelchair must travel, but the less effort required to propel the chair up the ramp. For example, if a porch is 2 feet from the ground and the ramp is 24 feet long, it would be fairly easy to propel the wheelchair up this fairly long ramp (Fig. 7-44A). If the ramp is only 12 feet long, it would be much steeper. The person would not have to propel the wheelchair as far, but would have to use more force to do so (Fig. 7-44B). Repeating the basic

rule of simple machines: what is gained in force is lost in distance.

Points to Remember

- The effect of forces can be linear, parallel, or concurrent.
- A force couple occurs when forces act together but in opposite directions to provide the same motion.
- A scalar quantity describes magnitude, whereas vector also includes direction.
- Forces can be a stabilizing, angular, or dislocating force.
- Gravity has an effect on all objects.
- Stability is affected by an object's COG, LOG, and BOS.
- The three classes of levers have different purposes and mechanical advantages depending on the relationship of the axis, the force, and the resistance.
- Changing the length of the FA or RA will make movement easier or harder.
- Fixed pulleys in the human body change the direction of force of a muscle.
- The wheel and axle, much like the lever, can increase the force.
- Inclined planes can exchange increased distance for decreased effort.

Review Questions

1. Putting a weight cuff in which position would require more effort at the shoulder joint to move the weight cuff through shoulder range of motion? Explain your answer.
   a. Cuff positioned at the wrist
   b. Cuff positioned at the the elbow

2. Two people have the same weight and BOS, but one is on stilts. Which person is more stable? Why?
   a. The person on stilts
   b. The person not on stilts

3. What is the resultant force of the following muscles:
   a. Two heads of the gastrocnemius

   b. Sternal and clavicular portions of the pectoralis major

4. You are given two different sets of instructions. The first instruction tells you to run 5 miles, and the second instruction tells you to walk 30 feet to the north. (circle correct answer)
   a. Running 5 miles is a vector/scalar quantity
   b. Walking 30 feet to the north is a vector/scalar quantity

5. A delivery person has several boxes stacked on a hand truck. Would the person have to use more force to push the hand truck when the hand truck is more horizontal or more vertical? Why?

6. Compare the push rims of a standard wheelchair and a racing wheelchair. Note that the racing wheelchair has much smaller push rims. What would be the advantage of smaller push rims to a wheelchair racer?

7. Label the BOS, COG, and LOG for the object shown here. The object is of uniform density throughout its shape.

   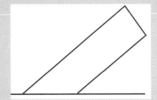

   a. Can this object remain upright without support? ____ Yes ____No. Why?

8. In terms of BOS, why is it more difficult for a person in a wheelchair to balance on the back wheels only ("wheelie") than on all four wheels?

Body Mechanics:

9. Two people are standing on the same side of a patient's bed. They plan to move the patient toward them by pulling on the draw sheet. This move would be what type of force: Linear, parallel, concurrent, or force couple?

10. Prior to moving the patient, what can the people do to increase their own stability?

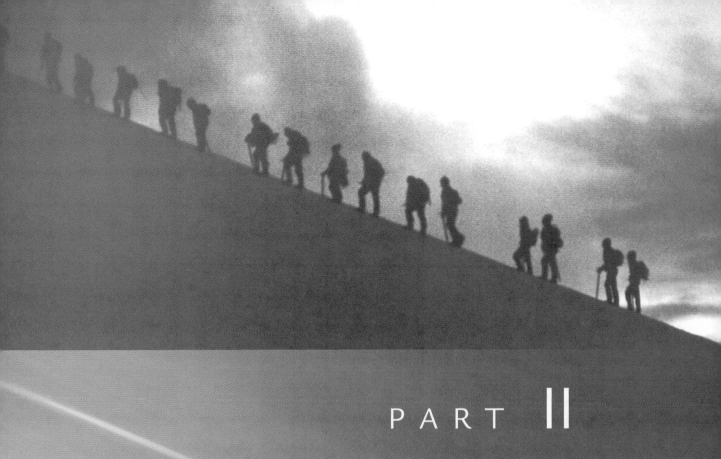

PART II

Clinical Kinesiology and Anatomy of the Upper Extremities

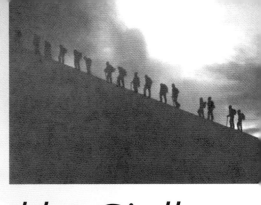

CHAPTER 8
Shoulder Girdle

Clarification of Terms

Bones and Landmarks

Joints and Ligaments

Joint Motions

Companion Motions of the Shoulder Joint and Shoulder Girdle

Scapulohumeral Rhythm

Angle of Pull

Muscles of the Shoulder Girdle

Muscle Descriptions

Force Couples

Reversal of Muscle Action

Summary of Muscle Innervation

Points to Remember

Review Questions

General Anatomy Questions

Functional Activity Questions

Clinical Exercise Questions

Clarification of Terms

The purpose of the shoulder and the entire upper extremity is to allow the hand to be placed in various positions to accomplish the multitude of tasks it is capable of performing. The shoulder, or glenohumeral joint, is the most mobile joint in the body and is capable of a great deal of motion. However, in talking about shoulder motion, we must recognize that motion also occurs at three other joints or areas. The shoulder complex is a term that is sometimes used to include all of the structures involved with motion of the shoulder. The **shoulder complex** consists of the scapula, clavicle, sternum, humerus, and rib cage and includes the sternoclavicular joint, acromioclavicular joint, glenohumeral joint, and "scapulothoracic articulation" (Fig. 8-1). In other words, it includes the shoulder girdle (scapula and clavicle) and the shoulder joint (scapula and humerus). The **scapulothoracic articulation** is not a joint in the pure sense of the word. Although the scapula and thorax do not have a point of fixation, the scapula does move over the rib cage of the thorax. The scapula and thorax are not directly attached but are connected indirectly by the clavicle and by several muscles. The scapulothoracic articulation does provide motion and flexibility to the body.

Shoulder girdle is a term often used to discuss the activities of the scapula and clavicle and, to a lesser degree, the sternum. The sternoclavicular and acromioclavicular joints allow shoulder girdle motions. These shoulder girdle motions are elevation and depression, protraction and retraction, and upward and downward rotation. There are five muscles that attach to the scapula, the clavicle, or both, providing motion of the shoulder girdle.

The **shoulder joint,** also called the glenohumeral joint, consists of the scapula and humerus. The motions

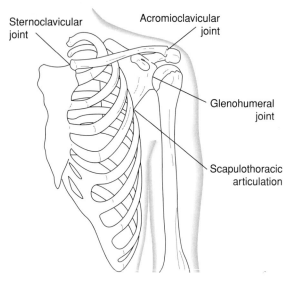

Figure 8-1.   The shoulder complex.

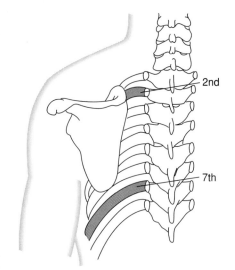

Figure 8-2.   Resting position of the scapula on the thorax.

of the shoulder joint are flexion, extension and hyper-extension, abduction and adduction, medial and lateral rotation, and horizontal abduction and adduction. Because the shoulder joint is such a mobile joint, there are few ligaments. There are nine muscles that cross the shoulder joint and are the prime movers in shoulder joint motion.

Now that the various terms connected with the shoulder complex have been defined, the shoulder girdle will be discussed in more detail. The shoulder joint will be addressed in the Chapter 9.

Bones and Landmarks

The scapula is a triangular-shaped bone located superficially on the posterior side of the thorax that, along with the clavicle, makes up the shoulder girdle. The scapula attaches to the trunk indirectly through its ligamentous attachment to the clavicle. The scapula is slightly concave anteriorly and glides over the convex posterior rib cage. Many muscles also connect the scapula to the trunk.

In the resting position, the scapula is located between the second and seventh ribs, with the vertebral border approximately 2 to 3 inches lateral from the spinous processes of the vertebra. The spine of the scapula is approximately level with the spinous process of the third and fourth thoracic vertebrae (Fig. 8-2).

Figures 8-1 and 8-2 show the position of the scapula on the body from an anterior and posterior view,

respectively. The important bony landmarks of the scapula (Fig. 8-3) in terms of shoulder girdle function are the following.

Superior angle
Superior medial aspect, providing attachment for the levator scapula muscle.

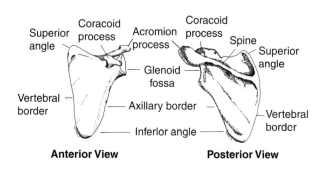

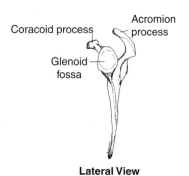

Figure 8-3.   Bony landmarks of the left scapula.

Inferior angle

Most inferior point and where vertebral and axillary border meet. This point determines scapular rotation.

Vertebral border

Between superior and inferior angles medially, and attachment of the rhomboid and serratus anterior muscles.

Axillary border

The lateral side between glenoid fossa and inferior angle.

Spine

Projection on posterior surface running from medial border laterally to the acromion process. It provides attachment for the middle and lower trapezius muscles.

Coracoid process

Projection on anterior surface, providing attachment for the pectoralis minor muscle.

Acromion process

Broad, flat area on superior lateral aspect, providing attachment for the upper trapezius muscle.

Glenoid fossa

Slightly concave surface that articulates with humerus on superior lateral side above the axillary border and below acromion process.

The **clavicle** is an S-shaped bone that connects the upper extremity to the axial skeleton at the sternoclavicular joint. Figure 8-1 shows the position of the clavicle in relation to the sternum, scapula, and rib cage. The important bony landmarks of the clavicle (Fig. 8-4) for shoulder girdle function are as follows:

Sternal end

Attaches medially to sternum

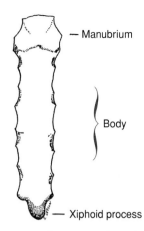

Figure 8-5.   The sternum (anterior view).

Acromial end

Attaches laterally to scapula, and provides attachment for the upper trapezius muscle

Body

Area between the two ends

The **sternum** is a flat bone located in the midline of the anterior thorax (Fig. 8-5). The position of the sternum in relation to the rib cage and clavicles is shown in Figure 8-1. At its superior end it provides attachment for the clavicle, followed beneath by attachments for the costal cartilages of the ribs. It is divided into three parts:

Manubrium

The superior end, providing attachment for the clavicle and the first rib

Body

The middle two-thirds of the sternum, providing attachment for the remaining ribs

Xiphoid process

Meaning "sword-shaped," the inferior tip

Joints and Ligaments

The **sternoclavicular joint** (Fig. 8-6) provides the shoulder girdle with its only direct attachment to the trunk. It is a synovial joint that is plane-shaped and has a double gliding motion. Motions occur in three planes and accompany the motions of the shoulder girdle. Although these motions are more subtle than those at most other joints, they are nonetheless important. Basically, the clavicle moves while the sternum remains stationary.

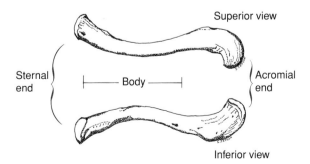

Figure 8-4.   The left clavicle.

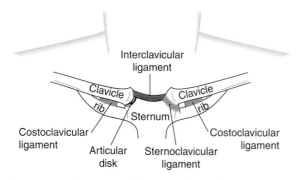

Figure 8-6.   Ligaments of the sternoclavicular joint (left side cut away to show the disk).

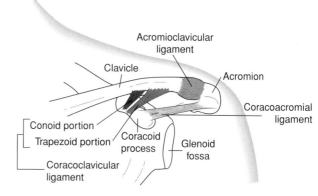

Figure 8-7.   Ligaments of the acromioclavicular joint.

The sternoclavicular joint, being a synovial joint, has a joint capsule. It also has three major ligaments and a joint disk. The joint capsule surrounds the joint and is reinforced by the anterior and posterior sternoclavicular ligaments. The articular disk serves as a shock absorber, especially from forces generated by falls on the outstretched hand. The disk and its ligamentous support are so effective that dislocation at the sternoclavicular joint is rare. This disk has a unique attachment that contributes to the motion of this joint. It has a double attachment much like that of a double-hung hinge found on doors that can swing in both directions. During shoulder girdle elevation and depression, motion occurs between the clavicle and the disk. During protraction and retraction motion occurs between the disk and the sternum.

The three major ligaments supporting this joint are the sternoclavicular, costoclavicular, and interclavicular ligaments. The sternoclavicular ligament connects the clavicle to the sternum on both the anterior and posterior surfaces and is therefore divided into the anterior and posterior sternoclavicular ligaments. As mentioned, it provides reinforcement to the joint capsule. The **costoclavicular ligament** is a short, flat, rhomboid-shaped ligament that connects the inferior surface of the clavicle to the superior surface of the costal cartilage of the first rib. The primary purpose of this ligament is to limit the amount of clavicular elevation. The **interclavicular ligament** is located on top of the manubrium, connecting the superior sternal ends of the clavicles. Its purpose is to limit the amount of clavicular depression.

The **acromioclavicular joint** (Fig. 8-7) connects the acromion process of the scapula with the lateral end of the clavicle. It is a plane-shaped synovial joint with three planes of motion. The motions are minimal but important to normal shoulder motion. The joint cap-

sule surrounds the articular borders of the joint. It is quite weak and is reinforced above and below by the superior and inferior acromioclavicular ligaments. These ligaments give support to the joint by holding the acromion process to the clavicle, thus preventing dislocation of the clavicle.

The coracoclavicular ligament and coracoacromial ligaments are two accessory ligaments of the acromioclavicular joint. Although the **coracoclavicular ligament** is not directly located at the joint, it does provide stability to that joint and allows the scapula to be suspended from the clavicle. It connects the scapula to the clavicle by attaching to the inferior surface of the lateral end of the clavicle and the superior surface of the coracoid process of the scapula. The ligament is divided into a lateral trapezoid portion and the deeper medial conoid portion. Together they prevent backward motion of the scapula, and individually they limit the rotation of the scapula.

The **coracoacromial ligament** does not actually cross the acromioclavicular joint, but rather forms an arch over the head of the humerus. It attaches laterally on the superior surface of the coracoid process and runs up and out to the inferior surface of the acromial process. It makes a roof over the head of the humerus and serves as a protective arch, providing support to the head when an upward force is transmitted along the humerus (Fig. 8-8).

Joint Motions

As mentioned, motions of the shoulder girdle are elevation and depression, protraction and retraction, and upward and downward rotation (Fig. 8-9). Because these motions can be seen best by looking at the scapula, these motions are commonly described as either *shoulder*

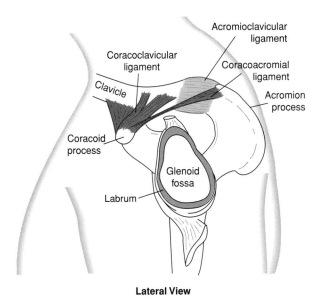

Lateral View

Figure 8-8. The coracoacromial ligament forms a roof over the shoulder joint.

girdle or *scapular motion.* For example, shoulder girdle protraction and retraction is synonymous with scapular abduction and adduction, and scapular rotation is the same as shoulder girdle rotation.

Elevation/depression and **protraction/retraction** are essentially linear motions. All points of the scapula move up and down along the thorax and away from and toward the vertebral column in parallel lines. Angular motion occurs during upward and downward rotation of the scapula. Because of the triangular shape of the scapula, one side moves one way while another side moves in an opposite or different direction. During **upward rotation,** the inferior angle of the scapula rotates up and away from the vertebral column, while **downward rotation** is the return to the resting anatomical position. For example, when the inferior angle rotates up and out, the superior angle moves down, and the glenoid fossa moves up and in. Therefore, it is important to have a point of reference to define this rotation. The inferior angle is that reference point (Fig. 8-10).

Another scapular motion should be mentioned—**scapular tilt** (see Fig. 8-9, lower right). Scapular tilt occurs when the shoulder joint goes into hyperextension. The superior end of the scapula tilts anteriorly and the inferior end tilts posteriorly. Examples of these combined motions are the "windup" or prerelease phase of a softball pitch, a bowling delivery, or a racing dive in swimming.

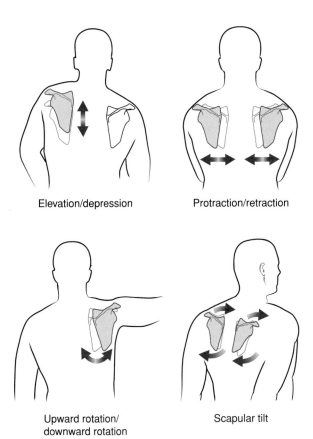

Elevation/depression   Protraction/retraction

Upward rotation/ downward rotation   Scapular tilt

Figure 8-9. Shoulder girdle motions.

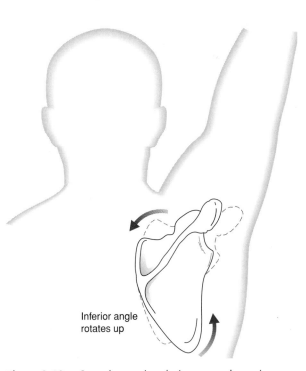

Inferior angle rotates up

Figure 8-10. Scapular motion during upward rotation.

Companion Motions of the Shoulder Joint and Shoulder Girdle

During the linear movements of elevation/depression and protraction/retraction, it is possible to move the shoulder girdle (clavicle and scapula) up, down, forward, or backward without moving the humerus. However, shoulder joint motions must accompany the angular motions of upward and downward rotation. To rotate the scapula upward, you must also flex or abduct the shoulder joint. Stated another way, when there is flexion or abduction of the shoulder joint, the scapula must also rotate upward. When there is extension or adduction of the shoulder joint, the scapula returns to anatomical position, or rotates downward. Because of the complex and interrelated activities of the shoulder girdle and the shoulder joint, it is difficult to discuss the function of one without discussing activities of the other. Impairment at one joint will also impair function at the other. The following list summarizes the shoulder girdle motions that must occur during various shoulder joint motions.

Shoulder Joint	Shoulder Girdle
Flexion	Upward rotation; protraction
Extension	Downward rotation; retraction
Hyperextension	Scapular tilt
Abduction	Upward rotation
Adduction	Downward rotation
Medial rotation	Protraction
Lateral rotation	Retraction
Horizontal abduction	Retraction
Horizontal adduction	Protraction

Scapulohumeral Rhythm

Scapulohumeral rhythm is a concept that further describes the movement relationship between the shoulder girdle and shoulder joint. The first 30 degrees of shoulder joint motion is pure shoulder joint motion. However, after that, for every 2 degrees of shoulder flexion or abduction that occurs, the scapula must upwardly rotate 1 degree. This 2:1 ratio is known as scapulohumeral rhythm.

It is possible to demonstrate that the first part of shoulder joint motion occurs only at the shoulder joint, but further motion must be accompanied by shoulder girdle motion. With a person in the anatomical position, stabilize the scapula by putting the heel of your hand against the axillary border to prevent rotation of the scapula. Instruct the person to abduct the

shoulder joint. Notice that the individual is only able to abduct a short distance before shoulder joint motion is impaired.

Angle of Pull

As discussed in Chapter 5, several factors determine the role that a muscle will play in a particular joint motion. Determining whether a muscle has a major role (prime mover), a minor role (assisting mover), or no role at all will depend on such factors as its size, angle of pull, the joint motions possible, and the location of the muscle in relation to the joint axis. Angle of pull is usually a major factor because most muscles pull at a diagonal. As discussed in Chapter 7 regarding torque, most muscles have a diagonal line of pull. That diagonal line of pull is the resultant force of a vertical force and a horizontal force. In the case of the shoulder girdle, muscles with a greater vertical angle of pull will be effective in pulling the scapula up or down (elevating or depressing the scapula). Muscles with a greater horizontal pull will be more effective in pulling the scapula in or out (protracting or retracting). Muscles with a more equal horizontal and vertical pull will have a role in both motions (see Fig. 5-12). For example, the levator scapula has a stronger vertical component, the middle trapezius has a stronger horizontal component, and the rhomboids have a more equal pull in both directions. As you will see when these muscles are described later in this chapter, the levator scapula is a prime mover in scapular elevation, the middle trapezius is a prime mover in retraction, and the rhomboids are a prime mover in both elevation and retraction.

Muscles of the Shoulder Girdle

Muscle Descriptions

There are five muscles primarily responsible for moving the scapula. Each muscle will be discussed with particular emphasis on its location and function. This will be followed by a summary of its proximal attachment origin **(O)**, distal attachment insertion **(I)**, and joint motions in which it is a prime mover action **(A)**. This listing is given for clarity and is not intended to be the only description. The student is encouraged to visualize the attachments and describe them using proper terminology instead of memorizing these listings. The nerve **(N),** which innervates the muscle, as well as the spinal cord level of that innervation, are also given.

The muscles of the shoulder girdle are the:

Trapezius
Levator scapulae
Rhomboids
Serratus anterior
Pectoralis minor

Trapezius

The **trapezius muscle** (Fig. 8-11) is a large superficial muscle, which is diamond-shaped when looking at both right and left sides. Functionally, it is usually divided into three parts: upper, middle, and lower. The reason for this separation is that there are three different lines of pull (up, in, down) resulting in different muscle actions.

The **upper trapezius muscle** (Fig. 8-12) originates from the occipital protuberance and the nuchal ligament of the upper cervical vertebra. The nuchal ligament attaches to the spinous processes of the cervical vertebra. The upper trapezius inserts on the lateral end of the clavicle and acromion process. Because its diagonal line of pull is more vertical (up) than horizontal (in), it is a prime mover in scapular elevation and upward rotation and only an assisting mover in scapular retraction.

The **middle trapezius muscle** (Fig. 8-13) originates from the nuchal ligament of the lower cervical vertebrae and spinous process of C7 and the upper thoracic ver-

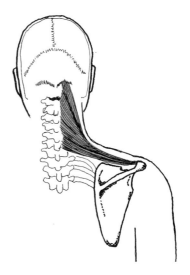

Figure 8-12. The upper trapezius muscle.

tebrae and inserts on the medial aspect of the acromion process and along the scapular spine. Its line of pull is horizontal, which makes it very effective at scapular retraction. Because the line of pull passes just above the axis for upward rotation, its role in scapular upward rotation is only assistive.

The **lower trapezius muscle** (Fig. 8-14) originates from the spinous processes of the middle and lower thoracic vertebrae and inserts on the base of the scapular spine. Its diagonal line of pull is more downward (vertical) than in (horizontal), making it effective in

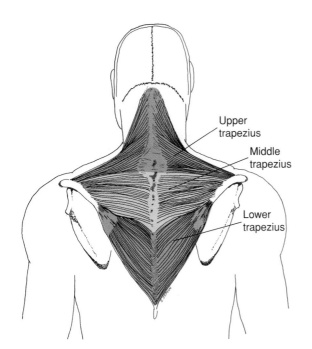

Upper
trapezius

Middle
trapezius

Lower
trapezius

Figure 8-11. The three parts of the trapezius muscle.

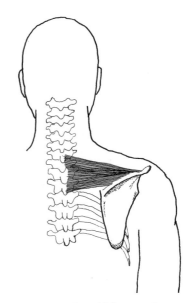

Figure 8-13. The middle trapezius muscle.

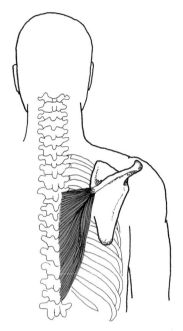

Figure 8-14. The lower trapezius muscle.

depression and upward rotation of the scapula and only assistive in retraction.

All three parts of the trapezius muscle work together (synergists) to retract the scapula. Remember, however, that the middle trapezius muscle is the prime mover and the upper and lower trapezius muscles can only assist. The upper and lower trapezius muscles are antagonistic to each other in elevation/depression and agonistic in upward rotation. To visualize the upward rotation component of these muscles, think of the scapula as a steering wheel (Fig. 8-15). In this example, a right scapula is used. Tie a ribbon at the bottom of

the wheel to represent the inferior angle of the scapula. Put your right hand at the 2-o'clock position representing the upper trapezius attachment, and put your left hand at the 10-o'clock position, representing the lower trapezius attachment. Turn the wheel to the left and note that the ribbon moves upward toward the right. In the case of the scapula, the upper trapezius muscle (right hand) moves up and in, the lower trapezius muscle (left hand) moves down and in. This combined effort causes the inferior angle to move up and out (upward rotation).

Upper Trapezius Muscle

O	Occipital bone, nuchal ligament on cervical spinous processes
I	Outer third of clavicle, acromion process
A	Scapular elevation and upward rotation
N	Spinal accessory (cranial nerve XI), C3 and C4 sensory component

Middle Trapezius Muscle

O	Spinous processes of C7 through T3
I	Scapular spine
A	Scapular retraction
N	Spinal accessory (cranial nerve XI), C3 and C4 sensory component

Lower Trapezius Muscle

O	Spinous processes of middle and lower thoracic vertebrae
I	Base of the scapular spine
A	Scapular depression and upward rotation
N	Spinal accessory (cranial nerve XI), C3 and C4 sensory component

The **levator scapula muscle** is named for its function of scapular elevation. It is covered entirely by the trapezius muscle. It arises from the transverse processes of C1 through C4 and attaches on the vertebral border of the scapula between the superior angle and the spine (Fig. 8-16). Its diagonal line of pull is mostly vertical. Therefore, it is a prime mover in scapular elevation and only an assisting mover in retraction. It is also a prime mover in downward rotation. Visualize the steering wheel with your left hand in the 10-o'clock position. Pull up (turning the wheel to the right) and notice that the inferior angle (ribbon) moves to the left (downward

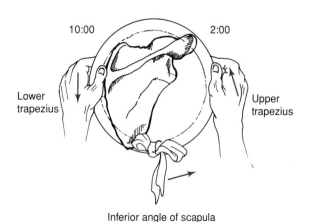

Figure 8-15. Rotational movement of the right scapula.

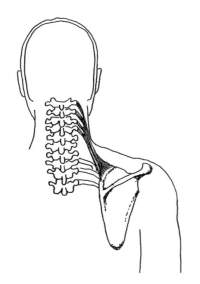

Figure 8-16. The levator scapula muscle.

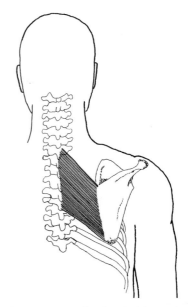

Figure 8-17. The rhomboid muscle.

rotation). Keep in mind that downward rotation is the return to anatomical position from an upwardly rotated position.

Levator Scapula Muscle

O	Transverse processes of first four cervical vertebrae
I	Vertebral border of scapula between the superior angle and spine
A	Scapular elevation and downward rotation
N	Third and fourth cervical nerves and dorsal scapular nerve (C5)

The **rhomboids** are actually two muscles: rhomboid major and rhomboid minor. They are commonly considered together as one muscle because it is anatomically difficult to separate these two muscles and functionally they have the same actions, They derive their name from their shape. This geometric shape is basically a rectangle that has been skewed so that the sides have oblique angles instead of right angles. The rhomboid muscles lie under the trapezius muscle and can be palpated when the trapezius muscle is relaxed. They originate from the nuchal ligament and spinous processes of C7 through T5 and insert on the vertebral border of the scapula below the levator scapula muscle between the spine and the inferior angle (Fig. 8-17). Because their oblique line of pull has a good horizontal and vertical component, they are a prime mover in retraction and elevation.

Like the levator scapula muscle, they downwardly rotate the scapula.

Rhomboid Muscles

O	Spinous processes of C7 through T5
I	Vertebral border of scapula between the spine and inferior angle
A	Scapular retraction, elevation, and downward rotation
N	Dorsal scapular nerve (C5)

It is impossible to raise your arm above your head without the action of the **serratus anterior muscle.** This muscle gets its name from the serrated, or sawtooth, pattern of attachment on the anterior lateral side of the thorax. It is superficial at this point and may be palpated when the arm is overhead. The muscle runs posteriorly to pass between the scapula and the rib cage. It attaches on the anterior surface of the scapula along the vertebral border between the superior and inferior angles (Fig. 8-18). Because it has a nearly horizontal line of pull outward, it is a prime mover in scapular protraction. Its lower fibers pulling outward on the lower part of the scapula are effective in upwardly rotating the scapula. These fibers join with the upper and lower trapezius muscles to form a force couple rotating the scapula upward. Another function of this muscle is to keep the vertebral border of the scapula against the rib cage. Without this muscle the vertebral border lifts away from the rib cage, which is called "winging of the scapula" (Fig. 8-19).

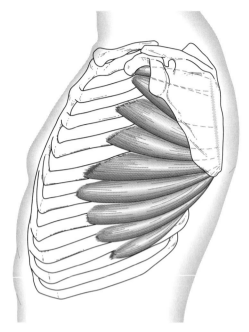

Figure 8-18. The serratus anterior muscle.

Serratus Anterior Muscle

O	Lateral surface of the upper eight ribs
I	Vertebral border of the scapula, anterior surface
A	Scapular protraction and upward rotation
N	Long thoracic nerve (C5, C6, C7)

The **pectoralis minor muscle** lies deep to the pectoralis major muscle and is the only shoulder girdle muscle located entirely on the anterior surface of the body. It arises from the anterior surface of the third through fifth ribs near the costal cartilages and runs upward to its attachment on the coracoid process of the scapula (Fig. 8-20). Its downward diagonal line of pull is mostly vertical, making it a prime mover in scapular depression, downward rotation, and scapular tilt. Although it is rather easy to see the depression action, the downward rotation is less obvious because the muscle is on the anterior surface while the scapula moves on the posterior surface. Visualize the steering wheel again with the ribbon (inferior angle of the scapula) rotated up to the right. Place your right hand in the 2-o'clock position (coracoid process) and pull down. Notice that the ribbon (inferior angle) moves downward toward the left (downward rotation). Because the pectoralis minor attaches on the anterior superior surface (coracoid process) of the scapula, and

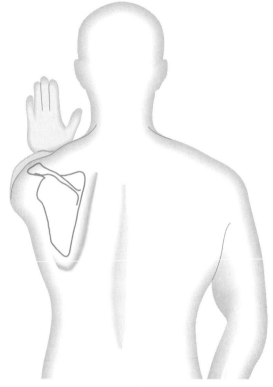

Figure 8-19. Winging of the scapula. This woman's left serratus anterior muscle is paralyzed. When she pushes against the wall with both hands, her left scapula rises away from the rib cage, standing out like a small wing.

moves vertically downward toward its attachment on the ribs, one can visualize the top part of the scapula being pulled down and forward, causing the bottom (inferior angle) to be tipped "out." In other words, the pectoralis minor causes scapular tilt.

Pectoralis Minor Muscle

O	Anterior surface, third through fifth ribs
I	Coracoid process of the scapula
A	Scapular depression, protraction, downward rotation, and tilt
N	Medial pectoral nerve (C8, T1)

The following list summarizes the actions of the prime movers of the shoulder girdle.

Action	Muscles
Retraction	Middle trapezius, rhomboids
Protraction	Serratus anterior, pectoralis minor

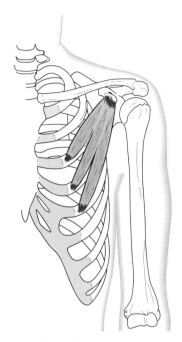

Figure 8-20.   The pectoralis minor muscle.

Elevation	Upper trapezius, levator scapula, rhomboids
Depression	Lower trapezius, pectoralis minor
Upward rotation	Upper and lower trapezius
	Serratus anterior (lower fibers)
Downward rotation	Rhomboids, levator scapulae, pectoralis minor
Scapular tilt	Pectoralis minor

Force Couples

A **force couple** is defined as muscles pulling in different directions to accomplish the same motion. In the case of the shoulder girdle, the upper trapezius muscle pulls up, the lower trapezius muscle pulls down, and the lower fibers of the serratus anterior muscle pull outwardly in a horizontal direction (Fig. 8-21). The net effect is that the scapula is rotated upwardly.

Downward rotation is another example of a force couple. The combined effect of the pectoralis minor muscle pulling down, the rhomboid muscles pulling in, and the levator scapular muscle pulling up is to downwardly rotate the scapula (Fig. 8-22). This motion

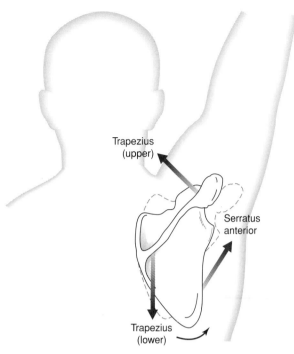

Figure 8-21.   The muscular force couple produces upward rotation of the scapula.

is accomplished when the shoulder joint is forcefully extended, as when chopping wood or paddling a canoe. Downward rotation of the scapula must accompany extension of the shoulder joint.

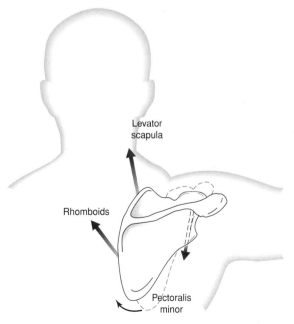

Figure 8-22.   The muscular force couple produces downward rotation of the scapula.

Table 8-1	Innervation of the Muscles of the Shoulder Girdle	
Muscle	**Nerve**	**Spinal Segment**
Trapezius	Cranial nerve XI	C3, C4
Levator scapula	Dorsal scapular	C3, C4, C5
Rhomboids	Dorsal scapular	C5
Serratus anterior	Long thoracic	C5, C6, C7
Pectoralis minor	Medial pectoral	C8, T1

Table 8-2	Segmental Innervation of Shoulder Girdle Muscles						
Spinal Cord Level	**C3**	**C4**	**C5**	**C6**	**C7**	**C8**	**T1**
Trapezius	X	X					
Levator scapula	X	X	X				
Rhomboids			X				
Serratus anterior			X	X	X		
Pectoralis minor						X	X

Reversal of Muscle Action

The actions of the shoulder girdle muscles have been described as moving insertion toward the origin. However, if the insertion is stabilized, the origin will move. As discussed in Chapter 5, this is called **reversal of muscle action.** This allows some of the shoulder girdle muscles to have assistive roles in other joints, primarily the head and neck.

Because of its attachment on the occiput and cervical vertebrae, the **upper trapezius** plays a role in moving the head and neck. When the shoulder girdle is stabilized, the upper trapezius can assist in extending the head and neck, laterally bending it to the same side (ipsilateral) and rotating it to the opposite side (contralateral).

With the shoulder girdle stabilized, the **lower trapezius** can reverse its action and assist in elevating the trunk. This is particularly useful during crutch walking. With the crutches planted on the floor in front, the person swings the body through. The lower origin on the vertebral column moves toward the higher attachment on the scapula, thus raising the body as it swings through the crutches.

When the scapula is stabilized, the **levator scapula** can move the neck. It can assist the splenius cervicis, a neck muscle, in rotating and laterally bending the neck ipsilaterally.

Summary of Muscle Innervation

The shoulder girdle gets its innervation fairly high off the spinal cord from a variety of sources proximal to the terminal nerves of the brachial plexus. The 11th cranial (spinal accessory) nerve innervates the trapezius muscle with sensory innervation from C3 and C4. The third and fourth cervical nerves innervate the levator scapula muscle with partial innervation by the dorsal scapular nerve coming from C5. The serratus anterior muscle is innervated by the long thoracic nerve, which is made up of branches of C5 through C7 and the rhomboid muscles are innervated by the dorsal scapular nerve via a branch of the anterior ramus to C5. The pectoralis minor muscle receives innervation from the medial pectoral nerve, which branches off the medial cord of the brachial plexus. Table 8-1 summarizes the innervation of these muscles and Table 8-2 gives the spinal cord level of innervation for each muscle.

Points to Remember

- The shoulder girdle has both linear and angular motions.
- The inferior angle is the point of reference for scapular rotation.
- Certain shoulder girdle and shoulder joint motions are connected.
- Scapulohumeral rhythm is an example of the combined motions of these joints.
- Muscles pulling in different directions to accomplish the same motion are a force couple.

Review Questions

General Anatomy Questions

1. Identify the structures that make up the shoulder girdle, shoulder joint, and shoulder complex.
2. Given that the scapula is shaped somewhat like a triangle—
   a. What landmark is commonly used to determine the direction the scapula is rotating?
   b. What direction is the landmark moving if the scapula is rotating upwardly?
3. Which shoulder girdle motions are mostly linear?
4. Which shoulder girdle motions are mostly angular?
5. What is scapulohumeral rhythm?
6. How is shoulder joint motion affected by the absence of scapulohumeral rhythm?
7. The trapezius muscle is usually referred to and described as consisting of three different muscles. The two rhomboid muscles (major and minor) are referred to and described as one. From a functional perspective:
   a. Why is the trapezius muscle separated into three muscles?
   b. Why are the rhomboid muscles described as one muscle?
8. Raising your hand over your head requires the combined action of which three shoulder girdle muscles?
9. Name and define the biomechanical term used to describe the combined action in question No. 8?
10. Starting at the inferior angle and going clockwise, name the shoulder girdle muscles that attach to the posterior surface of the scapula.

Functional Activity Questions

Identify the shoulder girdle motions that occur with the following actions. Accompanying shoulder joint motions have been provided in parentheses.

1. Closing a window by pulling down
   Shoulder girdle motion _____
   (Shoulder extension)
2. Opening a window by pulling up
   Shoulder girdle motion _____
   (Shoulder flexion)
3. Carrying a heavy suitcase
   Shoulder girdle motion _____
   (No shoulder motion)
4. Combing your hair in the back
   Shoulder girdle motion _____
   (Shoulder flexion, lateral rotation)
5. Reaching across the table
   Shoulder girdle motion _____
   (Shoulder flexion)

Clinical Exercise Questions

1. Lie prone on a table with your right arm hanging over the side of the table and holding a weight in your right hand (Fig. 8-23). Using only shoulder girdle motion and no shoulder joint motion, pull the weight straight up from the floor.
   a. What motion is occurring at the shoulder girdle?
   b. What muscles are prime movers of this shoulder girdle action?
   c. Is this an open-or closed-chain activity?

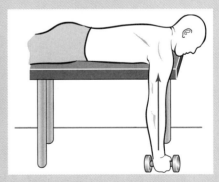

Figure 8-23. Starting position.

2. Stand with your back toward a corner, your shoulders abducted to 90 degrees, elbows flexed, with an elbow touching each wall. Using a shoulder horizontal adduction motion, push against

the wall with your elbows and move your body away from the corner.

   a. What shoulder girdle motion is accompanying the shoulder horizontal adduction?

   b. What muscles are prime movers in this shoulder girdle motion?

3. Sit in a chair that has arms; place your hands on the armrests in a position that puts your shoulders in hyperextension. Push down on the armrests and raise your buttock off the seat of the chair.

   a. What shoulder girdle motion is accompanying the shoulder flexion action (from hyperextension to neutral)?

   b. What muscles are prime movers in this shoulder girdle motion?

4. Lie in a prone position with your legs together, hands on the table next to your shoulders with your fingers pointing forward (Fig. 8-24). Push up with your hands as far as you can while straightening your elbows, bending your knees, and keeping your back straight.

   a. What shoulder girdle motion is occurring?

   b. What muscles are prime movers in this shoulder girdle motion?

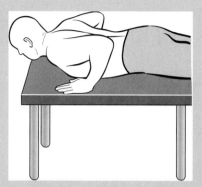

Figure 8-24.   Starting position.

5. Using the Lat Pull-down machine of the Universal Gym (or some other comparable apparatus), reach up and grasp the handles. Pull down while keeping your arms moving in the frontal plane.

   a. What shoulder girdle motions are accompanying the shoulder adduction and lateral rotation?

   b. What muscles are prime movers in this shoulder girdle motion?

CHAPTER 9

Shoulder Joint

Joint Motions

Bones and Landmarks

Ligaments and Other Structures

Common Shoulder Pathologies

Muscles of the Shoulder Joint

Glenohumeral Movement

Summary of Muscle Action

Summary of Muscle Innervation

Points to Remember

Review Questions

General Anatomy Questions

Functional Activity Questions

Clinical Exercise Questions

The **shoulder joint** is a ball-and-socket joint with movement in all three planes and around all three axes (Fig. 9-1). The humeral head articulating with the glenoid fossa of the scapula makes up the shoulder joint. The shoulder joint is one of the most movable joints in the body and, consequently, one of the least stable.

Joint Motions

There are four groups of motions possible at the shoulder joint (Fig. 9-2): flexion, extension, and hyperextension; abduction and adduction; medial and lateral rotation; and horizontal abduction and adduction. Flexion, extension, and hyperextension occur in the sagittal plane around the frontal axis. **Flexion** is from 0 to 180 degrees, and **extension** is the return to the anatomical position. There are approximately 45 degrees of **hyperextension** possible from anatomical position. **Abduction** and **adduction** occur in the frontal plane around the sagittal axis with 180 degrees of motion possible. **Medial** and **lateral rotation** occur in the transverse plane around the vertical axis. Sometimes the terms *internal* and *external* are used in place of *medial* and *lateral,* respectively. From a neutral position, it is possible to move 90 degrees in each direction. **Horizontal abduction** and **horizontal adduction** also occur in the transverse plane around the vertical axis. The starting position for these motions is at 90 degrees of shoulder abduction. There are approximately 30 degrees of horizontal abduction (backward motion) and approximately 120 degrees of horizontal adduction. *Circumduction* is a term used to describe the arc or circle of motion possible at the shoulder. Because it is really only a combination of all the shoulder motions, the term circumduction will not be used here.

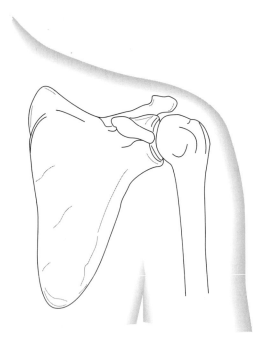

Figure 9-1.   The shoulder joint.

Another term frequently seen in the literature, especially regarding therapeutic exercise for shoulder conditions, is **scaption.** This motion is similar to flexion or abduction, but occurs in the **scapular plane** as opposed to the sagittal or frontal plane. The scapular plane is approximately 30 degrees forward of the frontal plane. It is not quite midway between flexion and abduction. With scaption of the shoulder, 180 degrees of up and down motion is possible. Most common functional activities occur in the scapular plane.

Bones and Landmarks

The **scapula** and many of its landmarks have been described earlier with the shoulder girdle. The following are landmarks of the scapula that you should know when talking about the shoulder joint (Fig. 9-3).

Glenoid fossa
A shallow, somewhat egg-shaped socket on the superior end, lateral side; articulates with the humerus

Glenoid labrum
Fibrocartilaginous ring attached to the rim of the glenoid fossa, which deepens the articular cavity

Subscapular fossa
Includes most of the area on the anterior (costal) surface, providing attachment for the subscapularis muscle

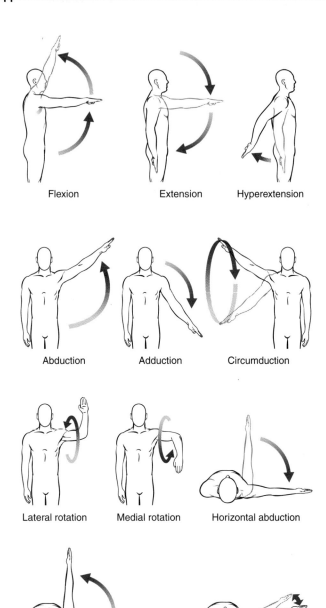

Figure 9-2.   Shoulder joint motions.

Infraspinous fossa
Below the spine, providing attachment for the infraspinatus muscle

Supraspinous fossa
Above the spine, providing attachment for the supraspinatus muscle

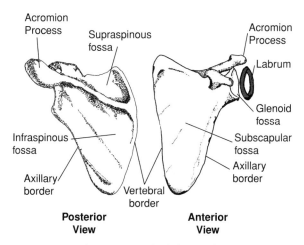

Figure 9-3.   The left scapula.

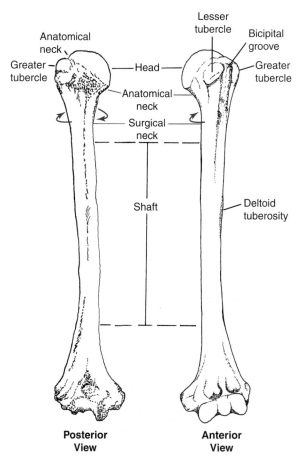

Figure 9-4.   The left humerus.

Axillary border
Providing attachment for the teres major and teres minor muscles

Acromion process
Broad, flat area on the superior lateral aspect, providing attachment for the middle deltoid muscle

The **humerus** is the longest and largest bone of the upper extremity (Fig. 9-4). The position of the humerus with the scapula is shown in an anterior view in Figure 9-1. The important landmarks are as follows:

Head
Semirounded proximal end; articulates with the scapula

Surgical neck
Slightly constricted area just below tubercles where the head meets the body

Anatomical neck
Circumferential groove separating the head from the tubercle

Shaft
Or "body"; the area between the surgical neck proximally and the epicondyles distally

Greater tubercle
Large projection lateral to head and lesser tubercle; provides attachment for the supraspinatus, infraspinatus, and teres minor muscles

Lesser tubercle
Smaller projection on the anterior surface, medial to the greater tubercle; provides attachment for the subscapularis muscle

Deltoid tuberosity
On the lateral side near the midpoint; not usually a well-defined landmark

Bicipital groove
Also called the "intertubercular groove"; the longitudinal groove between the tubercles, containing the tendon of the long head of the biceps

Bicipital ridges
Also called the lateral and medial lips of the bicipital groove, or the crests of the greater and lesser tubercles respectively. The lateral lip (crest of the greater tubercle) provides attachment for the pectoralis major, and the medial lip (crest of the lesser tubercle) provides attachment for the latissimus dorsi and teres major

Ligaments and Other Structures

The **joint capsule** is a thin-walled, spacious container that attaches around the rim of the glenoid fossa of the

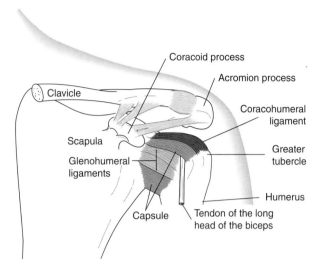

Figure 9-5. The shoulder joint capsule and ligaments that reinforce it.

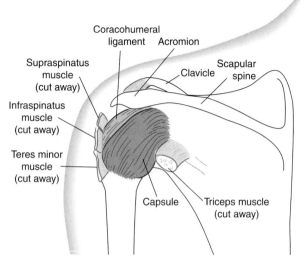

Figure 9-6. Left shoulder joint capsule and coracohumeral ligament. Posterior view, muscles cut away.

scapula and anatomical neck of the humerus (Figs. 9-5 and 9-6). It is formed by an outer fibrous membrane and an inner synovial membrane. With the arm hanging at the side, the superior portion of the capsule is taut, and the inferior part is slack. When the shoulder is abducted, the opposite occurs, with the inferior portion taut and the superior part slack. The superior, middle, and inferior **glenohumeral ligaments** reinforce the anterior portion of the capsule. These are not well-defined ligaments but actually pleated folds of the capsule.

The **coracohumeral ligament** attaches from the lateral side of the coracoid process and spans the joint anteriorly to the medial side of the greater tubercle (see Figs. 9-5 and 9-6). It strengthens the upper part of the joint capsule.

The **glenoid labrum** is a fibrous ring that surrounds the rim of the glenoid fossa (see Figs. 9-3 and 9-7). Its function is to deepen the articular cavity.

There are several bursae in the shoulder joint area. The subdeltoid bursa is large and located between the deltoid muscle and the joint capsule. The subacromial bursa lies below the acromion and coracoacromial ligament, between them and the joint capsule, and is frequently continuous with the subdeltoid bursa.

The **rotator cuff** is the tendinous band formed by the blending together of the tendinous insertions of the subscapularis, supraspinatus, infraspinatus, and teres minor muscles. These muscles help to keep the head of the humerus "rotating" against the glenoid fossa during joint motion. This rotating motion is what inspired the term rotator cuff, not the muscular action of medial or lateral rotation.

The **thoracolumbar fascia** (lumbar aponeurosis) is a superficial fibrous sheet attaching to the spinous processes of the lower thoracic and lumbar vertebra, the supraspinal ligament, and the posterior part of the iliac crest, covering the sacrospinalis muscle; it provides a very broad attachment for the latissimus dorsi muscle.

As mentioned, the shoulder joint allows a great deal of motion, which also makes it a rather unstable joint. Several features contribute to the stability that this

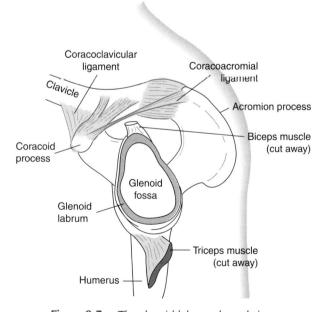

Figure 9-7. The glenoid labrum, lateral view.

joint does have. The fairly shallow glenoid fossa is made deeper by the glenoid labrum. The fossa is positioned in an anterior, lateral, and upward direction. This upward direction provides some stability to the joint. The joint is held intact by the joint capsule reinforced by the coracohumeral and glenohumeral ligaments. Because the capsule completely surrounds the joint, it creates a partial vacuum, which helps hold the head against the fossa. The rotator cuff muscles hold the joint surfaces together during joint motion. It is mostly the shoulder muscles that keep the joint from subluxing, or partially dislocating. An individual who has had a stroke and has lost function in the involved extremity often develops a subluxed shoulder. The lack of a deep socket for the humeral head to fit into, the loss of muscle tone, the weight of the extremity, and gravity all contribute to joint subluxation.

Common Shoulder Pathologies

Acromioclavicular separation is the term commonly used to describe the various amounts of ligament injury at the acromioclavicular joint. In a first-degree sprain, the acromioclavicular ligament is stretched. In a second-degree sprain, the acromioclavicular ligament is ruptured and the coracoclavicular ligament is stretched. In a third-degree sprain, both the acromioclavicular and coracoclavicular ligaments are ruptured.

Clavicular fractures account for the most frequently broken bone in children. They usually result from a fall on the lateral aspect of the shoulder or on the outstretched hand. The clavicle usually breaks in its midportion. Another fracture caused by a fall on the outstretched hand is a **humeral neck fracture.** It is common in the elderly and is usually an impacted fracture. **Midhumeral fractures** are often caused by a direct blow or a twisting force. Spiral fractures in this region increase the risk of a **radial nerve injury** as the nerve passes next to the bone. **Pathological fractures** of the humerus may be caused by benign tumors or metastatic carcinoma from primary sites such as the lung, breast, kidney, and prostate.

One of the most common joint dislocations involves the shoulder, and most of those are **anterior shoulder dislocations.** A forced shoulder abduction and lateral rotation tends to be the dislocating motion causing the humeral head to slide anteriorly out of the glenoid fossa. **Glenohumeral subluxation** is commonly seen in individuals who have hemiplegia, usually from a cardiovascular accident (stroke). Paralysis of the shoulder muscles leaves them no longer able to hold the head of the humerus in the glenoid fossa. This paralysis combined with the pull of gravity and the weight of the arm over time causes this partial dislocation.

Impingement syndrome is an overuse condition that involves compression between the acromial arch, humeral head, and coracoacromial ligament of soft tissue structures such as the rotator cuff muscles, long head of the biceps, and subacromial bursa. A type of impingement known as **swimmer's shoulder** is common with swimmers specializing in freestyle, butterfly, and backstroke. **Adhesive capsulitis** refers to the inflammation and fibrosis of the shoulder joint capsule leading to pain and loss of shoulder range of motion. It is also known as **frozen shoulder.** A **torn rotator cuff** involves the distal tendinous insertion of the supraspinatus, infraspinatus, teres minor, and subscapularis on the greater/lesser tubercle area of the humerus. Tears can be the result of acute trauma or gradual degeneration.

Chronic inflammation of the supraspinatus tendon can lead to an accumulation of mineral deposits and result in **calcific tendonitis,** which may be asymptomatic or quite painful. **Bicipital tendonitis** usually involves the long head of the biceps proximally as it crosses the humeral head, changes direction, and descends into the bicipital groove. This tendon commonly **ruptures** during repetitive and/or forceful overhead positions. Irritation as it slides in the groove can lead to **subluxing of the biceps long head tendon.** Overloading the muscle in an abducted and laterally rotated position tends to be the force subluxing the tendon out of the bicipital groove.

Muscles of the Shoulder Joint

The muscles that span the shoulder joint are as follows:

> Deltoid
> Supraspinatus
> Pectoralis major
> Latissimus dorsi
> Teres major
> Infraspinatus
> Teres minor
> Subscapularis
> Coracobrachialis
> Biceps brachii
> Triceps brachii, long head

The **deltoid muscle** is a superficial muscle covering the shoulder joint on three sides, giving the shoulder its characteristic rounded shape. The name "deltoid" describes its triangular shape (Fig. 9-8). Functionally,

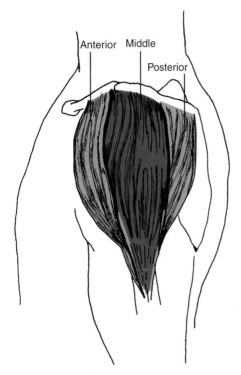

Figure 9-8.   The three parts of the deltoid muscle.

There is a concept called the "inchworm effect" that describes the action of the shoulder girdle and the deltoid muscles, especially the middle deltoid muscle, during shoulder abduction. If only the humerus moved during abduction, the middle deltoid muscle would quickly run out of contractile power as it approached 90 degrees. However, the middle deltoid muscle is effective throughout the entire range. Remember that for every 2 degrees the shoulder joint abducts, the shoulder girdle upwardly rotates 1 degree (scapulohumeral rhythm; see Chap. 8). With this upward rotation of the scapula, the origin of the deltoid muscle (the acromion process, lateral end of the clavicle, and the scapular spine) moves away from the insertion on the humerus. This lengthens the muscle, restoring its contractile potential, and allows it to continue to effectively contract throughout its entire range.

Anterior Deltoid Muscle

O	Lateral third of the clavicle
I	Deltoid tuberosity
A	Shoulder abduction, flexion, medial rotation, and horizontal adduction
N	Axillary nerve (C5, C6)

Middle Deltoid Muscle

O	Acromion process
I	Deltoid tuberosity (same as anterior deltoid muscle)
A	Shoulder abduction
N	Axillary nerve (C5, C6)

Posterior Deltoid Muscle

O	Spine of scapula
I	Deltoid tuberosity (same as anterior deltoid muscle)
A	Shoulder abduction, extension, hyperextension, lateral rotation, horizontal abduction
N	Axillary nerve (C5, C6)

this muscle is separated into three parts: anterior, middle, and posterior.

The **anterior deltoid muscle** attaches on the outer third of the clavicle and runs down and out to the deltoid tuberosity, which is located on the lateral aspect of the humerus near the midpoint. It spans the joint on the anterior surface at an oblique angle. Therefore, it is effective in abduction, flexion, and medial rotation. When the arm is at shoulder level, the line of pull is mostly horizontal and, therefore, an effective horizontal adductor.

The **middle deltoid muscle** attaches on the lateral side of the acromion process and runs directly down to the deltoid tuberosity. Because its vertical line of pull is lateral to the joint axis, it is most effective in abducting the shoulder joint.

The **posterior deltoid muscle** attaches to the spine of the scapula and runs obliquely down to its attachment with the anterior and middle fibers on the deltoid tuberosity. Because its oblique line of pull is posterior to the joint axis, it is strong in shoulder abduction, extension, hyperextension, and lateral rotation. When the arm is at shoulder level, the line of pull is mostly horizontal, making it effective in horizontal abduction.

As its name implies, the **supraspinatus muscle** (Fig. 9-9) lies above the spine of the scapula. It passes underneath the acromion process to attach on the greater tubercle of the humerus. The portion located in the supraspinous fossa is deep to the trapezius muscle above and to the deltoid muscle laterally. Early kinesiology studies suggested that the supraspinatus muscle

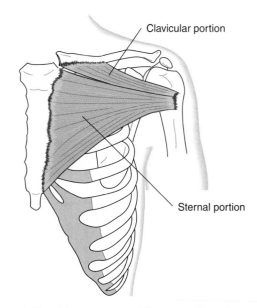

Figure 9-10.   The two parts of the pectoralis major muscle.

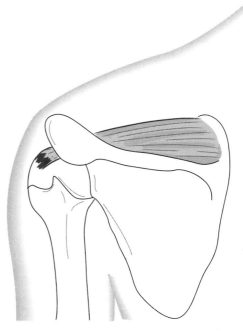

Figure 9-9.   The supraspinatus muscle.

was most effective in only initiating shoulder abduction. However, electromyography studies have since shown that it is active throughout abduction. In addition to its joint movement function, the supraspinatus muscle is very important in stabilizing the head of the humerus against the glenoid fossa.

Supraspinatus Muscle

O	Supraspinous fossa of the scapula
I	Greater tubercle of the humerus
A	Shoulder abduction
N	Suprascapular nerve (C5, C6)

The **pectoralis major muscle** (Fig. 9-10) is a large muscle of the chest as its name implies (*pectus* means "breast" or "chest"). It is superficial except for its distal attachment lying under the deltoid muscle. Because this muscle crosses the joint on the anterior surface from medial to lateral, it is effective in adduction and medial rotation of the shoulder joint.

This muscle, because of its proximal attachments and different lines of pull, is often separated into a clavicular and sternal portion. The **clavicular portion** attaches to the medial third of the clavicle. The clavicular portion has a more vertical line of pull when the shoulder is extended, making it very effective at flexing the shoulder during the first part of the range. As the shoulder approaches 90 degrees (shoulder level), the line of pull is no longer vertical but horizontal; thus,

this portion of the pectoralis major muscle is no longer effective. It is most effective in the early portion of the range (0–30 degrees) and becomes more ineffective toward the midpoint of the range (90 degrees). It is then safe to say that the clavicular portion of the pectoralis major acts as a prime mover in the first 60 degrees of shoulder flexion.

The **sternal portion** attaches to the sternum and costal cartilages of the first six ribs. It has a more vertical line of pull when the shoulder is in full flexion and loses effectiveness as the shoulder approaches 90 degrees of extension. Similar to, though in opposite directions of the clavicular portion, the sternal portion is most effective in the early portion of the range (180–150 degrees). It becomes more ineffective toward the midpoint of the range (90 degrees). Therefore, it is safe to say that the sternal portion of the pectoralis major acts as a prime mover in the first 60 degrees of shoulder extension. Since extension begins from a position of full flexion (180 degrees) and moves to anatomical position (0 degrees), the first 60 degrees of shoulder extension would be from 180 degrees to 120 degrees.

Both portions of the pectoralis major muscle are effective in the first parts of motion in the sagittal plane (clavicular portion for flexion, sternal portion for extension). They are, therefore, antagonistic to each other in flexion and extension, but agonists in shoulder adduction, medial rotation, and horizontal adduction.

Pectoralis Major Muscle, Clavicular Portion

O	Medial third of clavicle
I	Lateral lip of bicipital groove of humerus
A	Shoulder flexion—First 60 degrees

Pectoralis Major Muscle, Sternal Portion

O	Sternum, costal cartilage of first six ribs
I	Lateral lip of bicipital groove of humerus (same as clavicular portion)
A	Shoulder extension—First 60 degrees (from 180 degrees to 120 degrees)

Pectoralis Major Muscle, Clavicular and Sternal Portions

A	Shoulder adduction, medial rotation, and horizontal adduction
N	Lateral and medial pectoral nerve (C5, C6, C7, C8, T1)

The **latissimus dorsi muscle** (Fig. 9-11), as its name implies (in Latin *latissimus* means "widest," *dorsi* means "back" or "posterior"), is a broad, sheetlike muscle located on the back. It is mostly superficial except for a small portion covered posteriorly by the lower trapezius muscle and distally as it passes through the axilla to attach on the proximal, anterior, and medial surfaces of the humerus. Because of its attachment on the ilium and sacrum, it is able to elevate the pelvis if the arms are stabilized. This action occurs during crutch walking when the arms are stabilized on the crutch handles. This closed-chain activity is a good example of "reversal of muscle function" where the proximal (origin) attachment pulls toward the distal (insertion) attachment, instead of the more common distal attachment pulling toward the proximal. The larissimus dorsi muscle is a strong agonist in extension, hyperextension, adduction, and medial rotation of the shoulder because it crosses the shoulder joint inferior and medial to the joint axes.

Latissimus Dorsi Muscle

O	Spinous processes of T7 through L5 (via dorsolumbar fascia), posterior surface of sacrum, iliac crest, and lower three ribs
I	Medial lip of bicipital groove of humerus
A	Shoulder extension, adduction, medial rotation, hyperextension
N	Thoracodorsal nerve (C6, C7, C8)

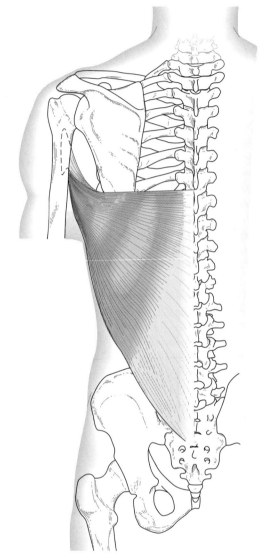

Figure 9-11. The latissimus dorsi muscle. Note that the humeral attachment is on the anterior surface, as indicated by the dotted line.

The **teres major muscle** (Fig. 9-12) has its proximal attachment on the axillary border the scapula just below the teres minor muscle. *Teres* means "long and round" in Latin. They are both superficial at this point. The teres major muscle travels with the latissimus dorsi muscle through the axilla, to where they attach close together on the anterior medial surface of the humerus near the proximal end. The teres major muscle is often referred to as the "little helper" of the latissimus dorsi muscle because it does everything that the latissimus dorsi muscle does except hyperextension, and because it is much smaller in size. Although the

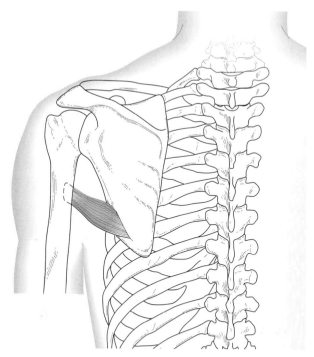

Figure 9-12.   The teres major muscle. Note that the humeral attachment is on the anterior surface, as indicated by the dotted lines.

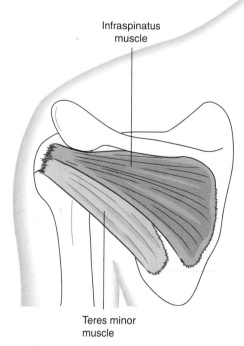

Infraspinatus muscle

Teres minor muscle

Figure 9-13.   The infraspinatus and teres minor muscles.

teres major muscle is a prime mover in extension, adduction, and medial rotation, its much smaller size makes it certainly less effective than the latissimus dorsi.

Teres Major Muscle

O	Axillary border of scapula near the inferior angle
I	Crest below lesser tubercle next to the latissimus dorsi muscle attachment
A	Shoulder extension, adduction, and medial rotation
N	Subscapular nerve (C5, C6)

As its name implies, the **infraspinatus muscle** (Fig. 9-13) lies below the spine of the scapula. Most of the muscle is superficial; however, the trapezius and deltoid muscles cover portions of it. The distal attachment of the infraspinatus muscle is just inferior to the attachment of the supraspinatus muscle on the greater tubercle of the humerus. Although some authors refer to the ability of the infraspinatus muscle to extend the shoulder joint, its more horizontal line of pull must be recognized. Therefore, its extension action is assistive at best.

Infraspinatus Muscle

O	Infraspinous fossa of scapula
I	Greater tubercle of humerus
A	Shoulder lateral rotation, horizontal abduction
N	Suprascapular nerve (C5, C6)

The **teres minor muscle** (see Fig. 9-13) is closely related to the infraspinatus muscle in both anatomical location and function. Both are mostly superficial with portions covered by the trapezius and the deltoid muscles. Both the teres major and teres minor muscles attach on the axillary border of the scapula and run obliquely up and outward to attach on the humerus. The teres minor muscle attaches posteriorly on the greater tubercle of the humerus, whereas the teres major muscle passes through the axilla to attach anteriorly below the lesser tubercle of the humerus. The long head of the triceps muscle passing between them in the axilla (Fig. 9-14) separates them.

Teres Minor Muscle

O	Axillary border of scapula
I	Greater tubercle of humerus
A	Shoulder lateral rotation, horizontal abduction
N	Axillary nerve (C5, C6)

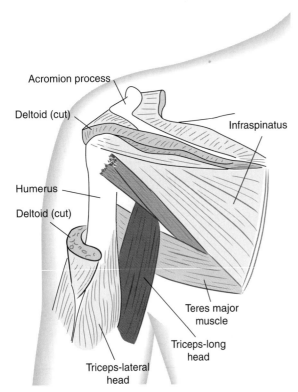

Figure 9-14. The long head of the triceps muscle separates the teres major and teres minor muscles at the axilla.

If you observe the distal attachments of the supraspinatus, infraspinatus, and teres minor muscles on the greater tubercle of the humerus, you will notice that they are essentially in a line (Fig. 9-15). For this reason, they are collectively referred to as the *SIT muscles,* taking the first letter from each muscle. These three muscles plus the subscapularis are referred to as the rotator cuff, or *SITS muscles.*

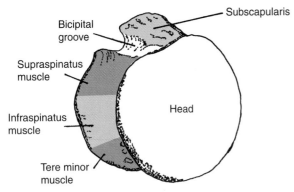

Figure 9-15. This superior view of the proximal end of the left humerus shows the attachments of the rotator cuff muscles.

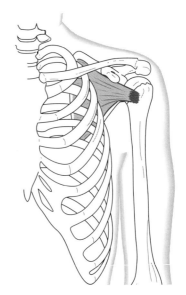

Figure 9-16. The subscapularis muscle.

The **subscapularis** muscle (Fig. 9-16) gets its name from its location, which can be slightly misleading. *Sub* means "under" in Latin. The subscapularis muscle is located deep on the "underside" of the scapula, lying next to the rib cage. This underside is actually the anterior, or costal, surface of the scapula. From this attachment on the anterior surface, the subscapularis muscle runs laterally to cross the shoulder joint anteriorly and attach on the lesser tubercle of the humerus. This distal attachment blends into a common tendinous sheath with the other rotator cuff muscles to cover the humeral head and hold the head against the glenoid fossa. Because the subscapularis has a horizontal line of pull and attaches anteriorly on the humerus, it is a prime mover in medial rotation of the shoulder.

Subscapularis Muscle

O	Subscapular fossa of the scapula
I	Lesser tubercle of the humerus
A	Shoulder medial rotation
N	Subscapular nerve (C5, C6)

The **coracobrachialis muscle** (Fig. 9-17) derives its name from its attachments on the coracoid process of the scapula and on the humerus, or arm (in Latin, "brachium"). It has an almost vertical line of pull quite close to the joint axis. Therefore, most of its force is directed back into the joint, stabilizing the head against the glenoid fossa. Some authors refer to the ability of this muscle to flex and adduct the shoulder. However, because its vertical line of

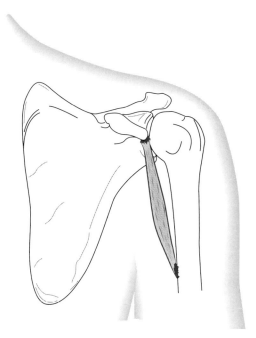

Figure 9-17. The coracobrachialis muscle.

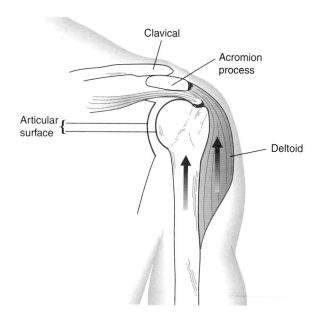

Figure 9-18. The articular surface of the glenohumeral joint and deltoid muscle. If the deltoid muscle acted alone, it would pull the humeral head upward and impinge it under the coracoacromial arch.

pull is so close to the joint axes, these actions are assistive at best.

Coracobrachialis Muscle

O	Coracoid process of the scapula
I	Medial surface of the humerus near the midpoint
A	Stabilizes the shoulder joint
N	Musculocutaneous nerve (C6, C7)

The biceps and triceps muscles are two-joint muscles that cross both the shoulder and the elbow. Their actions at the shoulder joint are assistive at best. Because their main functions are at the elbow, they will be discussed in Chapter 10.

Glenohumeral Movement

The movement of the humeral head on the glenoid fossa must be given some additional attention. Notice that the humeral head has more articular surface than does the glenoid fossa (Fig. 9-18). If the humeral head simply rotates in the glenoid fossa, it would run out of articular surface before much abduction has occurred. Also, the vertical pull of the deltoid muscle would pull the head up against the acromion process (Fig. 9-18).

It is the arthrokinematic motions of glide, spin, and roll that keep the head of the humerus articulating with the glenoid fossa (see Chap. 4 for a detailed description of these terms). As abduction occurs, the humeral head rolls across the glenoid fossa. At the same time, the head glides inferiorly, keeping the head of the humerus articulating with the glenoid fossa. This is accomplished by the rotator cuff muscles (Fig. 9-19). The supraspinatus muscle, in addition to abducting the shoulder joint, pulls the humeral head into the glenoid fossa. The other rotator cuff muscles

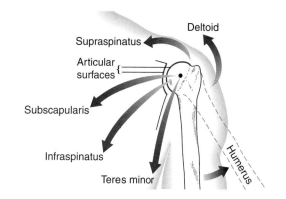

Figure 9-19. Force couple of the deltoid and rotator cuff muscles (SITS) rotating the humeral head in the glenoid fossa during shoulder abduction.

(subscapularis, infraspinatus, and teres minor) pull the head in and downward against the glenoid fossa. The glenoid labrum serves to slightly deepen the glenoid fossa, making the joint surfaces more congruent.

Another feature of shoulder abduction is that complete range of motion can be accomplished only if the shoulder joint is also laterally rotated. Try this on yourself. Start with your arm at your side (shoulder adduction) and in medial rotation; abduct your shoulder, keeping your thumb pointed down. This is also referred to as the "empty can" position. Notice how much motion you can comfortably achieve.

Next, repeat the motion with your shoulder in a neutral position between medial and lateral rotation (fundamental position) and your thumb pointed forward. Notice how much motion you can comfortably accomplish. Finally, repeat the motion with your shoulder in a laterally rotated position, keeping your thumb pointed up in the hitchhiking position. This is also referred to as the "full can" position. It is this laterally rotated position that should allow the most comfortable shoulder motion because the greater tubercle is being rotated from under the acromion process, allowing full abduction. The greater tubercle in the medially rotated or neutral position runs into the acromion process overhead.

Summary of Muscle Action

The prime mover actions of the shoulder joint muscles are summarized as follows:

Action	Muscles
Flexion	Anterior deltoid, pectoralis major (clavicular)*
Extension	Posterior deltoid, latissimus dorsi, teres major, pectoralis major (sternal)†
Hyperextension	Latissimus dorsi, posterior deltoid
Abduction	Deltoid, supraspinatus
Adduction	Pectoralis major, teres major, latissimus dorsi
Horizontal abduction	Posterior deltoid, infraspinatus, teres minor
Horizontal adduction	Pectoralis major, anterior deltoid
Lateral rotation	Infraspinatus, teres minor, posterior deltoid
Medial rotation	Latissimus dorsi, teres major, subscapularis, pectoralis major, anterior deltoid

*To approximately 60 degrees.
†To approximately 120 degrees

Summary of Muscle Innervation

Muscles of the shoulder joint receive innervation from various branches high on the brachial plexus (see Fig. 6-19). Tables 9-1 and 9-2 summarize the segmental and nerve innervation of the muscles of the shoulder joint. It should be noted that there is some discrepancy among various sources regarding the spinal cord level of innervation.

Table 9-1	Innervation of the Muscles of the Shoulder Joint		
Muscle	**Nerve**	**Plexus Portion**	**Segment**
Subscapularis	Upper subscapular	Superior trunk	C5, C6
Teres major	Lower subscapular	Posterior cord	C5, C6, C7
Pectoralis major	Lateral pectoral	Lateral cord	C5, C6, C7
	Medial pectoral	Medial cord	C8, T1
Latissimus dorsi	Thoracodorsal	Posterior cord	C6, C7, C8
Supraspinatus	Suprascapular	Superior trunk	C5, C6
Infraspinatus	Suprascapular	Superior trunk	C5, C6
Deltoid	Axillary		C5, C6
Teres minor	Axillary		C5, C6
Coracobrachialis	Musculocutaneous		C6, C7
Biceps	Musculocutaneous		C5, C6
Triceps	Radial		C7, C8

| Table 9-2 | Segmental Innervation of Shoulder Joint | | | | | |
Spinal Cord Level	C4	C5	C6	C7	C8	T1
Supraspinatus		X	X			
Infraspinatus		X	X			
Teres minor		X	X			
Subscapularis		X	X			
Teres major		X	X			
Deltoid		X	X			
Biceps		X	X			
Pectoralis major		X	X	X	X	X
Coracobrachialis			X	X		
Latissimus dorsi			X	X	X	
Triceps				X	X	

Points to Remember

- The shoulder is a triaxial ball-and-socket joint.
- The close-packed position is abduction and lateral rotation.
- Concave joint surfaces move in the same direction as the joint motion.
- Convex joint surfaces move in the opposite direction as the joint motion.
- A force couple has muscles pulling in different directions to achieve the same motion.

Review Questions

General Anatomy Questions

1. There are four sets of motions that occur at the shoulder joint. Which motions occur:
   a. In the frontal plane around the sagittal axis?
   b. In the transverse plane around the vertical axis?
   c. In the sagittal plane around the frontal axis?
2. Describe circumduction and the shoulder joint motions involved.
3. Which fossa is located on the anterior surface of the scapula?
4. The spine of the scapula divides the posterior surface into which two fossas?
5. What landmarks can be used to determine if a model of an unattached bone is a right or left humerus?
6. What are the SITS muscles, and why are they called "rotator cuff muscles"?
7. Name the shoulder joint muscles attaching on the anterior surface of the scapula.
8. Name the shoulder joint muscles attaching on the posterior surface of the scapula.
9. Which shoulder joint muscles do not attach on the scapula?

10. Regarding the pectoralis major:
   a. Which portion of it is effective in shoulder flexion?
   b. What part of the range is it more effective?
   c. Why?

Functional Activity Questions

Identify the shoulder joint motions and the accompanying shoulder girdle motions in the following actions.

1. Putting your billfold in your left back pocket with your left hand.
   a. Shoulder joint motion _____
   b. Shoulder girdle motion _____
2. Reaching up to get hold of your seat belt (driver's side with left hand).
   a. Shoulder joint motion _____
   b. Shoulder girdle motion _____
3. Fastening your seat belt with your left hand.
   a. Shoulder joint motion _____
   b. Shoulder girdle motion _____
4. Placing a book on the upper bookshelf.
   a. Shoulder joint motion _____
   b. Shoulder girdle motion _____

5. Tucking a book under your arm.
   a. Shoulder joint motion _____
   b. Shoulder girdle motion _____

Clinical Exercise Questions

1. Lie prone with your arm over edge of table with your shoulder flexed 90 degrees, elbow extended, and with a weight in your hand (Fig. 9-20A). Lift the weight away from the table in a sideward motion(Fig. 9-20B).
   a. What is the shoulder joint motion?
   b. What type of contraction (isometric, concentric, eccentric) is occurring?
   c. What muscles are prime movers in this shoulder joint motion?

2. Repeat exercise No. 1, except flex the elbow to 90 degrees as you lift the weight up.
   a. Does flexing the elbow shorten the force arm?
   b. Does flexing the elbow shorten the resistance arm?
   c. Why is this exercise easier than No. 1?

3. Stand with your arm adducted at the side of your body, elbow flexed to 90 degrees, holding a loop of elastic tubing with the other end anchored in front of you at the same level as your hand. In a sawing motion (back and forth motion like you are sawing wood), pull back on the tubing.
   a. What is the shoulder joint motion?
   b. What type of contraction (isometric, concentric, eccentric) is occurring?
   c. What muscles are prime movers in this shoulder joint motion?

4. Return to the starting position of No. 3.
   a. What is the shoulder joint motion?

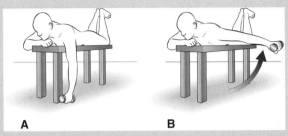

A   **B**

Figure 9-20.   *(A)* Starting position. *(B)* Ending position.

   b. What type of contraction (isometric, concentric, eccentric) is occurring?
   c. What muscles are prime movers in this shoulder joint motion?

5. Lie on your right side with your left elbow flexed to 90 degrees and holding a weight in your hand. Keep your left elbow resting on the left side of your body. First part: roll the weight up toward the ceiling.
   a. What is the shoulder joint motion?
   b. What type of contraction (isometric, concentric, eccentric) is occurring?
   c. What muscles are prime movers in this shoulder joint motion?

Second part: hold for the count of five.
   a. What is the shoulder joint motion?
   b. What type of contraction (isometric, concentric, eccentric) is occurring?
   c. What muscles are prime movers in this shoulder joint motion?

Third part: slowly return to the starting position.
   a. What is the shoulder joint motion?
   b. What type of contraction (isometric, concentric, eccentric) is occurring?
   c. What muscles are prime movers in this shoulder joint motion?

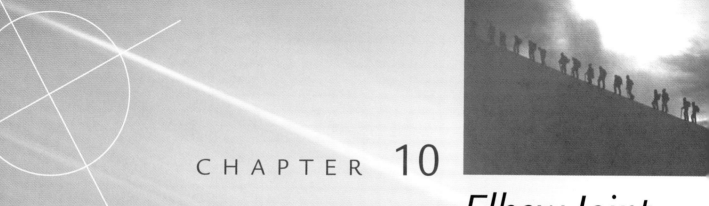

CHAPTER 10

Elbow Joint

Joint Structure and Motions

Bones and Landmarks

Ligaments and Other Structures

Common Elbow Pathologies

Muscles of the Elbow and Forearm

Summary of Muscle Action

Summary of Muscle Innervation

Points to Remember

Review Questions

General Anatomy Questions

Functional Activity Questions

Clinical Exercise Questions

Joint Structure and Motions

The elbow complex is made of three bones, three ligaments, two joints, and one capsule. The articulation of the humerus with the ulna and radius is commonly called the **elbow joint** (Fig. 10-1). On the humerus, the trochlea articulates with the trochlear notch of the ulna and the capitulum articulates with the head of the radius. The elbow is a uniaxial hinge joint that allows only **flexion** and **extension** (Fig. 10-2). There are approximately 145 degrees of flexion measured from the 0-degree position of extension (Lehmkuhl, p 403).

There is no active hyperextension at the elbow as there is at the shoulder joint. This motion is blocked by the olecranon process of the ulna fitting into the olecranon fossa of the humerus. Some individuals may be able to hyperextend a few degrees, but this is due to a laxity of ligaments rather than bony structure.

The articulation between the radius and ulna is known as the **radioulnar joint** (Fig. 10-3). They articulate with each other at both ends. At the proximal end, the head of the radius pivots within the radial notch of the ulna, forming the **superior** or **proximal radioulnar joint.** At the distal end, the ulnar notch of the radius rotating around the head of the ulna forms the **inferior** or **distal radioulnar joint.** They are considered together as one joint (Brunnstrom, 1983, p 403). The radioulnar joint is a uniaxial pivot joint, allowing only **pronation** and **supination** of the forearm (Fig. 10-4). Measured from the neutral or midposition, there are approximately 90 degrees of supination and 80 degrees of pronation.

When pronation and supination occur, the radius moves around the ulna (Fig. 10-5). The ulna does not rotate. It is locked in place by its bony shape at the proximal end. You can confirm this on yourself. With

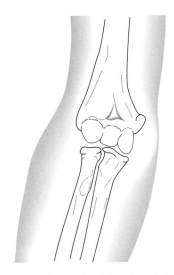

Figure 10-1.   The right elbow joint.

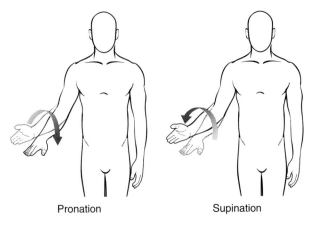

Pronation   Supination

Figure 10-4.   Forearm motions.

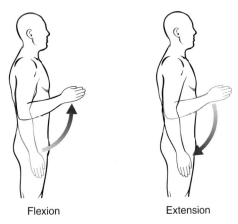

Flexion   Extension

Figure 10-2.   Elbow motions.

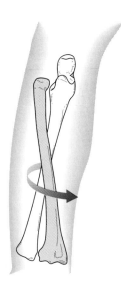

Figure 10-5.   The radius moves around the ulna.

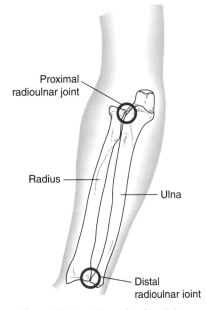

Proximal
radioulnar joint

Radius

Ulna

Distal
radioulnar joint

Figure 10-3.   The radioulnar joints.

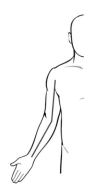

Figure 10-6.   The carrying angle.

your elbow flexed, place the fingers of your other hand on either side of the olecranon process, and then pronate and supinate your forearm. Note that the olecranon process does not move. If you put your fingers on the shaft of the ulna, you again will notice that the ulna does not move. Remember this when figuring out muscle action. The radius moves and the ulna does not. Therefore, a muscle must attach on the radius to be able either to pronate or supinate the forearm.

In the anatomical position, the longitudinal axes of the humerus and forearm form an angle called the **carrying angle** (Fig. 10-6). This angle tends to be greater in women than in men. Normal carrying angle measures approximately 5 degrees in males and between 10 and 15 degrees in females (Hoppenfeld, 1976, p 36). This angle occurs because the distal end of the humerus is not level. The medial side (trochlea) is lower than the lateral side (capitulum). Therefore, as the ulna and radius rotate about the trochlea and capitulum of the humerus, they do not do so in a straight line like a typical hinge joint, in which the long axis of the lower segment is in line with the long axis of the upper segment. The effect of this carrying angle can be seen if a line is drawn along the long axis of the humerus and extended down the forearm. You will notice that during elbow extension the hand is on the outside of that imaginary line. When the elbow is flexed, the hand moves to the inside of the imaginary line. This angle is quite functional in getting your hand to your mouth.

Bones and Landmarks

The bony landmarks of the **scapula** were covered in Chapter 9, but those important to elbow function are as follows (Fig. 10-7):

Infraglenoid tubercle
The raised portion on the inferior lip of the glenoid fossa providing attachment of the long head of the triceps muscle

Supraglenoid tubercle
Raised portion on the superior lip of the glenoid fossa providing attachment for the long head of the biceps muscle

Coracoid process
Projection on the anterior surface, providing attachment for the short head of the biceps muscle (Described in Chap. 8)

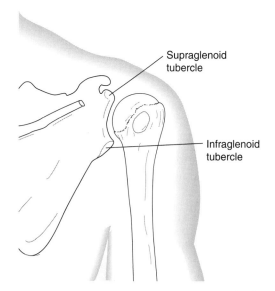

Figure 10-7.   Attachments for the biceps and triceps muscles. A posterior view with the scapular spine cut away.

The distal end of the **humerus** (Fig. 10-8) provides the bony landmarks important to elbow function.

Trochlea
Located on the medial side of the distal end; articulates with the ulna

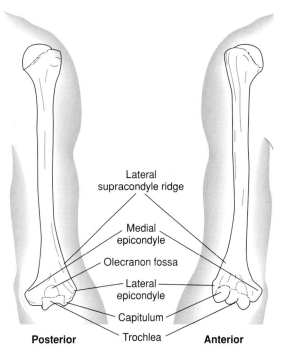

Figure 10-8.   The right humerus.

Capitulum

On the lateral side next to the trochlea; articulates with head of radius

Medial epicondyle

Located on the medial side of the distal end above the trochlea; larger and more prominent than the lateral epicondyle. It provides attachment for the pronator teres muscle

Lateral epicondyle

Located on the lateral sides of the distal end above the capitulum; provides attachment for the anconeus and supinator muscles

Lateral supracondylar ridge

Located above the lateral epicondyle; provides attachment for the brachioradialis muscle

Olecranon fossa

Located on the posterior surface between the medial and lateral epicondyles; articulates with the olecranon process of the ulna

The **ulna** is the medial bone of the forearm lying parallel to the radius. The bony landmarks important to elbow function are as follows (Fig. 10-9):

Olecranon process

Located at the proximal end of the ulna, on posterior surface; forms the prominent point of the elbow and provides attachment for the triceps muscle

Trochlear notch

Also called the *semilunar notch;* articulates with the trochlea of the humerus; makes up the anterior surface at the proximal end

Coronoid process

Located just below the trochlear notch; with the ulnar tuberosity, provides attachment for the brachialis muscle

Radial notch

Located at the proximal end on the lateral side just distal to the trochlear notch; articulation point for the head of the radius

Ulnar tuberosity

Located below the coronoid process; provides an attachment for the brachialis muscle

Styloid process

At the distal end on the posterior medial surface

Head

At the distal end on the lateral surface; the ulnar notch of the radius pivots around it during pronation and supination

The **radius,** located lateral to the ulna, provides many important bony landmarks for elbow function. They are as follows (Fig. 10-10):

Head

Proximal end; has a cylinder shape with a depression in the superior surface where it articulates with the capitulum of the humerus

Radial tuberosity

Located on the medial side near the proximal end; provides attachment for the biceps muscle

Styloid process

Located on the posterior lateral side of the radius at the distal end; provides attachment for the brachioradialis muscle

Ligaments and Other Structures

The three ligaments of the elbow are the medial and lateral collateral ligaments and the annular ligament (Fig. 10-11). The **medial collateral ligament** is triangular shaped and spans the medial side of the elbow. It attaches on the medial epicondyle of the humerus and

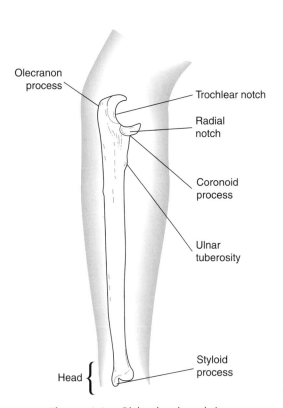

Figure 10-9.   Right ulna, lateral view.

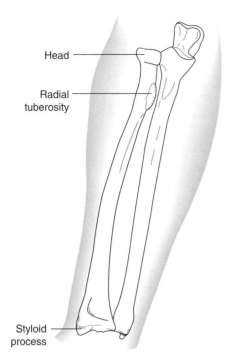

Figure 10-10. Right radius, anterior view.

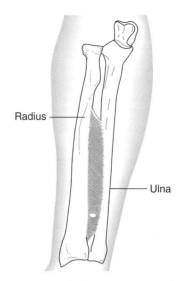

Figure 10-12. The interosseous membrane.

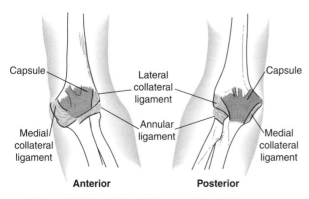

Figure 10-11. Elbow joint capsule and ligaments.

runs obliquely to the medial sides of the coronoid process and olecranon process of the ulna. The **lateral collateral ligament** is also triangular shaped. It attaches proximally on the lateral epicondyle of the humerus and distally on the annular ligament and the lateral side of the ulna. These two ligaments provide a great deal of medial and lateral stability to the elbow. The **annular ligament** attaches anteriorly and posteriorly to the radial notch of the ulna, encompassing the head of the radius and holding it against the ulna.

The **joint capsule** attaches around the distal end of the humerus, encompassing the trochlea and capitulum and the fossas located above them. It attaches around the proximal end of the ulna under the radial notch and coronoid process and around the trochlear notch. It attaches around the radius just under the head. The capsule is strengthened anteriorly and somewhat posteriorly by the annular ligament. The collateral ligaments reinforce the capsule on the sides of the joint.

In addition to the annular ligament, the radioulnar articulations are held together by the **interosseous membrane** (Fig. 10-12). This broad, flat membrane is located between the radius and ulna for most of their length. Not only does this membrane keep the two bones from separating, but it also provides more surface area for attachment of the forearm and wrist muscles.

Common Elbow Pathologies

Lateral epicondylitis, also know as **tennis elbow,** is a very common overuse condition of the common extensor tendon where it inserts into the lateral epicondyle of the humerus. The extensor carpi radialis brevis is particularly affected. It is common in racquet sports and other repetitive wrist extension activities. **Medial epicondylitis,** also know as **golfer's elbow,** is an inflammation of the common flexor tendon that inserts into the medial epicondyle. It is an overuse condition that results in tenderness over the medial epicondyle and pain on resisted wrist flexion.

Little league elbow is an overuse injury of the medial epicondyle usually caused by a repetitive throwing motion. It is seen in young baseball players who have not reached skeletal maturity. The throwing motion places a valgus stress on the elbow causing lateral compression and medial distraction. **Pulled elbow** or **nursemaid's elbow** is seen in young children under the age of 5 years when there is a sudden strong traction force on the child's arm. This often occurs when an adult suddenly pulls on the child's arm, or the child falls away from an adult while being held by the arm. This results in the radial head subluxing out from under the annular ligament.

Elbow dislocation requires a great deal of force in a slightly flexed position. This causes the ulna to slide posterior to the distal end of the humerus. Because of the close proximity of the brachial artery, Volkmann's ischemic contracture, a rare but potentially devastating complication, can result. **Supracondylar fractures** are one of the most common fractures in children and are caused by a fall on the outstretched hand. The distal end of the humerus fractures just above the condyles. The great danger of this fracture is the potential damage to the brachial artery, which can lead to Volkmann's ischemic contracture. **Volkmann's ischemic contracture** is the result of ischemic necrosis of the forearm muscles caused by trauma to the brachial artery.

Muscles of the Elbow and Forearm

Muscles of the elbow and forearm are as follows:

Brachialis
Brachioradialis
Biceps
Supinator
Triceps
Anconeus
Pronator teres
Pronator quadratus

The **brachialis muscle** (Fig. 10-13) gets its name from its location (Latin for "arm"). It attaches to the distal half of the humerus on the anterior surface and spans the elbow joint anteriorly to attach on the coronoid process and ulnar tuberosity of the ulna. It lies deep to the biceps muscle. Because the brachialis muscle has no attachment on the radius, it has no role in pronation or supination. This muscle is, however, a very strong elbow flexor regardless of the position of the forearm and is therefore sometimes referred to as the "workhorse of the elbow joint."

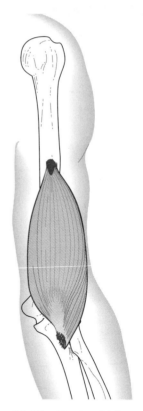

Figure 10-13.   The brachialis muscle.

Brachialis Muscle

O	Distal half of humerus, anterior surface
I	Coronoid process and ulnar tuberosity of the ulna
A	Elbow flexion
N	Musculocutaneous nerve (C5, C6)

As the name of the **biceps brachii muscle** implies, it has two heads and is located on the arm (Fig. 10-14). The muscle is commonly referred to as simply the *biceps*. Both heads attach on the scapula. The **long head** arises from the supraglenoid tubercle and runs over the head of the humerus and out of the joint capsule to descend through the intertubercular (bicipital) groove to join with the **short head** that has come from the coracoid process. Because tendons of both heads cross the shoulder joint anteriorly, the biceps assists in shoulder flexion. However, its main function is at the elbow. After joining, the two heads form a common muscle belly covering the anterior surface of the arm. The biceps muscle tendon crosses the elbow joint to attach on the radial tuberosity. It is the superficial muscle of the anterior

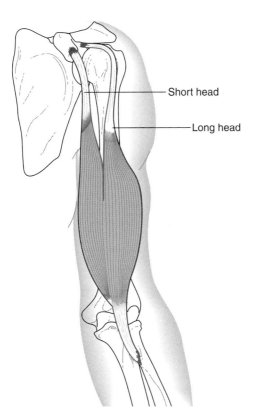

Figure 10-14. The biceps brachii muscle, commonly referred to as the biceps, has two heads.

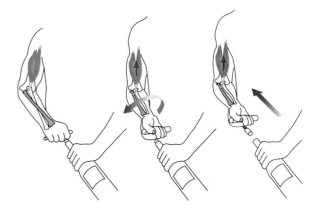

Figure 10-15. Supination action of biceps. The action of the biceps as a forearm supinator and elbow flexor is used when pulling a cork out of a bottle with a corkscrew. First, it unscrews the cork (supination), then it pulls on the cork (flexion).

Biceps Brachii Muscle

O	Long head, supraglenoid tubercle of scapula Short head, coracoid process of scapula
I	Radial tuberosity of radius
A	Elbow flexion, forearm supination
N	Musculocutaneous nerve (C5, C6)

The **brachioradialis muscle** gets its name from its two attachments: one on the humerus (brachii) and the other on the radius (Fig. 10-16). Proximally, it is attached slightly above the lateral epicondyle of the

arm. Because the biceps brachii muscle spans the elbow joint anteriorly, it is a good elbow flexor, especially in the midrange. Because it attaches obliquely on the radius, it contributes to supination of the forearm.

To understand the supination component of the biceps muscle, think of it as a corkscrew. The tendon crosses the elbow joint anteriorly to attach medially on the radial tuberosity. When the forearm is in pronation, the radial tuberosity is rotated further medially toward the posterior side. In effect, the tendon of the biceps muscle wraps partially around the radius in the pronated position. During supination, the biceps muscle contracts and essentially "unwraps" or "untwists" the forearm (Fig. 10-15). It is most effective in supination when the elbow is in approximately 90 degrees of flexion, and it loses its effectiveness as the elbow is extended. This is because at 90 degrees the moment arm of the muscle is greatest; therefore, its angular force is also greatest. As the elbow is extended, the moment arm decreases, as does angular force, while the stabilizing force increases (see Chap. 7 for a discussion of torque).

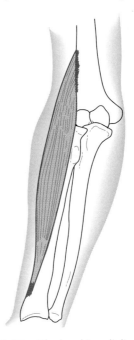

Figure 10-16. The brachioradialis muscle.

humerus on the supracondylar ridge. It crosses the elbow anteriorly and laterally to attach distally near the styloid process of the radius. It is a superficial muscle and easy to identify. Place your hand in your lap in a neutral position between supination and pronation; then give resistance to elbow flexion. The brachioradialis muscle should be quite prominent on the top of your forearm near the elbow. Because of its more lateral attachment, it is most effective as an elbow flexor when the forearm is in a neutral position. This is because its line of pull is vertical with essentially no diagonal component and goes through the axis for pronation and supination. Therefore, the brachioradialis muscle has no real effect in pronation or supination, even though it has an attachment on the radius.

Brachioradialis Muscle

O	Lateral supracondylar ridge on the humerus
I	Styloid process of the radius
A	Elbow flexion
N	Radial nerve (C5, C6)

The **triceps brachii muscle,** commonly called the **triceps,** derives its name from its three heads. This muscle is located posteriorly and makes up the entire muscle mass of the posterior arm. (Fig. 10-17). The **long head** comes from the inferior rim of the glenoid fossa of the scapula and descends between the teres minor muscle and teres major muscle to join the other two heads. The **lateral head** is attached laterally on the posterior surface of the humerus below the greater tubercle. The **medial head** lies deep to the long and lateral heads and is attached below the lateral head to most of the posterior surface. The three heads come together to form the muscle belly. The triceps muscle tendon crosses the elbow posteriorly to attach to the olecranon process of the ulna. Because it spans the elbow quite vertically, it is very effective in elbow extension. Because it has no attachment on the radius, it can play no role in pronation or supination.

Triceps Muscle

O	Long head: Infraglenoid tubercle of scapula Lateral head: Inferior to greater tubercle on posterior humerus Medial head: Posterior surface of humerus
I	Olecranon process of ulna
A	Elbow extension
N	Radial nerve (C7, C8)

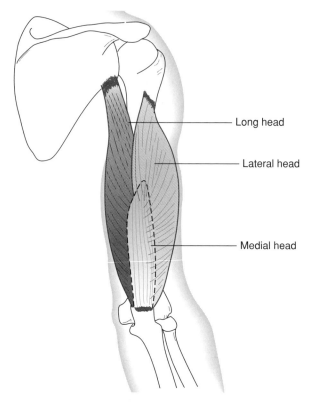

Figure 10-17. The triceps brachii muscle, commonly referred to as the triceps, has three heads. The dotted line indicates the portion of the muscle that lies deep.

The **anconeus muscle** is a very small muscle that attaches next to the much larger triceps muscle (Fig. 10-18). It attaches proximally to the posterior surface of the lateral epicondyle and then spans the elbow posteriorly to attach laterally and inferior to the olecranon process. It is a small muscle in comparison to the triceps muscle, and it would therefore be foolish to say that the anconeus plays any significant role in elbow extension. Perhaps Carlin has explained its role best: the anconeus lies on top of the annular ligament and attaches to part of it. When the anconeus contracts, it pulls on the ligament and keeps the ligament from being pinched in the olecranon fossa during elbow extension.

Anconeus Muscle

O	Lateral epicondyle of humerus
I	Lateral and inferior to olecranon process of ulna
A	Not a prime mover in any joint action; assists in elbow extension
N	Radial nerve (C7, C8)

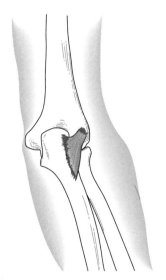

Figure 10-18.   The anconeus muscle.

The **pronator teres muscle** (Fig. 10-19) gets its name partially from its action (pronation) and partially from its cordlike shape (*teres,* from the Latin). It is a superficial muscle as it crosses the elbow, but is covered by the brachioradialis muscle at its distal attachment. Proximally, it attaches on the medial epicondyle of the humerus and the medial aspect of the coronoid process of the ulna. It crosses the anterior surface of the elbow, running diagonally to attach

distally on the lateral surface of the radius at about the midpoint. Because it crosses the elbow anteriorly, it has the ability to flex the elbow. This role is only as an assisting mover because of its smaller size and diagonal line of pull.

Pronator Teres Muscle

O	Medial epicondyle of humerus and coronoid process of ulna
I	Lateral aspect of radius at its midpoint
A	Forearm pronation, assistive in elbow flexion
N	Median nerve (C6, C7)

The **pronator quadratus muscle** (see Fig. 10-19) also gets its name from its action (pronation) and partially from its shape (quadratus). It is a small, flat, quadrilateral muscle located deep on the anterior surface of the distal forearm; therefore, it cannot be palpated. It attaches from the distal one-fourth of the ulna to the distal one-fourth of the radius. It has a horizontal line of pull, and it works with the pronator teres muscle to pronate the forearm.

Pronator Quadratus Muscle

O	Distal one-fourth of ulna
I	Distal one-fourth of radius
A	Forearm pronation
N	Median nerve (C8, T1)

The **supinator muscle** (Fig. 10-20) is a deep muscle that wraps around the elbow joint laterally from the

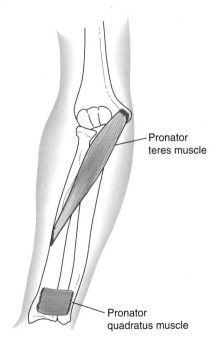

Pronator teres muscle

Pronator quadratus muscle

Figure 10-19.   The pronator muscles.

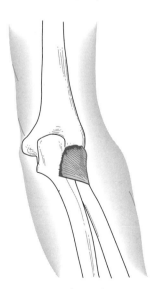

Figure 10-20.   The supinator muscle.

posterior surface to the anterior surface. It attaches posteriorly to the lateral epicondyle and adjacent surface of the ulna. It crosses the elbow joint laterally to wrap around the proximal end of the radius to attach distally on the proximal anterior surface of the radius. It combines with the biceps muscle to be a prime mover in forearm supination (Fig. 10-21).

Supinator Muscle

O	Lateral epicondyle of humerus and adjacent ulna
I	Anterior surface of the proximal radius
A	Forearm supination
N	Radial nerve (C6)

Summary of Muscle Action

The following list summarizes the muscle action of the prime movers of the elbow and forearm:

Flexion	Biceps, brachialis, and brachioradialis
Extension	Triceps
Pronation	Pronator teres and pronator quadratus
Supination	Biceps and supinator

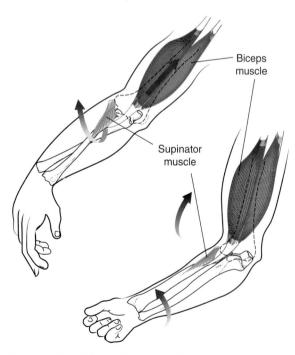

Figure 10-21. The supinator and biceps muscles combine in a force couple action to move the radius around the ulna from a pronated forearm to a supinated forearm.

Table 10-1 Innervation of the Muscles of the Elbow Joint

Muscle	Nerve	Spinal Segment
Brachialis	Musculocutaneous	C5, C6
Biceps	Musculocutaneous	C5, C6
Brachioradialis	Radial	C5, C6, C7
Triceps	Radial	C6, C7, C8
Anconeus	Radial	C7, C8, T1
Pronator teres	Median	C7, C8, T1
Pronator quadratus	Median	C8, T1
Supinator	Radial	C6

Summary of Muscle Innervation

Terminal nerves of the brachial plexus innervate all muscles of the elbow. The musculocutaneous nerve innervates muscles of the anterior arm involved with elbow flexion. The radial nerve travels through the axilla and around the middle portion of the humerus to innervate the posterior surface of the arm, forearm, and hand. It is responsible for all elbow extension. The median nerve descends the arm anteriorly, sending branches to the pronator muscles. Table 10-1 summarizes the innervation of elbow joint musculature. Table 10-2 summarizes the segmental innervation. Please note that there is some discrepancy among various sources regarding the spinal cord level of innervation.

Table 10-2 Segmental Innervation of the Elbow Joint

Spinal Cord Level	C5	C6	C7	C8	T1
Biceps	X	X			
Brachialis	X	X			
Brachioradialis	X	X			
Supinator		X			
Pronator teres		X	X		
Triceps			X	X	
Anconeus			X	X	X
Pronator quadratus				X	X

Points to Remember

- Synovial joint shapes can be irregular (plane), hinge, pivot, condyloid, saddle, and ball-and-socket.
- Synovial joints can have zero to three axes.
- When a muscle has contracted (shortened) over all its joints as far as it can, it has become actively insufficient.
- When a muscle has elongated (stretched) over all of its joints as far as possible, it has become passively insufficient.
- An activity can be an open or closed kinetic chain movement depending on whether or not the distal segment is fixed.

Review Questions

General Anatomy Questions

1. In terms of the elbow and forearm joints, identify the following:
   a. Name of bones involved
      Forearm _____
      Elbow _____
   b. Number of axes:
      Forearm _____
      Elbow _____
   c. Shape of joint:
      Forearm _____
      Elbow _____
   d. Joint motion allowed:
      Forearm _____
      Elbow _____

2. If you were handed an unattached model of an ulna, how could you orient landmarks to determine on which side of the body it belonged?

3. Name the ligament that:
   a. Stabilizes the lateral side of the elbow.
   b. Stabilizes the medial side of the elbow.
   c. Stabilizes the radius and allows it to rotate.

4. Which muscles of the elbow and/or forearm are two-joint muscles?

5. To which bone must a muscle attach to do forearm supination or pronation?

6. Which elbow or forearm muscles do not attach to the humerus?

7. Which muscles connect the scapula to the ulna and/or radius?

8. Which muscles connect the humerus and ulna?

9. The only part of the triceps that crosses the shoulder joint is _____.

10. What positions would you put the upper extremity in to achieve:
    a. Active insufficiency of the biceps?
    b. Passive insufficiency of the biceps?

Functional Activity Questions

Identify the elbow and forearm motion in each of the following activities:

1. Place a dinner plate in an upper kitchen cabinet.
   a. Elbow _____
   b. Forearm _____

2. Bring a spoonful of soup to your mouth.
   a. Elbow _____
   b. Forearm _____

3. When answering the telephone—reach for the receiver (Fig. 10-22A).
   a. Elbow _____
   b. Forearm _____

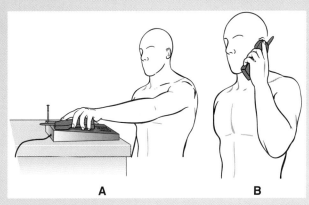

A   **B**

Figure 10-22. Elbow and forearm motion when answering the telephone. *(A)* Starting position. *(B)* Ending position.

4. Next, put the receiver to your ear (Fig. 10-22B).
   a. Elbow _____
   b. Forearm _____

5. With a hammer in your hand, pound on a nail midposition that has been set in the wall.
   a. Elbow _____
   b. Forearm _____

Clinical Exercise Questions

1. In the sitting position, place your right forearm on the table palm down with your elbow flexed as necessary (Fig. 10-23A). Using your left hand, push against the radial side of the right forearm just proximal to the wrist until the right palm is facing up (Fig. 10-23B). The right forearm remains relaxed.
   a. What joint motion is occurring in the right forearm?
   b. What muscles are being stretched?

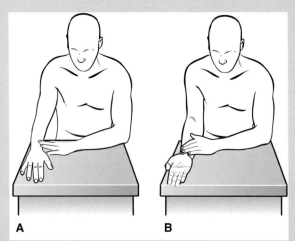

Figure 10-23. Self-stretch at the forearm. *(A)* Starting position. *(B)* Ending position.

2. Stand with your right arm extended straight up toward the ceiling. Using your left hand, push your right hand down behind your head (Fig. 10-24). Allow your left elbow to bend.
   a. What joint motion is occurring in the right elbow?
   b. What muscles are being stretched?

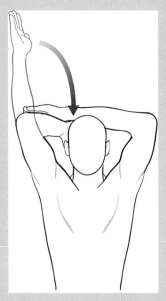

Figure 10-24. Self-stretch at the elbow.

3. Sit in a chair with armrests and place your hands on the arms of the chair. Do a "chair" push-up, lifting your buttock off of the seat.
   a. What joint motion is occurring in the right elbow?
   b. What type of contraction is occurring? (isometric, concentric, eccentric)
   c. What muscles are being strengthened?
   d. Is this an open or closed kinetic chain activity?

4. In a sitting position, place your hands and forearms on the table. Push down on the table as if you are trying to hold down the table.
   a. What joint motion is occurring in the right elbow?
   b. What type of contraction is occurring? (isometric, concentric, eccentric)
   c. What muscles are being strengthened?

5. Standing with your right hand up to your right shoulder, holding a small weight. Move your hand to anatomical position.
   a. What joint motion is occurring in the right elbow?
   b. What type of contraction is occurring? (isometric, concentric, eccentric)
   c. What muscles are being strengthened?
   d. Is this an open or closed kinetic chain activity?

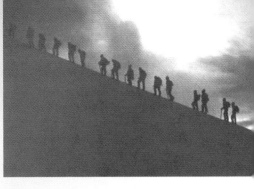

CHAPTER 11

Wrist Joint

Joint Structure

Joint Motions

Bones and Landmarks

Ligaments and Other Structures

Muscles of the Wrist

Summary of Muscle Action

Summary of Muscle Innervation

Points to Remember

Review Questions

General Anatomy Questions

Functional Activity Questions

Clinical Exercise Questions

Joint Structure

The wrist joint is perhaps one of the most complex joints of the body. The wrist joint is actually made up of two joints: the radiocarpal joint and the midcarpal joint. The **radiocarpal joint** (Fig. 11-1) consists of the distal end of the radius and the radioulnar disk proximally and the scaphoid, lunate, and triquetrum distally. Because an articular disk is located between the ulna and the proximal row of carpals, the ulna is not considered part of this joint. The pisiform, located in the proximal row of carpal bones, does not articulate with the disk because it is more anterior to the triquetrum. Therefore, it is not considered part of this joint, either. As a synovial joint, the radiocarpal joint is classified as a **condyloid joint,** with the concave distal end of the radius and the articular disk articulating with the convex scaphoid, lunate, and triquetrum.

The radiocarpal joint is also classified as a biaxial joint allowing flexion and extension, plus radial deviation and ulnar deviation. The combination of all four of these motions is called *circumduction.* There is no rotation at the wrist.

The **midcarpal,** or **intercarpal, joints** (see Fig. 11-1) occur between the two rows of carpal bones and contribute to wrist motion. Their shape is **irregular** and they are classified as **plane joints.** They are nonaxial joints that allow gliding motions, which collectively contribute to radiocarpal joint motion.

The **carpometacarpal (CMC) joints** occur between the distal row of carpal bones and the proximal end of the metacarpal bones (see Fig. 11-1). Because they have a more direct function in the movement of the hand, they will be discussed in more detail in Chapter 12.

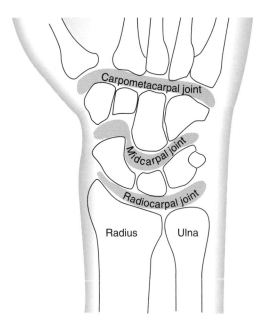

Figure 11-1. The joints of the left wrist, anterior view.

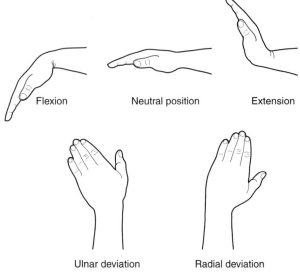

Figure 11-2. Joint motions of the wrist.

Joint Motions

When discussing wrist motion, several terms are frequently used. *Wrist flexion* and *palmar flexion* are synonymous terms, as are *extension, hyperextension,* and *dorsiflexion.* Approximately midway between flexion and extension, putting the hand in a straight line with the forearm, is referred to as *neutral position.* This is the position of the wrist joint in anatomical position. *Extension* is the return from *flexion.* Movement beyond the neutral position would be *hyperextension.* However, the most commonly used terms are **flexion, neutral,** and **extension,** and will be used here. You should, nevertheless, be familiar with these other terms, which are summarized in Table 11-1.

Flexion and extension occur in the sagittal plane around the frontal axis. There are approximately 90 degrees of flexion and 70 degrees of extension. **Radial** and **ulnar deviation** occur in the frontal plane around the sagittal axis. There are approximately 25 degrees of radial deviation and 35 degrees of ulnar deviation. These motions are illustrated in Figure 11-2.

Bones and Landmarks

The carpal bones consist of two rows of four bones each (Fig. 11-3). Starting on the thumb side of the proximal row are the **scaphoid, lunate, triquetrum,** and **pisiform.** In the distal row, lateral to medial, are the **trapezium, trapezoid, capitate,** and **hamate.** These are short bones arranged in an arch with the concavity on the anterior (palmar surface) side, and the convexity on the posterior side. This arched arrangement contributes greatly to the ability of the thumb to oppose.

The bony landmarks for the wrist are as follows:

Styloid process
Distal projection on the lateral side of the radius and distal medial posterior side of the ulna, providing attachment for the collateral ligaments

Table 11-1	Comparison of Wrist Joint Terminology*	
Preferred Terminology	**Alternate Terminology**	**Motion or Position**
Flexion	Flexion, palmar flexion	Anterior from anatomical position
Neutral	Extension, neutral	Anatomical position
Extension	Hyperextension, dorsiflexion	Posterior from anatomical position
Radial deviation	Abduction	Lateral from anatomical position
Ulnar deviation	Adduction	Medial from anatomical position

*__Bold print__ indicates which terms are used in this book.

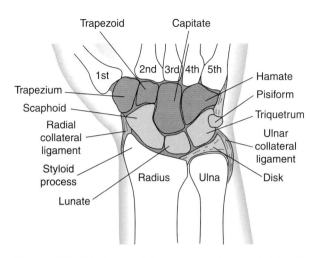

Figure 11-3. The bones of the wrist, anterior view, left hand.

Hook of the hamate
Projection on the anterior surface of the hamate, providing attachment for the transverse carpal ligament

Medial epicondyle
Located on the distal medial side of the humerus; attachment for the common flexor tendon (see Fig. 10-8)

Lateral epicondyle
Located on the distal lateral side of the humerus; attachment for the common extensor tendon

Supracondylar ridge
Located just proximal to the lateral epicondyle; attachment for the extensor carpi radialis longus muscle (see Fig. 10-8)

Ligaments and Other Structures

There are basically four ligaments of the radiocarpal joint that provide the major support of the wrist. In addition, there are numerous smaller ligaments supporting the intercarpal joints. The **radial collateral ligament** attaches to the styloid process of the radius and to the scaphoid and trapezium bones. The **ulnar collateral ligament** attaches to the styloid process of the ulna and to the pisiform and triquetrum. These ligaments provide lateral and medial support respectively to the wrist joint. They are illustrated in Figures 11-3, 11-4, and 11-5.

The **palmar radiocarpal ligament** is a thick, tough ligament that limits wrist extension. It is a broad band attaching from the anterior surface of the distal radius and ulna to the anterior surface of the of the proximal

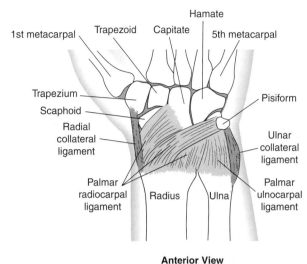

Anterior View

Figure 11-4. Palmar radiocarpal ligament, left hand.

carpal bones, and to the capitate bone in the distal row (see Fig. 11-4). It is perhaps more important to wrist function than its counterpart, the dorsal radiocarpal ligament, because most activities of the hand occur with the wrist extended, as opposed to being flexed. Therefore, the palmar radiocarpal ligament is also more apt to be stretched or sprained. It should be noted that some sources separate the radiocarpal ligament from the ulnocarpal ligament, and some do not. Functionally, they essentially act as one.

The **dorsal radiocarpal ligament** attaches from the posterior surface of the distal radius to the same surface of the scaphoid, lunate, and triquetrum (see Fig. 11-5). This ligament limits the amount of flexion allowed at the wrist. Because forces causing excessive

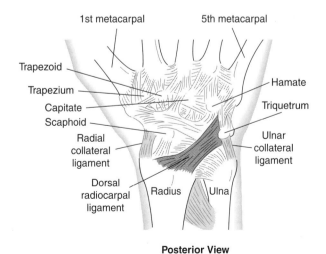

Posterior View

Figure 11-5. Dorsal radiocarpal ligament, left hand.

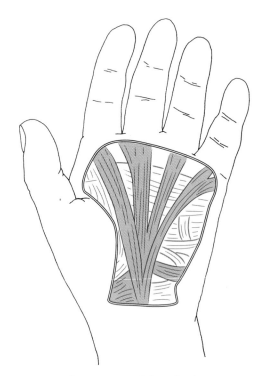

Figure 11-6.   Palmar fascia.

flexion are not as great as those causing excessive extension, this ligament is not as strong as the palmar radiocarpal ligament.

A **joint capsule,** which encloses the radiocarpal joint, is reinforced by the radial and ulnar collateral ligaments and by the palmar and dorsal radiocarpal ligaments. The **articular disk** (see Fig. 11-3) is located on the distal end of the ulna and articulates with the triquetrum and lunate bones. It not only acts as a shock absorber, but also as filler between the distal ulna and its adjacent carpal bones—the triquetrum and lunate. The disk fills the gap created because the ulna and its styloid process do not extend as far distally as the radius and its styloid process.

The **palmar fascia** is a relatively thick, triangular-shaped fascia located superficially in the palm of the hand (Fig. 11-6). It is also called the *palmar aponeurosis.* It covers the tendons of the extrinsic muscles and provides some protection to the structures in the palm. The palmar fascia serves as the distal attachment of the palmaris longus, which blends into this fascia, as does the flexor retinaculum.

Muscles of the Wrist

The muscles spanning and having a primary function at the wrist will be discussed here; the muscles that cross the wrist but have a more significant function at the thumb or fingers will be discussed in Chapter 12. The muscles to be discussed in this section are as follows:

Anterior	Posterior
Flexor carpi ulnaris	Extensor carpi radialis longus
Flexor carpi radialis	Extensor carpi radialis brevis
Palmaris longus	Extensor carpi ulnaris

Some general statements can be made about the proximal muscle attachments of the wrist muscles. First, the flexors attach on the medial epicondyle and the extensors attach on the lateral epicondyle. Second, the distal attachment for all the wrist muscles is a metacarpal. Third, the names of the muscles tell generally what their action is (flexor, extensor), that they act on the wrist (*carpi* means "wrist"), and on what side of the wrist the distal attachment (*radialis* means "radial," *ulnaris* means "ulnar") is located. Their names will also describe if the muscle functions in ulnar or radial deviation.

The **flexor carpi ulnaris muscle** is a superficial muscle running along the ulnar, slightly anterior, side of the forearm (Fig. 11-7). Its proximal attachment is mostly on the medial epicondyle of the humerus, and its distal attachment is the base of the fifth metacarpal and pisiform bone. It is the only wrist muscle attaching to a carpal bone. It is a prime mover in wrist flexion and ulnar deviation.

Flexor Carpi Ulnaris Muscle

O	Medial epicondyle of humerus
I	Pisiform and base of fifth metacarpal
A	Wrist flexion, ulnar deviation
N	Ulnar nerve (C8, T1)

The **flexor carpi radialis muscle** is also a relatively superficial muscle running from the medial epicondyle diagonally across the anterior forearm to attach laterally at the base of the second and third metacarpals (Fig. 11-8). It is a prime mover in wrist flexion and radial deviation.

Flexor Carpi Radialis Muscle

O	Medial epicondyle of the humerus
I	Base of second and third metacarpals
A	Wrist flexion, radial deviation
N	Median nerve (C6, C7)

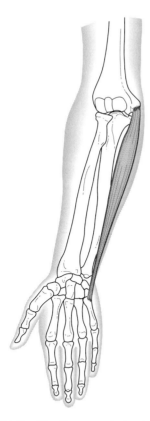

Figure 11-7.   The flexor carpi ulnaris muscle.

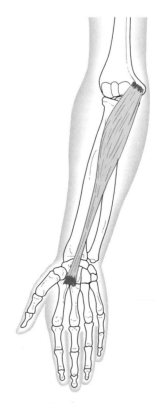

Figure 11-8.   The flexor carpi radialis muscle.

The **palmaris longus muscle** is also a superficial muscle running down the anterior surface of the fore-arm from the common flexor attachment of the medial epicondyle to attach in the midline to the palmar fascia (Fig. 11-9). It is easily identified in the midline at the base of the wrist, especially against slight resistance to wrist flexion. This muscle is rather unique because it only has one bony attachment, which is at the proximal end. This muscle is missing in approximately 21 percent of individuals, either unilaterally or bilaterally (Moore, 1985, p 698). Because the palmaris longus muscle is quite small, its absence does not result in any real loss of strength. Although it is in an ideal position to flex the wrist, because of its size, it is assistive at best.

Palmaris Longus Muscle

O	Medial epicondyle of humerus
I	Palmar fascia
A	Assistive in wrist flexion
N	Median nerve (C6, C7)

On the posterior side of the wrist is the **extensor carpi radialis longus muscle.** This muscle is mostly

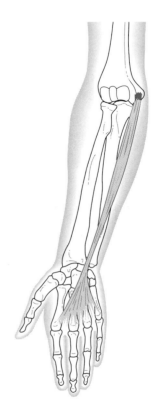

Figure 11-9.   The palmaris longus muscle.

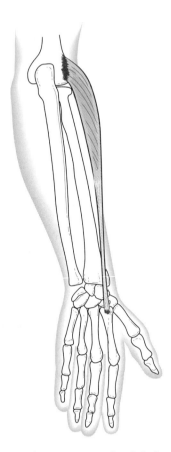

Figure 11-10. The extensor carpi radialis longus muscle.

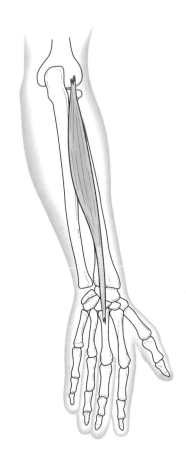

Figure 11-11. The extensor carpi radialis brevis muscle.

superficial (Fig. 11-10). It attaches proximally just above the lateral epicondyle on the lateral supracondylar ridge. It then runs down the lateral posterior side of the forearm, under two tendons that go to the thumb, and then under the extensor retinaculum to attach at the base of the second metacarpal. It is a prime mover in wrist extension and radial deviation.

Extensor Carpi Radialis Longus Muscle

O	Supracondylar ridge of humerus
I	Base of second metacarpal
A	Wrist extension, radial deviation
N	Radial nerve (C6, C7)

Because the extensor carpi radialis muscle also has "longus" in its name, this implies that there is a "brevis." The **extensor carpi radialis brevis muscle** lies next to the extensor carpi radialis longus muscle (Fig. 11-11). It arises from the common extensor tendon on the lateral epicondyle. Like the "longus," it

passes under two tendons that go to the thumb and then under the extensor retinaculum. Its distal attachment is at the base of the third metacarpal. Because its attachment is close to the axis of motion for radial and ulnar deviation, it is only assistive in radial deviation. It is, however, a prime mover in wrist extension.

Extensor Carpi Radialis Brevis Muscle

O	Lateral epicondyle of humerus
I	Base of third metacarpal
A	Wrist extension
N	Radial nerve (C6, C7)

The **extensor carpi ulnaris muscle** is also a superficial muscle arising from the common extensor tendon on the lateral epicondyle (Fig. 11-12). It runs down the medial side of the posterior forearm to attach at the base of the fifth metacarpal. It is a prime mover in wrist extension and ulnar deviation.

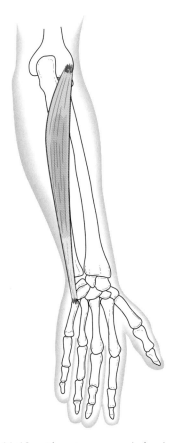

Figure 11-12. The extensor carpi ulnaris muscle.

Extensor Carpi Ulnaris Muscle

O	Lateral epicondyle of humerus
I	Base of fifth metacarpal
A	Wrist extension, ulnar deviation
N	Radial nerve (C6, C7, C8)

Table 11-2	Innervation of the Muscles of the Wrist	
Muscle	**Nerve**	**Spinal Segment**
Extensor carpi radialis longus	Radial	C6, C7
Extensor carpi radialis brevis	Radial	C6, C7
Extensor carpi ulnaris	Radial	C6, C7, C8
Flexor carpi radialis	Median	C6, C7
Palmaris longus	Median	C6, C7
Flexor carpi ulnaris	Ulnar	C8, T1

Table 11-3	Segmental Innervation of the Wrist Joint			
Spinal Cord Level	**C6**	**C7**	**C8**	**T1**
Extensor carpi radialis longus	X	X		
Extensor carpi radialis brevis	X	X		
Extensor carpi ulnaris	X	X	X	
Palmaris longus	X	X		
Flexor carpi radialis	X	X		
Flexor carpi ulnaris			X	X

Summary of Muscle Action

The following list is a summary of the muscle action of the prime movers of the wrist.

Action	Muscles (prime movers)
Flexion	Flexor carpi radialis, flexor carpi ulnaris
Extension	Extensor carpi radialis longus and brevis, extensor carpi ulnaris
Radial deviation	Flexor carpi radialis, extensor carpi radialis longus
Ulnar deviation	Flexor carpi ulnaris, extensor carpi ulnaris

Summary of Muscle Innervation

Innervation of the wrist muscles is quite straightforward. If it is a posterior muscle, the radial nerve innervates it. If it is an anterior muscle on the thumb side, the median nerve innervates it, and if on the ulnar side, it is innervated by the ulnar nerve. Tables 11-2 and 11-3 summarize the innervation of the muscles of the wrist. There is some variation among sources regarding segmental innervation.

Points to Remember

- An isometric contraction has relatively no joint motion.
- The muscle attachments move closer together with a concentric contraction.
- An eccentric contraction is a deceleration activity.

Review Questions

General Anatomy Questions

1. Name the bones of the wrist joint starting laterally on the proximal row and going medially. Use the same order for the distal row.

2. Which wrist motions occur in:
   a. The sagittal plane around the frontal axis?
   b. The frontal plane around the sagittal axis?
   c. The transverse plane around the vertical axis?

3. Describe the wrist joints:
   a. Number of axes
      Radiocarpal _____
      Intercarpal _____
   b. Shape of joint
      Radiocarpal _____
      Intercarpal _____
   c. Type of motion allowed
      Radiocarpal _____
      Intercarpal _____

4. Which muscles attach on the medial epicondyle of the humerus?

5. Which muscles attach on the lateral epicondyle of the humerus?

6. If you were shown a drawing of only a wrist joint, what landmarks could tell you if the drawing were a posterior or anterior view?

7. Which muscles cross the wrist on the radial side?

8. Which muscles cross the wrist on the ulnar side?

9. Which muscle, if present, is very easy to identify but has little functional importance?

10. Starting on the anterior surface of the ulnar side and moving in the direction of the radial side, name the muscles that cross the wrist. Go completely around the wrist.

Functional Activity Questions

Many, but not all, functional activities have the wrist in a neutral position. Often an isometric contraction is required to maintain that position. In the following activities, identify the wrist joint position, and the muscle group contracting isometrically.

1. Holding a cup of coffee
   a. Wrist position _____
   b. Wrist muscle group _____

2. Brushing long hair with a comb (with right hand brushing on left side as illustrated)
   a. Wrist position _____
   b. Wrist muscle group _____

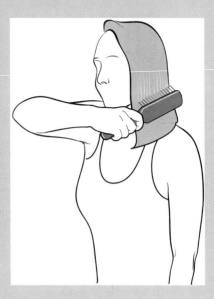

3. Pushing down on a stapler
   a. Wrist position _____
   b. Wrist muscle group _____

4. Typing on a conventional computer keyboard
   a. Wrist position _____
   b. Wrist muscle group _____

5. Holding a box from the bottom (as illustrated)
   a. Wrist position _____
   b. Wrist muscle group _____

Clinical Exercise Questions

Remember that elastic tubing loses its recoil quickly and is not as effective in the end range of an eccentric contraction. There may be more effective ways to perform eccentric contractions than examples given here. You should be able to recognize an eccentric contraction regardless of an exercise's effectiveness.

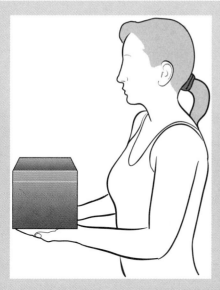

1. Sit, with your forearm resting on your thigh, your palm up, and holding a weight in your hand. Bend your wrist up.
   a. What joint motion is occurring in the wrist?
   b. What type of contraction is occurring? (isometric, concentric, eccentric)
   c. What muscles are being strengthened?

2. Slowly lower the weight to the starting position described in exercise No. 1.
   a. What joint motion is occurring in the wrist?
   b. What type of contraction is occurring? (isometric, concentric, eccentric)
   c. What muscles are being strengthened?

3. Standing with your arm at your side, elbow flexed, palm down, holding on to a loop of elastic tubing that has the other end anchored under your foot. Curl your wrist up.
   a. What joint motion is occurring in the wrist?
   b. What type of contraction is occurring? (isometric, concentric, eccentric)
   c. What muscles are being strengthened?

4. Slowly lower your wrist to the starting position described in exercise No. 3.
   a. What joint motion is occurring in the wrist?
   b. What type of contraction is occurring? (isometric, concentric, eccentric)
   c. What muscles are being strengthened?

5. Standing with your arm at your side, elbow flexed, forearm in a neutral position, holding on to a loop of elastic tubing that has the other end anchored above your head to some stationary object. Bend your wrist down.
   a. What joint motion is occurring in the wrist?
   b. What type of contraction is occurring? (isometric, concentric, eccentric)
   c. What muscles are being strengthened?

6. Slowly return to the starting position described in exercise No. 5.
   a. What joint motion is occurring in the wrist?
   b. What type of contraction is occurring? (isometric, concentric, eccentric)
   c. Explain why it is this type of contraction.
   d. What muscles are being strengthened?

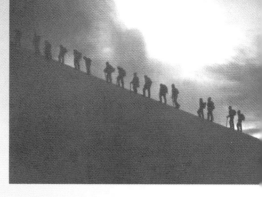

CHAPTER 12

Hand

Joints and Motions of the Thumb

Joints and Motions of the Fingers

Bones and Landmarks

Ligaments and Other Structures

   Common Wrist and Hand Pathologies

Muscles of the Thumb and Fingers

   Extrinsic Muscles

   Intrinsic Muscles

   Summary of Muscle Actions

   Summary of Muscle Innervation

Hand Function

   Grasps

Points to Remember

Review Questions

   General Anatomy Questions

   Functional Activity Questions

   Clinical Exercise Questions

The hand is the distal end of the upper extremity. It is made up of the thumb and finger metacarpals and phalanges. The hand is the key point of function for the upper extremity. We use our hand to accomplish an inexhaustible number of activities, ranging from very simple to quite complex tasks. The main purpose of the other joints of the upper extremity is to place the hand in various positions to accomplish these tasks. Not only is the hand extremely useful and versatile, it is also quite complex. This chapter will deal only with the hand's more basic structures and functions.

Joints and Motions of the Thumb

The first digit, the thumb, has three joints: the carpometacarpal (CMC) joint, metacarpophalangeal (MCP) joint, and interphalangeal (IP) joint (Fig. 12-1). The **CMC joint** is made up of the trapezium bone articulating with the base of the first metacarpal (Fig. 12-2). It is a saddle joint with both joint surfaces being both concave and convex. The shape and relationship of these joint surfaces can be compared to two Pringles potato chips stacked one on top of the other. The shape of the inferior surface of the top chip is similar to the shape of the first metacarpal; the shape of the superior surface of the bottom surface is similar to the trapezium bone. Each surface is concave in one direction and convex in the other direction. Sometimes the CMC joint is described as a modified ball-and-socket joint, implying that it has motion in all three planes. If you look at your thumb in anatomical position, you will notice that the pad is perpendicular to the palm. When you oppose your thumb, the pad is now facing, or parallel to, the palm. Clearly, rotation has occurred. However, if you try to rotate the thumb

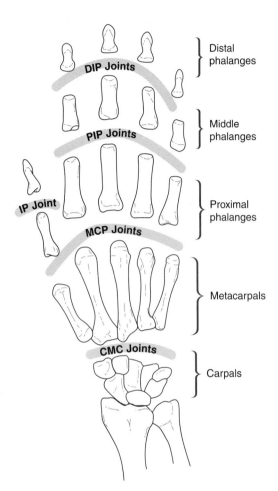

Figure 12-1. Joints and bones of the fingers and thumb. Note that each finger has a DIP and PIP joint, whereas the thumb only has an IP joint.

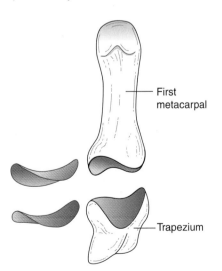

Figure 12-2. The saddle shape of the carpometacarpal (CMC) joint of the thumb can be compared to the shape of two Pringles potato chips.

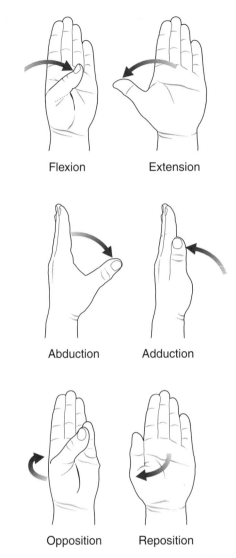

Figure 12-3. Motions of the CMC joint of the thumb.

without any other joint movement, you will find it impossible to do so. The rotation at the CMC joint is a passive motion, not a voluntary one, which occurs as a result of the shape of the joint. This type of motion is commonly referred to as an **accessory movement** (a movement that accompanies the active movement and is essential to normal motion).

The CMC joint of the thumb allows more mobility than the CMC joints of the other four fingers, yet it also provides as much stability. This is unusual. It allows flexion and extension, abduction and adduction, and opposition and reposition (Fig. 12-3). Thumb motions differ from the usual way we name joint motions. **Flexion** and **extension** occur in a plane *parallel* to the palm. **Abduction** and **adduction** occur in a plane *perpendicular* to the palm. In other words, with the forearm supinated and the palm facing up, the thumb moving side to side across the palm is flexion and extension. The thumb moving up toward the ceiling, away from the palm, is abduction, and its return is adduction. **Opposition** is a combination of flexion, abduction, with "built in" accessory motion of rotation; **reposition** is the return to anatomical position. It is because of this accessory rotation, that the CMC joint is usually considered a "modified" biaxial joint.

Although the CMC joint of the thumb is quite mobile, the MCP and IP joints are not. The MCP joint is a hinge joint that allows only **flexion and extension** and is therefore a uniaxial joint. The IP joint, the only phalangeal joint, also allows only **flexion and extension.**

Joints and Motions of the Fingers

The second, third, fourth, and fifth digits, commonly known as the *index, middle, ring,* and *little fingers,* respectively, have four joints each. These joints are the CMC joint, MCP joint, proximal interphalangeal (PIP) joint, and distal interphalangeal (DIP) joint (see Fig. 12-1).

The **carpometacarpal joints** are classified as nonaxial plane (irregular) synovial joints that provide more stability than mobility. The trapezium articulates with

the base of the first metacarpal as described previously in the discussion of the thumb joint. The trapezoid articulates with the second metacarpal, the capitate with the third metacarpal, and the hamate with the fourth and fifth metacarpals (Fig. 12-4). The fifth CMC joint is the most mobile of the fingers and allows for a small amount of **fifth finger opposition.** It does not allow as much opposition as the thumb (the first CMC joint). The fourth CMC joint is slightly mobile, but the second and third CMC joints are not.

This can be demonstrated by looking at your knuckles with your forearm supinated and your elbow flexed. Note that with a relaxed fist, the MCP joints are essentially in a straight line. When you make a tight fist, the fifth MCP joint moves a great deal and the fourth MCP joint moves to a lesser extent, while the second and third MCP joints remain stationary. This MCP movement actually is initiated at the CMC joints.

The **metacarpophalangeal joints (MCP)** of the fingers are biaxial condyloid joints. The rounded heads of the metacarpals articulate with the base of the proximal phalanges, which have a concave shape (see Fig. 12-1). These are commonly referred to as the "knuckles." The motions allowed at these joints are **flexion, extension,** and **hyperextension** plus abduction and adduction (Fig. 12-5). The middle finger is the point

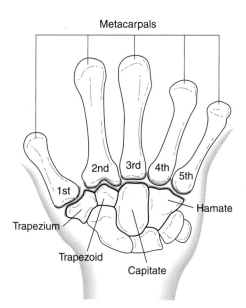

Figure 12-4. The carpometacarpal (CMC) joints of the thumb and fingers. Note that the trapezium articulates with the first metacarpal, the trapezoid with the second metacarpal, the capitate with the third metacarpal, and the hamate with the fourth and fifth metacarpals.

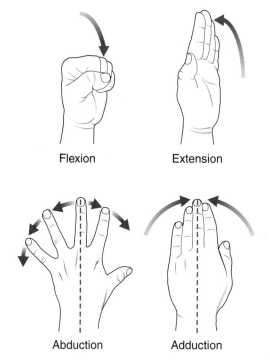

Figure 12-5. Motions of the metacarpophalangeal (MCP) joints and fingers.

of reference for abduction and adduction. **Abduction** occurs when the second, fourth, and fifth fingers move away from the middle (third) finger, and when the middle finger moves in either direction. **Adduction** is the return from abduction and occurs with the second, fourth, and fifth fingers. There is no adduction of the middle finger, only abduction occurring in either direction.

There are two **interphalangeal joints** in the fingers. The PIP joint occurs between the proximal and middle phalange, and the DIP joint occurs between the middle and distal phalanges. They are uniaxial hinge joints and allow only **flexion** and **extension.**

Bones and Landmarks

Although the thumb and fingers have essentially the same bony structure, there is one major difference. The thumb has two phalanges, whereas the fingers each have three. This feature makes the thumb shorter, allowing opposition to be more functional.

Therefore, the hand, made up of the thumb and four fingers, has five metacarpals, five proximal phalanges, five distal phalanges, but only four middle phalanges (see Fig. 12-1). There are no significant landmarks on these bones other than the bone ends. The proximal end of the metacarpals and phalanges is called the base, and the distal end is called the head. There is one landmark on the forearm, which, although not distinct, is sometimes referred to when describing muscle attachments.

Oblique line
Located on the anterior surface of the radius from below the tuberosity, running diagonally to approximately midradius

Ligaments and Other Structures

Although there are numerous structures in the hand, only a few of those more commonly referred to will be described here. The **flexor retinaculum** ligament is a fibrous band that spans the wrist on the anterior surface of the wrist in a mediolateral (horizontal) direction (Fig. 12-6). Its main function is to hold these tendons close to the wrist, thus preventing the tendons from pulling away from the wrist (bow-stringing) when the wrist flexes. It also prevents the two sides of the carpal bones from spreading apart or separating. In construction, this horizontal structure is called a "tie beam." The flexor retinaculum is made up of two parts that for-

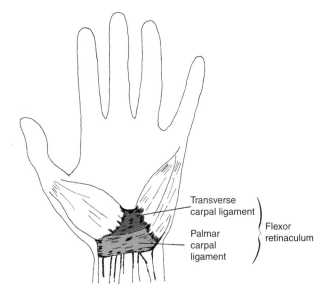

Figure 12-6.   The flexor retinaculum is made up of the palmar and transverse carpal ligaments.

merly were known as the *palmar carpal ligament* and the *transverse carpal ligament.* Currently, they are grouped together as the *flexor retinaculum.* Because of their clinical significance, they will be described individually.

The **palmar carpal ligament** is more proximal and superficial than the transverse carpal ligament. Its distal fibers do blend with the transverse carpal ligament. The palmar carpal ligament attaches to the styloid process of the radius and ulna and crosses over the flexor muscles.

The **transverse carpal ligament** lies deeper and more distally. It attaches to the pisiform and hook of the hamate on the medial side and to the scaphoid and trapezium bones laterally. It arches over the carpal bones forming a tunnel through which the median nerve and nine extrinsic flexor tendons of the fingers and thumb (four tendons each of the flexor digitorum superficialis and flexor digitorum profundus, and one tendon for the flexor pollicis longus) pass. Figure 12-7 shows the bony floor of the carpal bones, the fibrous ceiling of the transverse carpal ligament. Together they form the tunnel through which the tendons and nerve pass. It also shows the area of the hand innervated by the medial nerve.

The **extensor retinaculum ligament** is a fibrous band traversing the wrist on the posterior side in a horizontal mediolateral direction (Fig. 12-8). It attaches to the styloid process of the ulna medially, and to the triquetrum, pisiform, and lateral side of the radius. It holds the extensor tendons close to the wrist, especially during wrist extension.

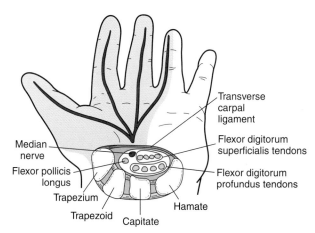

Figure 12-7. The bony floor of the carpal bones and fibrous ceiling of the transverse carpal ligament form the carpal tunnel. The median nerve and several tendons pass through this tunnel. Note the area of the hand innervated by this nerve.

The **extensor expansion ligament,** also called the extensor hood, (Fig. 12-9) is a small triangular-shaped flat aponeurosis covering the dorsum and sides of the proximal phalanx of the fingers. The extensor digitorum tendon blends into the expansion. It is wider at its base over the MCP joint, actually

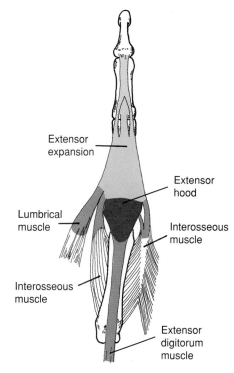

Figure 12-9. The extensor expansion provides an attachment on the middle and/or distal phalanx for several muscles.

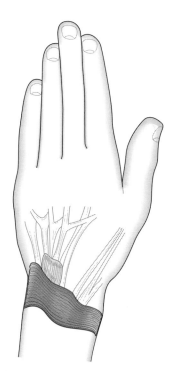

Figure 12-8. Extensor retinaculum.

wrapping over the sides somewhat. As it approaches the PIP joint, it is joined by tendons of the lumbricales and interossei muscles. It narrows toward its distal end at the base of the distal phalanx. The extensor digitorum, lumbricales, and interossei muscles form an attachment to the middle and/or distal phalanx by way of this expansion. The **extensor hood** area, formed by the extensor expansion proximally, covers the head of the metacarpal and keeps the extensor tendon in the midline.

When the hand is relaxed, the palm assumes a cupped position. This palmar concavity is due to the arrangement of the bony skeleton reinforced by ligaments. There are three arches that are responsible for this shape (Fig. 12-10). The **proximal carpal arch** is formed by the proximal end of the metacarpals (base) and carpal bones and is maintained by the flexor retinaculum (see Fig. 12-7). The shallower **distal carpal arch** is made up of the metacarpal heads. The **longitudinal arch** begins at the wrist and runs the length of the metacarpal and phalanges for each digit. It is perpendicular to the other two arches. These arches contribute to the function of various types of grasp described at the end of this chapter.

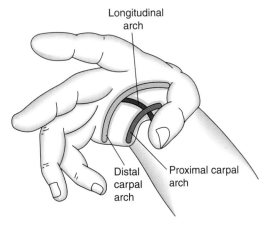

Figure 12-10.   The three arches of the hand.

Common Wrist and Hand Pathologies

A **Colles' fracture** is a common injury of elderly people resulting from a fall on the outstretched hand. It is a transverse fracture of the distal radius with posterior displacement of the distal fragment. With a **Smith's fracture,** the distal fragment is displaced anteriorly (reverse Colles') and is caused by a fall on the back of the hand. A **"greenstick" fracture** refers to the incomplete fracture usually of the radius, more proximal than a Colles' fracture. It is more common in children than adults. This fracture is similar to the breaking of a young or new tree limb. If you try to break the limb, you will find that it does not break completely in half like an older, more brittle limb. **Ganglion cyst** is a benign tumor mass commonly seen as a bump on the dorsal surface of the wrist.

Carpal tunnel syndrome is an extremely common condition caused by compression on the medial nerve within the carpal tunnel. The symptoms are numbness and tingling in the hand, which often begins at night. There is often tingling, pain, and weakness in the hand, particularly in the thumb, index, and middle fingers. Tapping over the carpal tunnel often produces symptoms. The transverse carpal ligament is frequently surgically cut to relieve the symptoms. **De Quervain's disease** is caused by an inflammation and thickening of the sheath containing the extensor pollicis brevis and abductor pollicis longus, resulting in pain on the radial side of the wrist. Because it is an inflammation of tendons and their surrounding sheaths, it is called a **tenosynovitis.** Making a fist with your thumb inside and then moving the wrist into ulnar deviation can elicit pain in those tendons and is considered a positive test. Care should be exercised in doing this test because it often causes some discomfort in a normal wrist.

Dupuytren's contracture occurs when the palmar aponeurosis undergoes a nodular thickening. It is most common in the area of the palm in line with the ring and little fingers. Often those fingers will develop flexion contractures. **Stenosing tenosynovitis,** commonly known as **trigger finger,** is a problem with the sliding mechanism of a tendon in its sheath. When a nodule or swelling of the lining of the sheath or of the tendon develops, the tendon can no longer slide in and out smoothly. It may pass into the sheath when the finger flexes, but becomes stuck as the finger attempts to extend. The finger can become locked in that position, and must be manually extended. The flexor tendons of the middle and ring fingers are most commonly involved. **Skier's thumb,** a common hand injury among athletes, involves an acute tear of the ulnar collateral ligament of the thumb. **Gamekeeper's thumb** is an old term referring to the same injury sustained by English gamekeepers as they twisted the necks of small game.

Swan neck deformity is characterized by flexion of the MCP joint, (hyper) extension of the PIP joint, and flexion of the DIP joint. With a **boutonnière deformity,** the deformity is in the opposite direction. There is extension of the MCP joint, flexion of the PIP joint, and extension of the DIP joint. **Ulnar drift** results in the ulnar deviation of the fingers at the MCP joints. **Mallet finger** is caused by disruption of the extensor mechanism of the DIP joint either because the tendon was severed, or because the portion of bone where the tendon attached has avulsed from the distal phalanx. In either case, the distal phalanx remains in a flexed position and cannot be extended. The scaphoid is the most frequently injured carpal bone. A **scaphoid fracture** usually is the result of a fall on the outstretched hand of a younger person. Because of a poor vascular supply, it has a high incidence of avascular necrosis. **Kienböck's disease** refers to the necrosis of the lunate, which may develop after trauma.

Muscles of the Thumb and Fingers

Extrinsic Muscles

In addition to the wrist muscles previously described, several other muscles not only span the wrist but also cross the joints in the hand as well. These muscles are called **extrinsic muscles** of the hand because their proximal attachment is above, or proximal to, the wrist joint. They have an assistive role in wrist function, but

The **flexor digitorum superficialis** muscle lies deep to the wrist flexors and palmaris longus muscle (Fig. 12-11). Its broad proximal attachment is part of the common flexor tendon on the medial epicondyle of the humerus. It also has an attachment on the coronoid process of the ulna and the oblique line of the radius. It divides into four tendons and crosses the wrist with one tendon then going to each finger (Fig. 12-12). Its distal attachment splits into two parts and attaches on each side of the middle phalanx of each finger. Its action is to flex the MCP and PIP joints of the second through fifth fingers.

Flexor Digitorum Superficialis Muscle

O	Common flexor tendon, coronoid process, and radius
I	Sides of the middle phalanx of the four fingers
A	Flexes the MCP and PIP joints of the fingers
N	Median nerve (C7, C8, T1)

The **flexor digitorum profundus muscle** lies deep to the flexor digitorum superficialis muscle as they traverse the forearm and hand together (Fig. 12-13). The profundus muscle has its proximal attachment on the ulna on the anterior and medial surfaces from the coronoid process to approximately three-fourths of the way down the ulna. It runs beneath the flexor digitorum superficialis muscle until the superficialis tendon splits into two parts at its distal attachment. The profundus muscle passes through this split and continues distally to attach at the base of the distal phalanx of the second through fifth fingers (see Fig. 12-12). Its action is to flex the MCP, PIP, and DIP joints of the second through fifth fingers.

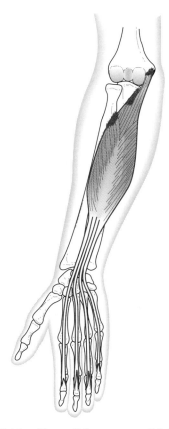

Figure 12-11.   Flexor digitorum superficialis muscle.

their primary function is at the thumb or finger. The extrinsic muscles of the finger are as follows:

Anterior	**Posterior**
Flexor digitorum superficialis	Extensor digitorum
Flexor digitorum profundus	Extensor digiti minimi
	Extensor indicis

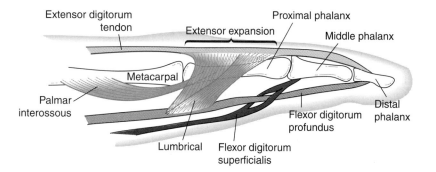

Figure 12-12.   Side view of a digit showing tendon relationship of the flexor digitorum superficialis with the flexor digitorum profundus, and the two flexor tendons with the extensor digitorum tendon.

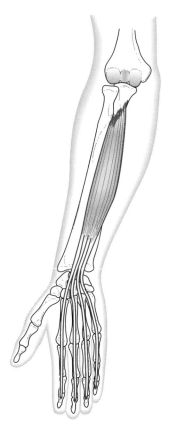

Figure 12-13. Flexor digitorum profundus muscle.

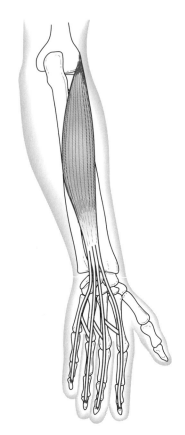

Figure 12-14. Extensor digitorum muscle.

Flexor Digitorum Profundus Muscle

O	Upper three-fourths of the ulna
I	Distal phalanx of the four fingers
A	Flexes all three joints of the fingers
N	Median and ulnar nerves (C8, T1)

The **extensor digitorum muscle** is a superficial muscle on the posterior forearm and hand (Fig. 12-14). It attaches proximally to the lateral epicondyle of the humerus as part of the common extensor tendon. It passes under the extensor retinaculum to attach distally on the distal phalanx of the second through fifth fingers via the extensor expansion (see Fig. 12-12). In the area of the metacarpals are interconnecting bands joining the four extensor digitorum tendons. These interconnecting bands limit independent finger extension. The extensor digitorum muscle is the only common extensor muscle of the fingers. It extends the

MCP, PIP, and DIP joints of the second, third, fourth, and fifth fingers.

Extensor Digitorum Muscle

O	Lateral epicondyle of the humerus
I	Base of distal phalanx of the second through fifth fingers
A	Extends all three joints of the fingers
N	Radial nerve (C6, C7, C8)

The **extensor indicis muscle** is a deep muscle that has its proximal attachment on the posterior surface of the distal ulna (Fig. 12-15). It crosses the wrist under the extensor retinaculum medial to the extensor digitorum muscle and attaches into the extensor expansion, with the extensor digitorum muscle. It extends the MCP, PIP, and DIP joints of the index finger.

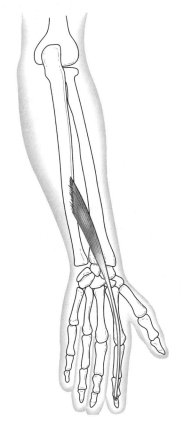

Figure 12-15. Extensor indicis muscle.

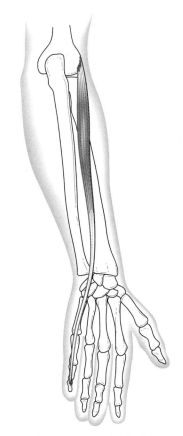

Figure 12-16. Extensor digiti minimi muscle.

Extensor Indicis Muscle

O	Distal ulna
I	Base of distal phalanx of the second finger
A	Extends all three joints of the second finger
N	Radial nerve (C6, C7, C8)

Extensor Digiti Minimi Muscle

O	Lateral epicondyle of humerus
I	Base of distal phalanx of fifth finger
A	Extends all three joints of fifth finger
N	Radial nerve (C6, C7, C8)

The **extensor digiti minimi muscle** is a long, narrow muscle (Fig. 12-16) that is deep to the extensor digitorum and extensor carpi ulnaris muscles near its proximal attachment. It becomes superficial before crossing the wrist. It comes off the common extensor tendon on the lateral epicondyle of the humerus, crosses the wrist under the extensor retinaculum, and attaches to the base of the distal phalanx of the fifth finger via the extensor expansion. It is a prime mover in extending the MCP, PIP, and DIP joints of the fifth finger.

It is rather easy to distinguish the muscles having a function on the thumb because *pollicis* means "thumb" in Latin. The extrinsic muscles of the thumb are the following:

Flexor pollicis longus
Abductor pollicis longus
Extensor pollicis longus
Extensor pollicis brevis

The **flexor pollicis longus muscle** is a deep muscle that has its proximal attachment on the anterior surface of the radius and interosseous membrane and its distal attachment at the base of the distal phalanx of

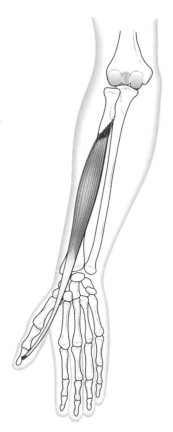

Figure 12-17.   Flexor pollicis longus muscle.

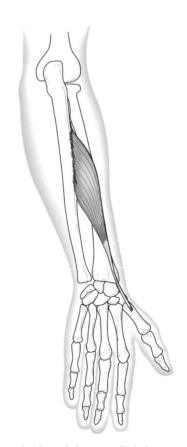

Figure 12-18.   Abductor pollicis longus muscle.

the thumb (Fig. 12-17). It is a prime mover in flexion of the CMC, MCP, and IP joints of the thumb.

Flexor Pollicis Longus Muscle

O	Radius, anterior surface
I	Distal phalanx of thumb
A	Flexes all three joints of the thumb
N	Median nerve (C8, T1)

The **abductor pollicis longus muscle** is located deep on the posterior forearm (Fig. 12-18). It attaches to the radius just distal to the supinator, the interosseous membrane, and the middle portion of the ulna. It becomes superficial just proximal to crossing the wrist and attaches to the base of the first metacarpal on the radial side. It effectively abducts the thumb at the CMC joint even though it is attached only to the metacarpal, because the distal joints (MCP and IP) allow only flexion and extension. Therefore, the thumb moves as one unit in the direction of abduction and

adduction. Similarly, adducting the metacarpal also adducts the entire thumb. Therefore, in this text, when referring to thumb abduction, adduction, opposition, and reposition, it is implied that the action occurs at the CMC joint.

Abductor Pollicis Longus Muscle

O	Posterior radius, interosseous membrane, middle ulna
I	Base of the first metacarpal
A	Abducts thumb
N	Radial nerve

The **extensor pollicis brevis muscle** is also located deep on the posterior forearm and spans the wrist just medial to the abductor pollicis longus muscle. Its proximal attachment is on the posterior radius near the distal end and just below the abductor pollicis longus muscle. Its distal attachment is on the posterior surface at the base of the thumb's proximal phalanx

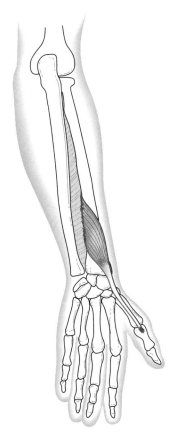

Figure 12-19.   Extensor pollicis brevis muscle.

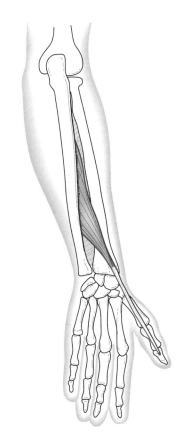

Figure 12-20.   Extensor pollicis longus muscle.

(Fig. 12-19). It functions to extend the MCP joint of the thumb.

Extensor Pollicis Brevis Muscle

O	Posterior distal radius
I	Base of the proximal phalanx of thumb
A	Extends CMC and MCP joints of thumb
N	Radial nerve (C6, C7)

The **extensor pollicis longus muscle** is located near the two previously mentioned muscles deep on the posterior forearm. Its proximal attachment is on the middle third of the ulna and interosseous membrane (Fig. 12-20). Like the other two muscles, it becomes superficial just before crossing the wrist. Its distal attachment is at the base of the distal phalanx of the thumb on the posterior side. It functions to extend the CMC, MCP, and IP joints of the thumb.

Extensor Pollicis Longus Muscle

O	Middle posterior ulna and interosseous membrane
I	Base of distal phalanx of thumb
A	Extends all three joints of the thumb
N	Radial nerve (C6, C7, C8)

If you extend your thumb, you will notice that a depression is formed between what appears to be two tendons. Actually, there are three tendons. The abductor pollicis longus and extensor pollicis brevis muscles form the lateral border, and the extensor pollicis longus muscle forms the medial border. This depression is called the **anatomical snuffbox** (Fig. 12-21).

In review, the extrinsic muscles have their proximal attachment above the wrist and their distal attachment on the hand. Because they cross the wrist, they could have a function there; however, any wrist function is usually assistive at best. Their prime function is in moving the fingers or thumb.

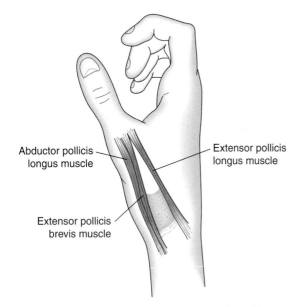

Figure 12-21. The borders of the anatomical snuffbox are defined by the tendon of the extensor pollicis longus muscle on one side, and the tendons of the abductor pollicis longus and brevis muscles on the other side.

Intrinsic Muscles

Intrinsic muscles have their proximal attachment at, or distal to, the carpal bones, and have a function on the thumb or fingers. These muscles are responsible for the fine motor control and precision movement of the hand. The intrinsic muscles can be further divided into the thenar, hypothenar, and palm muscles. The **thenar muscles** are those muscles that function to move the thumb. They form the thenar eminence, or ball of the thumb. The **hypothenar muscles,** forming the hypothenar eminence, act primarily on the little finger. The **deep palm muscles** are located deep in the palm of the hand between the thenar and hypothenar muscles. They have some of the more intricate motions that usually involve multiple muscles. These muscles are the adductor pollicis, the interossei (of which there are four dorsal and four palmar), and the lumbricales (of which there are also four muscles). Table 12-1 summarizes the three groups of intrinsic muscles.

In the thenar group, the **flexor pollicis brevis muscle** is a relatively superficial muscle. It attaches proximally to the trapezium and the flexor retinaculum, and distally to the base of the proximal phalanx of the thumb (Fig. 12-22). In older texts, this muscle is described as having two parts: a lateral superficial part (described here) and a medial deep part. In more recent literature, this medial part is often considered a separate muscle—the first palmar interossei—and this is the terminology

Table 12-1	Intrinsic Muscles of the Hand	
Thenar	**Hypothenar**	**Deep Palm**
Flexor pollicis brevis	Flexor digiti minimi	Adductor pollicis
Abductor pollicis brevis	Abductor digiti minimi	Interossei
Opponens pollicis	Opponens digiti minimi	Lumbricales

used here. Thus, the flexor pollicis muscle has one part, and its primary actions are to flex the CMC and MCP joints of the thumb.

Flexor Pollicis Brevis Muscle

O	Trapezium and flexor retinaculum
I	Proximal phalanx
A	Flexes the CMC and MCP joints of thumb
N	Median nerve (C6, C7)

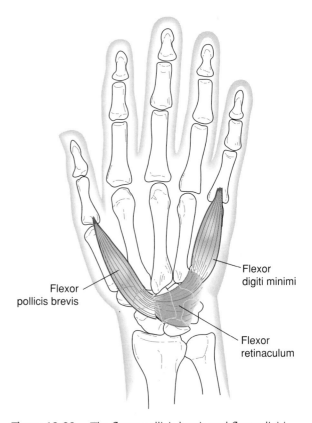

Figure 12-22. The flexor pollicis brevis and flexor digiti minimi muscles.

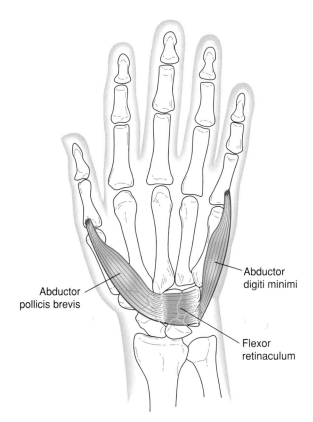

Figure 12-23.   The abductor pollicis brevis and abductor digiti minimi muscles.

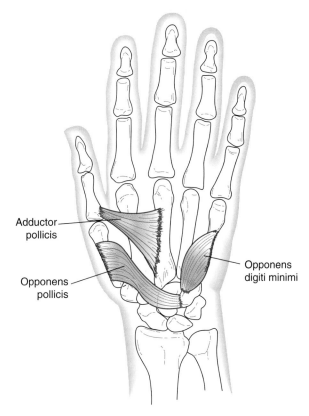

Figure 12-24.   The opponens pollicis, adductor pollicis, and opponens digiti minimi muscles.

The **abductor pollicis brevis muscle** lies just lateral to the flexor pollicis brevis muscle. It attaches proximally to the flexor retinaculum, scaphoid, and trapezium, and distally to the base of the proximal phalanx of the thumb (Fig. 12-23). It acts to abduct the CMC joint of the thumb.

Abductor Pollicis Brevis Muscle

O	Scaphoid, trapezium, and flexor retinaculum
I	Proximal phalanx
A	Abducts the thumb (CMC joint)
N	Median nerve (C6, C7)

The **opponens pollicis muscle** lies deep to the abductor pollicis brevis muscle. It attaches proximally to the trapezium and flexor retinaculum and distally to the entire lateral surface of the first metacarpal (Fig. 12-24). Its primary function is to oppose the thumb. Remember, this action occurs at the CMC joint.

Opponens Pollicis Muscle

O	Trapezium and flexor retinaculum
I	First metacarpal
A	Opposes the thumb (CMC joint)
N	Median nerve (C6, C7)

Thumb opposition is perhaps the most important function of the hand. Because it is a combination of flexion, abduction, and rotation of the thumb, other muscles, such as the flexor pollicis brevis and abductor pollicis muscles, assist in this function.

The **adductor pollicis muscle** is a thumb muscle, although it is not usually considered part of the thenar group. This is probably because it is located deep and does not make up the muscle bulk of the thenar eminence. This concept will be discussed in more detail later in this chapter. It has its proximal attachments on the capitate, base of the second metacarpal, and the palmar surface of the third metacarpal. Its distal attachment is at the base of the proximal phalanx of the thumb (see Fig. 12-24). As its name implies, its function is to adduct the thumb (at the CMC joint).

Adductor Pollicis Muscle

O	Capitate, base of the second metacarpal, palmar surface of the third metacarpal
I	Base of proximal phalanx of thumb
A	Adducts thumb (CMC joint)
N	Ulnar nerve (C8, T1)

The counterpart to the thenar muscle group is the hypothenar group. The **flexor digiti minimi muscle** serves the same function on the little finger as the flexor pollicis brevis does on the thumb. It is attached proximally to the hook of the hamate and the flexor retinaculum, and distally to the base of the proximal phalanx of the little finger (see Fig. 12-22). It flexes the MCP joint of that finger. Remember, although most thumb motion occurs at the CMC joint, most finger motion occurs at the MCP joint.

Flexor Digiti Minimi Muscle

O	Hamate and flexor retinaculum
I	Base of proximal phalanx of the fifth finger
A	Flexes CMC and MCP joints of the fifth finger
N	Ulnar nerve (C8, T1)

The **abductor digiti minimi muscle** lies superficially just medial to the flexor digiti minimi muscle on the ulnar border of the hypothenar eminence. It attaches proximally to the pisiform and to the tendon of the flexor carpi ulnaris muscle and distally to the base of the proximal phalanx of the fifth finger (see Fig. 12-23). It abducts the MCP joint of that finger.

Abductor Digiti Minimi Muscle

O	Pisiform and tendon of flexor carpi ulnaris
I	Proximal phalanx of fifth finger
A	Abducts the MCP joint of the fifth finger
N	Ulnar nerve (C8, T1)

The **opponens digiti minimi muscle** lies deep to the other hypothenar muscles. Its proximal attach-

ments, the hook of the hamate and the flexor retinaculum, are similar to the proximal attachments of the flexor digiti minimi muscle. Distally, it attaches to the ulnar border of the fifth metacarpal (see Fig. 12-24). Its primary action is in opposition of the fifth finger. This occurs at the CMC joint.

Opponens Digiti Minimi Muscle

O	Hamate and flexor retinaculum
I	Fifth metacarpal
A	Opposes the fifth finger (CMC joint)
N	Ulnar nerve (C8, T1)

The **palmaris brevis** is a small, thin, square muscle with no bony attachments and little importance in hand function. It attaches at the ulnar border of the palmar aponeurosis and inserts into the skin along the ulnar border of the hand. It wrinkles the skin over the hypothenar eminence deepening the hollow of the palm, which improves grasp somewhat. It is not part of

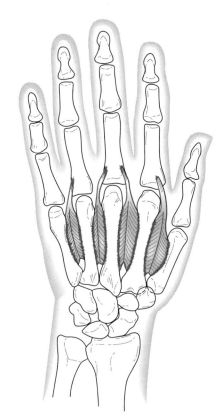

Figure 12-25.   Dorsal interossei muscles. Note that the middle finger has two attachments.

the hypothenar muscles and does not have an action on the little finger. It receives innervation from the ulnar nerve.

The muscles located in the area between the thenar and hypothenar muscle groups are often called the **deep palm group,** or the *intermediate group.* The adductor pollicis muscle is sometimes placed in this group because it is located deep within the palm. Other sources place it with the thenar group because of its action on the thumb. Here it is placed in the deep palm group for perhaps no other reason than to discuss the intrinsic muscles in groups of three. In any event, it was described with the thenar muscles.

There are four **dorsal interossei** muscles. They each attach proximally to two adjacent metacarpals and distally at the base of the proximal phalanx (Fig. 12-25). Table 12-2 summarizes the attachments and actions of each of the dorsal interossei muscles. Their action is to abduct the second, third, and fourth fingers at the MCP joint. Remember that the third finger abducts in both directions. The fifth finger is abducted by the abductor digiti minimi. The ulnar nerve innervates all dorsal interossei muscles.

Dorsal Interossei

O	Adjacent metacarpals
I	Base of proximal phalanx
A	Abduct fingers at MCP joint
N	Ulnar nerve (C8, T1)

The **palmar interossei** muscles are an interesting group of muscles with some controversy as to whether there are three or four of them. Most of the older texts describe three. These texts also describe the flexor pollicis brevis muscle as having two parts: a medial part coming from the flexor retinaculum and attaching to the base of the proximal phalanx of the thumb, and a lateral part coming from the first metacarpal bone and

attaching on the proximal phalanx. Each part has a different innervation. A branch of the median nerve innervates the lateral portion. The medial portion gets its nerve supply from a branch of the ulnar nerve, as do the palmar interossei muscles.

More recent texts, however, list the flexor pollicis brevis muscle as having only one part (lateral part), with innervation from the median nerve. These sources have renamed the medial head as the first palmar interosseous muscle. This muscle has the same attachments and nerve supply as the other palmar interossei muscles, so it makes sense to group these muscles together. Although this appears to be a logical way to present these muscles (and how they will be presented here), you should be aware of the discrepancies.

The palmar interossei muscles, like the dorsal interossei muscles, are four in number. They attach proximally to the palmar surface of the first, second, fourth, and fifth metacarpals. They do not attach, or have a function on, the middle finger. Distally, they attach to the base of the proximal phalanx of the same finger as the proximal attachment (Fig. 12-26). These attachments are summarized in Table 12-3. Like the dorsal interossei muscles, the palmar interossei muscles are innervated by the ulnar nerve.

Palmar Interossei Muscles

O	Respective metacarpal
I	Base of respective proximal phalanx
A	Adduct fingers at MCP joint
N	Ulnar nerve (C8, T1)

As mentioned, the middle finger is the point of reference for abduction and adduction. Movement away from the middle finger is abduction, and movement toward it is adduction. Note that the middle finger abducts in two directions and therefore does not adduct.

Table 12-2	Dorsal Interossei Muscles of the Hand		
Muscle	**Proximal Attachment**	**Distal Attachment**	**Action**
First	First and second metacarpals	Lateral side of index finger	Abduct index finger
Second	Second and third metacarpals	Lateral side of middle finger	Abduct middle finger laterally
Third	Third and fourth metacarpals	Medial side of middle finger	Abduct middle finger medially
Fourth	Fourth and fifth metacarpals	Medial side of ring finger	Abduct ring finger

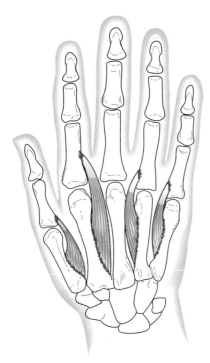

Figure 12-26. Palmar interossei muscles. Note that the middle finger has no attachments.

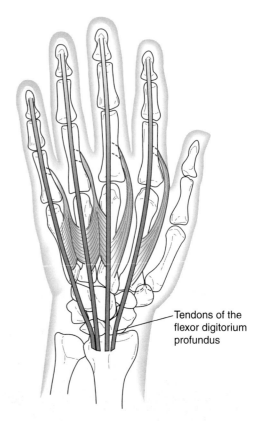

Tendons of the flexor digitorium profundus

Figure 12-27. The lumbrical muscles, palmar view.

The last muscle group to be discussed is rather unique. The **lumbrical muscles,** of which there are four, have no bony attachment. They are located quite deep and attach only to tendons. Proximally, they attach to the tendon of the flexor digitorum profundus muscle, spanning the MCP joint anteriorly (Fig. 12-27). This allows them to flex the MCP joint. They then pass posteriorly at the proximal phalange to attach to the tendinous expansion of the extensor digitorum muscle (Fig. 12-28). This allows them to extend the PIP and DIP joint. Therefore, their action is to flex the MCP joint and extend the PIP and DIP joints of the second through fifth fingers. This combined motion is referred to as the "tabletop position."

Lumbrical Muscles

O	Tendon of the flexor digitorium profundus muscle
I	Tendon of the extensor digitorium muscle
A	Flex the MCP joint while extending the PIP and DIP joints
N	First and second lumbricales: medial nerve Third and fourth lumbricales: ulnar nerve (C6, C7, C8)

Table 12-3	Palmar Interossei Muscles		
Muscles	**Proximal Attachment**	**Distal Attachment**	**Action**
First	First metacarpal	Medial side of thumb	Adduct thumb
Second	Second metacarpal	Medial side of index finger	Adduct index finger
Third	Fourth metacarpal	Lateral side of ring finger	Adduct ring finger
Fourth	Fifth metacarpal	Lateral side of little finger	Adduct little finger

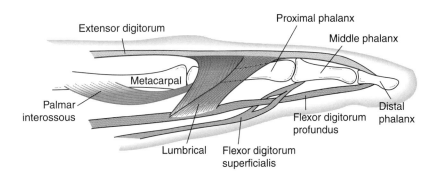

Figure 12-28. The lumbrical muscles, side view.

Summary of Muscle Actions

The actions of the prime movers of the hand are summarized in Table 12-4.

Summary of Muscle Innervation

Innervation of the hand is almost as straightforward as the wrist; however, a few exceptions must be discussed. As with the wrist, muscles on the posterior surface of the hand are innervated mostly by the radial nerve. Muscles on the thumb side are supplied primarily by the median nerve, and muscles on the ulnar side by the ulnar nerve.

The adductor pollicis muscle appears to be the exception; it is innervated by the ulnar nerve instead of the median nerve like all the other thumb (pollicis) muscles. However, remember that the adductor pollicis muscle attaches in the middle of the palm to the third metacarpal (see Fig. 12-24). It is here that the ulnar nerve changes direction and runs toward the thumb. As it does, it sends branches to the adductor pollicis and dorsal and palmar interossei muscles (see Fig. 6-28). The flexor digitorum profundus muscle receives its innervation from both the median and ulnar nerve, as do the lumbrical muscles. This does not seem surprising, because the lumbrical muscles have their proximal attachment on the tendons of the flexor digitorum

Table 12-4	Prime Movers of the Hand	
Action	**Joint**	**Muscle**
Thumb		
Flexion	CMC, MCP	Flexor pollicis brevis
	IP (MCP, CMC)	Flexor pollicis longus
Extension	CMC, MCP	Extensor pollicis brevis
	IP (MCP, CMC)	Extensor pollicis longus
Abduction	CMC	Abductor pollicis brevis, Abductor pollicis longus
Adduction	CMC	Adductor pollicis
Opposition	CMC	Opponens pollicis
Reposition	CMC	Adductor pollicis, extensor pollicis longus, extensor pollicis brevis
Action	**Joint**	**Muscle**
Finger		
Flexion	MCP	Lumbricales, flexor digitorum superficialis, flexor digitorum profundus
	PIP	Flexor digitorum superficialis, flexor digitorum profundus
	DIP	Flexor digitorum profundus
Extension	MCP	Extensor digitorum, extensor indicis, extensor digiti minimi
	PIP and DIP	Lumbricales, extensor digitorum, extensor digiti minimi, extensor indicis
Abduction	MCP	Dorsal interossei, abductor digiti minimi
Adduction	MCP	Palmar interossei
Opposition (fifth)	CMC	Opponens digiti minimi

Table 12-5	Innervation of the Muscles of the Hand	
Muscle	**Nerve**	**Spinal Segment**
Extensor digitorum	Radial	C6, C7, C8
Extensor indicis	Radial	C6, C7, C8
Extensor digiti minimi	Radial	C6, C7, C8
Extensor pollicis longus	Radial	C6, C7, C8
Extensor pollicis brevis	Radial	C6, C7
Abductor pollicis longus	Radial	C6, C7
Flexor digitorum superficialis	Median	C7, C8, T1
Flexor digitorum profundus	Median	C8, T1
	Ulnar	C8, T1
Flexor pollicis longus	Median	C8, T1
Flexor pollicis brevis	Median	C6, C7
Abductor pollicis brevis	Median	C6, C7
Opponens pollicis	Median	C6, C7
Lumbricales 1 and 2	Median	C6, C7
Lumbricales 3 and 4	Ulnar	C8
Flexor digiti minimi	Ulnar	C8, T1
Abductor digiti minimi	Ulnar	C8, T1
Opponens digiti minimi	Ulnar	C8, T1
Adductor pollicis	Ulnar	C8, T1
Dorsal and palmar interossei	Ulnar	C8, T1

profundus muscle. Table 12–5 further summarizes hand muscle innervation. One can see from the table that injury to the lower cervical vertebrae will affect all hand function. Table 12–6 summarizes the segmental innervation. Note that there is some discrepancy among various sources regarding the spinal cord level of innervation.

Hand Function

The human hand performs many functions. The primary function of the hand is grasp, or *prehension*. This means the hand is adapted to hold or manipulate objects. There are also many nonprehensile hand functions, such as expressing emotions, scratching, using a fist as a club, and using the open palm, as in pushing down on an armrest to assist in standing. Because no manipulative movement occurs with these types of activities, no further description of nonprehensile function will be made here.

With prehension (grasping or holding an object), how the hand is used depends on the size, shape, and weight of the object, how that object will be used, and the involvement of the proximal segments of the upper extremity. Generally speaking, the shoulder girdle and shoulder joint place the hand in space. The elbow allows the hand to move closer or farther away from the body, especially the face. The wrist provides stability while the hand is manipulating objects and is important in the tenodesis action described in Chapter 5. Although much attention tends to be placed on the grasping aspect of hand function, release is equally important. Release is the role of the MP, PIP, and DIP extensors. Without the ability to release, the hand's grasp function is greatly diminished.

Of paramount importance to hand function is sensation. Without intact sensation, an individual must compensate with visual clues to find items, know what is being held, and how hard the object is being grasped. For example, if you were presented with a laundry bag full of clothes and told to find the small box of soap, you could feel around inside the bag until locating the soap. However, if your hand's sensation were not intact, you would have to empty the bag and visually search for the box. A person with an upper extremity amputation who uses a prosthetic device is a good example of having hand function without sensation. That person would need visual feedback to find the soap and to know if the terminal device had grasped it. Hand sensation is provided by the radial, ulnar, and median nerves. Figure 12–29 shows the pattern of

Table 12-6	Segmental Innervation of the Hand			
Spinal cord level	C6	C7	C8	T1
Extensor digitorum	X	X	X	
Extensor indicis	X	X	X	
Extensor digiti minimi	X	X	X	
Extensor pollicis longus	X	X	X	
Extensor pollicis brevis	X	X		
Abductor pollicis longus	X	X		
Abductor pollicis brevis	X	X		
Flexor pollicis brevis	X	X		
Opponens pollicis	X	X		
Flexor digitorum superficialis		X	X	X
Flexor digitorum profundus			X	X
Flexor pollicis longus			X	X
Lumbricales			X	X
Flexor digiti minimi			X	X
Abductor digiti minimi			X	X
Opponens digiti minimi			X	X
Adductor pollicis			X	X
Dorsal and palmar interossei			X	X

sensory distribution. This distribution varies somewhat among authors.

There is an optimal position for the wrist and hand for the hand to be most effective in terms of strength and precision. This position is called the **functional position of the hand.** In this position, the wrist is in a slightly extended position, the MCP and PIP joints of the fingers are slightly flexed, and the thumb is in opposition. Figure 12-30 illustrates this position. Maintenance of the thenar web is vital to thumb opposition.

Grasps

There are basically two types of prehension: power grips and precision grips. The activity dictates which grip is needed. A **power grip** is used when an object needs to be held forcefully while being moved about by more proximal joint muscles (holding a hammer or doorknob) (Fig. 12-31). Often a power grip involves an isometric contraction with no movement occurring between the hand and the object being held. A **precision grip,** often referred to as *precision prehension,* is used when an object needs to be manipulated in a finer type movement such as holding a pen or threading a needle (Fig. 12-32).

Power Grips

A power grip usually involves a significant amount of force and is considered the most powerful grip. The

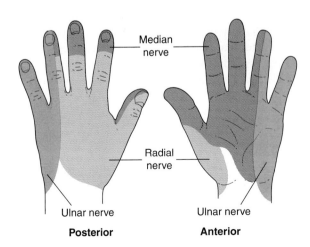

Figure 12-29. Sensory innervation of the hand.

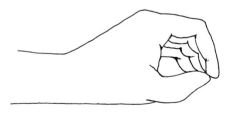

Figure 12-30. Functional position of the wrist and hand. The wrist is in slight extension, the MCP and PIP joints are in some degree of flexion, and the thumb is in opposition.

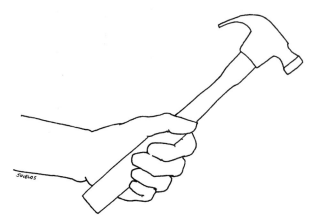

Figure 12-31.   Power grip.

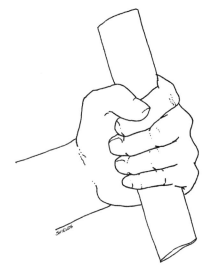

Figure 12-33.   Cylindrical grip.

fingers tend to flex around the object in one direction and the thumb wraps around in the opposite direction, providing a counterforce to keep the object in contact with the palm and/or fingers. Once the object is firmly set in the hand, it can be moved about in space by more proximal joint musculature. The long finger flexors (extrinsics) grip the object, and the long finger extensors (also extrinsics) assist in holding the wrist in a neutral or slightly extended position. When the thumb is involved, it tends to be in an adducted position.

The three commonly described power grips are cylindrical, spherical, and hook. The **cylindrical grip** (Fig. 12-33) has all the fingers flexed around the object, which usually lies at a right angle to the forearm. The thumb is wrapped around the object in the opposite direction, often overlapping the fingers. Examples of a cylindrical grip would be holding a hammer, racquet, or wheelbarrow handle.

A variation of the cylindrical grip has the fingers flexed around a handle in a graded fashion (Fig. 12-34). The fifth finger joints are flexed the most, and the second finger joints are only partly flexed. The

thumb lies parallel and against the handle, and the wrist is in slight ulnar deviation. The advantage of this grip over a cylindrical grip is that it allows a forceful but more controlled use of the tool. Examples of this type of grip would involve holding a golf club or screwdriver.

A **spherical grip** has all the fingers and thumb adducted around an object, and unlike the cylindrical grip, the fingers are more spread apart. The palm of the hand is often not involved (Fig. 12-35). Activities involving a spherical grip would be holding an apple or doorknob, or picking up a glass by its top.

The **hook grip** involves the second through fifth fingers flexed around an object in a hooklike manner (Fig. 12-36). The MCP joints are extended, and the PIP and DIP joints are in some degree of flexion. The thumb is usually not involved. Therefore, this is the only power grip possible if a person has a median nerve injury and loses the ability to oppose the thumb. Examples of a hook grip are seen when holding on to a handle, like a suitcase, wagon, or bucket.

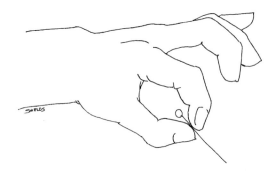

Figure 12-32.   Precision grip.

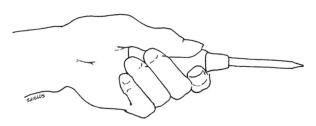

Figure 12-34.   Cylindrical grip variation.

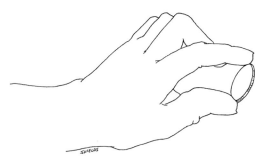

Figure 12-37. Pinch grip.

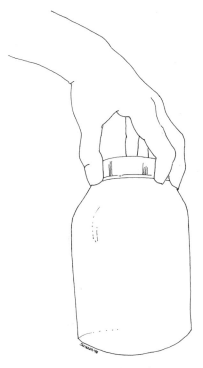

Figure 12-35. Spherical grip.

Precision Grips

Precision grips tend to hold the object between the tips of the fingers and thumb. The intrinsic muscles are involved along with the extrinsics. The thumb tends to be abducted. These grips provide more fine movement

and accuracy. The object is usually small, even fragile. The palm does not tend to be involved, and the proximal joints do not tend to move. There are four commonly recognized types of precision grip.

With the **pad-to-pad grip,** the MCP and PIP joints of the finger(s) are flexed, the thumb is abducted, and the distal joints of both are extended, bringing the pads of the finger(s) and thumb together. It may involve the thumb and one finger, usually the index finger, which is called a **pinch grip** (Fig. 12-37). It may also involve the thumb and two fingers, usually the index and middle fingers. This is called a **three-jaw chuck.** If you observe how a power drill holds the drill bit in place, you will see the similarity to this grip (Fig. 12-38). There are three "jaws" pinching in on the drill bit and the entire holding mechanism is called a "chuck." Holding a pen or pencil would be an example of this grip. This is by far the most common precision grip.

Similar to the pad-to-pad grip, the **tip-to-tip grip** involves bringing the tip of the thumb up against the tip of another digit, usually the index finger, to pick up a small object such as a coin or pin (see Fig. 12-32). It is also called **pincer grip.** This type of grip becomes difficult, if not impossible, with very long fingernails.

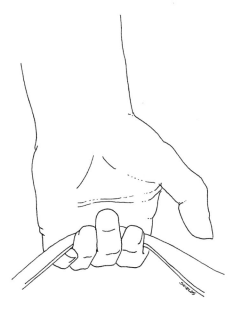

Figure 12-36. Hook grip.

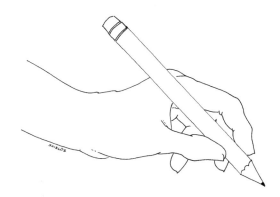

Figure 12-38. Three-jaw chuck grip.

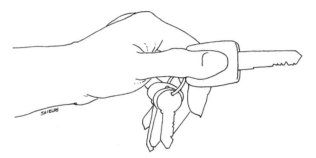

Figure 12-39.   Pad-to-side grip.

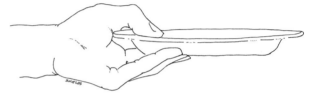

Figure 12-41.   Lumbrical grip.

The **pad-to-side grip,** also called lateral prehension, has the pad of the extended thumb pressing an object against the radial side of the index finger (Fig. 12-39). This is a strong grip, but allows less fine movements than the other two types. The terminal device of upper extremity prostheses adapts this type of grip. Also, because this grip does not require an opposed thumb, a person who has lost opposition but has retained thumb adduction can grasp and hold small objects.

The **side-to-side grip,** somewhat similar to pad-to-side grip, requires adduction of two fingers, usually the index or middle fingers (Fig. 12-40). It is a weak grip and does not permit much precision. It is perhaps most frequently used to hold a cigarette. It is also used to hold an object, like a pencil, between two fingers while using another pencil or pen. Because the

thumb is not involved, this grip could be used in the absence of the thumb.

Lumbrical grip, sometimes referred to as the **plate grip,** has the MCP and PIP joints flexed and the DIP joints extended. The thumb opposes the fingers holding an object horizontal (Fig. 12-41). This grip is usually used when something needs to be kept horizontal such as a plate or tray. It is called a lumbrical grip because the action of the lumbrical muscles is to flex the MCP joints while extending the IP joints.

Points to Remember

- Isometric contractions are used to stabilize or hold a body part in position.
- Cylindrical, spherical, and hook grips are used for power hand movements.
- Pad-to-pad, pinch, three-jaw chuck, tip-to-tip, pad-to-side, side-to-side, and lumbrical grips are used for precision hand movements.

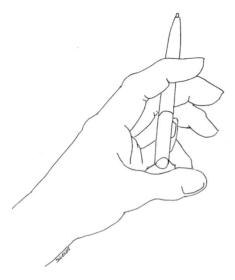

Figure 12-40.   Side-to-side grip.

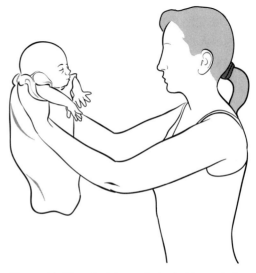

Figure 12-42.   Activity analysis: holding a baby.

Review Questions

General Anatomy Questions

1. Which finger and thumb motions occur in:
   a. the frontal plane around the sagittal axis?
   b. the sagittal plane around the frontal axis?
   c. the transverse plane around the vertical axis?

2. Compare the thumb and fingers:
   a. Number of bones
      Thumb _____
      Finger _____
   b. Number of joints
      Thumb _____
      Finger _____
   c. Names of the joints
      Thumb _____
      Finger _____

3. Thumb opposition is a combination of what motions?

4. Which of the thumb opposition motions is an accessory motion?

5. What is the purpose of the retinaculum?

6. What structures make up the carpal tunnel? Which tendons and nerve run through the carpal tunnel?

7. What is an extrinsic muscle? List the extrinsic muscles of the hand.

8. What is an intrinsic muscle? List the intrinsic muscles of the hand.

9. Explain the difference between thenar muscles and hypothenar muscles, and give an example of each.

10. What is the "anatomical snuffbox"? Which muscles act as the borders of this area?

11. What hand muscle does not have a bony attachment? To what two tendons does it attach?

Functional Activity Questions

Identify the type of power or precision grip used in the following activities:

1. Holding the handle of a skillet

2. Pulling a little red wagon

3. Turning pages of a book

4. Fastening a snap or button

5. Carrying a coffee mug by its handle

6. Holding a hand of playing cards

7. Holding an apple

8. Holding on to a barbell

9. Analyze the following activity in terms of the entire upper extremity action. Hold an infant with your hands on either side of the infant's trunk so that you are looking eye-to-eye (Fig.12–42).
   a. A combination of what two types of grasp is used?
   b. The wrist is being held in a neutral position by isometric contractions occurring in two different planes. What are the two muscle groups involved?
   c. Name the wrist muscle prime movers of these two muscles groups.
   d. The forearm is in midposition between pronation and supination. What muscle group is holding the elbow in position isometrically?
   e. Name the elbow prime movers of this muscle group.
   f. The shoulder joint is being held in position by isometric contractions occurring in two different planes. What are the two muscle groups involved?
   g. Name the shoulder prime movers of these two muscle groups
   h. What shoulder girdle positions occur with the shoulder joint positions?
   i. Name the shoulder girdle prime movers.

Clinical Exercise Questions

Identify the joint motion and prime movers involved in the following exercises:

1. Keeping the fingers straight, spread them wide apart; bring them together.

2. With your forearm supinated and the thumb next to the radial side of the index finger, raise it straight up from the palm.

3. Touch the tip of your thumb to the tip of the little finger.

4. Keep the fingers straight and bend at the knuckles.

5. Starting with the thumb next to the radial side of the index finger, move it across the palm toward the little finger.

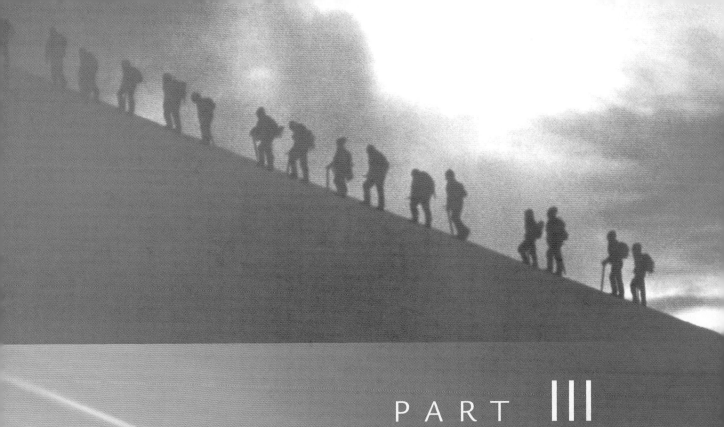

PART III

Clinical Kinesiology and Anatomy of the Trunk

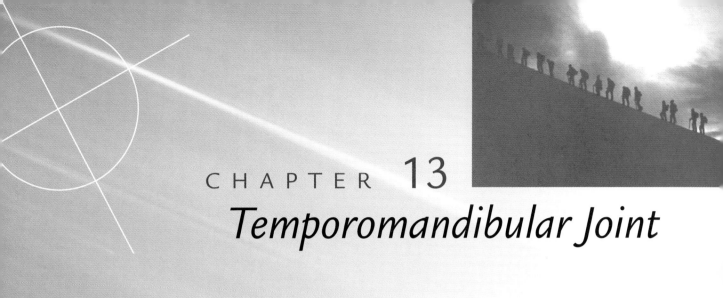

CHAPTER 13
Temporomandibular Joint

Joint Structure and Motions

Bones and Landmarks

Ligaments and Other Structures

Mechanics of Movement

Muscles of the TMJ

Summary of Muscle Action

Summary of Muscle Innervation

Points to Remember

Review Questions

General Anatomy Questions

Functional Activity Questions

Clinical Exercise Questions

Joint Structure and Motions

The temporomandibular joint, often referred to as the TMJ, is one of the most frequently used joints in the body. It is used during chewing, swallowing, yawning, talking, and any other activity involving jaw motion. The TMJ is located anterior to the ear and at the posterior superior end of the jaw (Fig. 13-1). It is made up of the articular fossa of the temporal bone superiorly, articulating with the condyle of the mandible inferiorly. It is a synovial joint and is best described as having a hingelike shape. It is not a pure hinge joint because it also allows some gliding motion.

The TMJ is made up of two bones, a disk that divides the joint into two joint spaces, a joint capsule, four ligaments, and four main muscles that create five motions. The joint motions are **depression** (opening the mouth), **mandibular elevation** (closing the mouth), **lateral deviation** (side-to-side jaw movement), **protrusion,** or *protraction,* (moving the jaw forward), and **retrusion,** or *retraction,* (moving the jaw posteriorly) (Fig. 13-2). Retrusion is basically the return to anatomical position from a protruded position.

When the mandible is at rest, the condyle of the mandible is seated in the mandibular fossa of the temporal bone. The normal resting position of the mandible is with the lips closed and teeth several millimeters apart. This is maintained by low levels of activity of the temporalis muscles (Basmajian, 1978). The mouth should open far enough for you to be able to put two to three fingers between the front upper and lower teeth.

Bones and Landmarks

The skull consists of two parts: the bones of the large cranium cavity, which encases the brain, and the bones

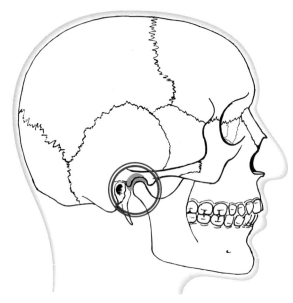

Figure 13-1.   The temporomandibular joint (TMJ) is highlighted within the circle.

of the face (Fig. 13-3). The TMJ is made up of the mandible, a facial bone articulating with the temporal bone, a cranial bone. Surrounding bones provide an area for muscle and ligament attachment. The following is a description of the bones and landmarks significant to the TMJ.

The **mandible,** or **mandibular bone** (Figs. 13-4 and 13-5) is shaped somewhat like a horseshoe and it articulates with the temporal bone on each side of the face. It consists of a body and two upwardly projecting rami Therefore, although the mandible is considered one bone, each lateral end articulates with a temporal bone, forming two identical joints on either side of the face. The mandible makes up the inferior part of the face and is often referred to as the jaw or lower jaw. Its significant landmarks are as follows:

Angle
Located between the body and ramus, and the joining point of the two landmarks.

Body
The horizontal portion of the mandible; the superior surface of the body holds the lower teeth.

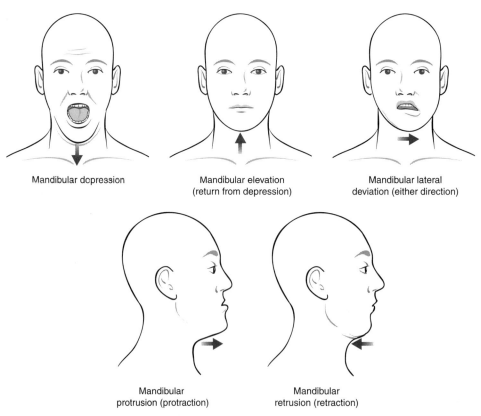

Mandibular depression

Mandibular elevation
(return from depression)

Mandibular lateral
deviation (either direction)

Mandibular
protrusion (protraction)

Mandibular
retrusion (retraction)

Figure 13-2.   TMJ motions.

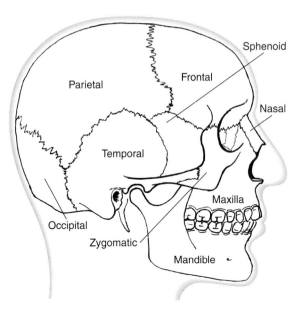

Figure 13-3. Bones of the skull.

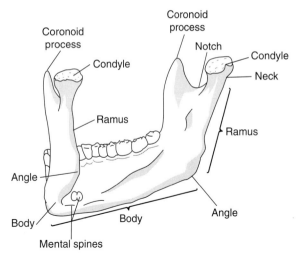

Figure 13-5. The bony landmarks of the mandible, posterior and slightly lateral view.

Condyle

Also called the condylar process. It is the posterior projection on the ramus and it articulates with the temporal bone.

Coronoid process

Located anterior to the condyle on the ramus. It serves as an attachment for the masseter muscle.

Mental spine

Located on the interior side (inside) of the mandible near the midline. It serves as an attachment for the geniohyoid muscle.

Neck

Located just inferior to the condyle.

Notch

Located between the condyle and coronoid process on the ramus.

Ramus

The vertical portion of the mandible from the angle to the condyle.

The **temporal bone** is located on the side of the skull posterior to the zygomatic bone, inferior to the parietal bone, posterior to the greater wing of the sphenoid, and anterior to the occipital bone (see Fig. 13-3). The articular portion of the temporal bone is made up of the concave articular (mandibular) fossa in the middle, with the convex articular tubercle located anteriorly and the convex postglenoid tubercle located posteriorly (Fig. 13-6). Its main landmarks consist of:

Articular tubercle

Makes up the anterior portion of the articulating surface of the temporal bone. When the mandible is depressed, the condyle of the mandible rests under this landmark.

Articular fossa

Also called the mandibular fossa, it lies anterior to the external auditory meatus and articulates with the condyle of the mandible.

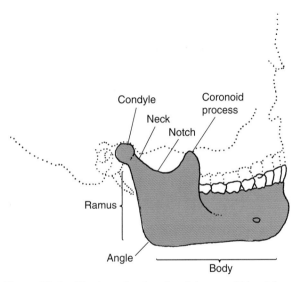

Figure 13-4. The bony landmarks of the mandible, right lateral view.

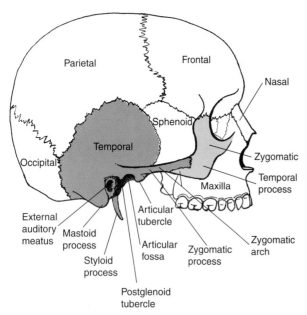

Figure 13-6. The bony landmarks of the temporal and zygomatic bones, Right lateral view of skull with mandible removed.

Postglenoid tubercle

Makes up the posterior wall of the fossa, and is located just anterior to the external auditory meatus.

Styloid process.

A slender projection positioned down and forward from the temporal bone on the inferior, slightly interior, surface. It serves as attachment for various muscles and ligaments.

Mastoid process

Bony prominence posterior and inferior to the ear to which the digastric muscle attaches.

External auditory meatus

The external opening for the ear, located posterior to the TMJ.

Zygomatic process

Makes up the posterior portion of the zygomatic arch. It serves as the attachment for the masseter.

The **sphenoid bone** is located at the lateral base of the skull anterior to the temporal bone. It resembles a bat with extended wings (Fig. 13-7). Because of its location, the sphenoid bone connects with six other cranial bones and two facial bones. Only the following external surface features are relevant to TMJ function:

Greater wing

A large bony process located medial to the zygomatic bone and arch, and anterior to the rest of the temporal bone. As part of the temporal fossa, it provides attachment for the temporalis and lateral pterygoid muscles.

Lateral pterygoid plate

Lies deep to the zygomatic arch. It serves as an attachment for the lateral and medial pterygoid muscles.

Spine

Lies deep to the articular fossa of the temporal bone and provides attachment for the sphenomandibular ligament.

The **zygomatic bone** forms the prominence of the cheek and contributes the lateral wall and floor of the eye orbit (see Fig. 13-6). The frontal, maxilla, sphenoid, and temporal bones border it. The zygomatic bone, along with the zygomatic process of the temporal bone, forms the zygomatic arch, to which the masseter attaches. Only the following feature is relevant to TMJ function:

Temporal process

Lies posterior and inferior and joins with the zygomatic process of the temporal bone to form the zygomatic arch.

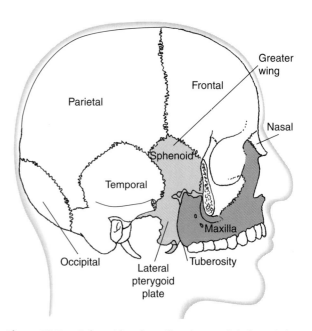

Figure 13-7. Sphenoid and maxillary bones, right lateral view with zygomatic arch removed.

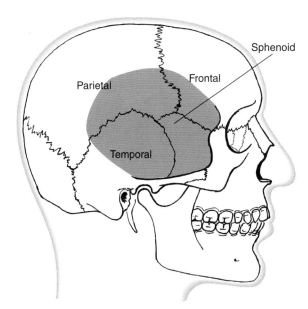

Figure 13-8. Temporal fossa includes portions of the temporal, parietal, frontal, and sphenoid bones.

The following are made up of combinations of skull bones (Fig. 13-8):

Temporal fossa
Bony floor formed by the zygomatic, frontal, parietal, sphenoid, and temporal bones. It contains the attachment of the temporalis muscle.

Zygomatic arch
Formed by two bones; the zygomatic process of the temporal bone posteriorly and the temporal process of the zygomatic bone anteriorly.

The **maxilla** or **maxillary bone** is commonly called the upper jaw. It is located in the upper part of the face and houses the upper teeth. It connects with the nasal bone superiorly and the zygomatic bone laterally (see Fig. 13-7).

Tuberosity
A rounded projection located on the inferior posterior angle. It serves as attachment for the medial pterygoid.

The **hyoid bone** is a horseshoe-shaped bone lying just superior to the thyroid cartilage at about the level of C3. It has no bony articulation, but is suspended from the styloid processes of the temporal bones by the stylohoid ligaments (Fig. 13-9). Its main function is to provide attachment for the tongue muscles. However, it also provides attachment for the suprahyoid and infrahyoid muscles that have an assisting role in mandibular depression.

The **thyroid cartilage** is the largest of the nine cartilages of larynx. It is commonly called the "Adam's apple" and tends to be more prominent in males. It lies just inferior to the hyoid bone at about the level of C3 to C4 (see Fig. 13-9). It provides attachment for the infrahyoid muscles.

Ligaments and Other Structures

The **lateral ligament** is also known as the **temporomandibular ligament.** Anteriorly, it attaches on the neck of the mandibular condyle and disk, and then runs superiorly to the articular tubercle of the temporal bone (Fig. 13-10). It limits downward, posterior, and lateral motions of the mandible.

The **sphenomandibular ligament** attaches to the spine of the sphenoid bone and runs to the middle of the ramus on the internal surface of the mandible (see Figs. 13-10 and 13-11). It suspends the mandible and limits excessive anterior motion.

The **stylomandibular ligament** runs from the styloid process of the temporal bone to the posterior inferior border of the ramus of the mandible (see Figs. 13-10 and 13-11). It lies between the masseter and

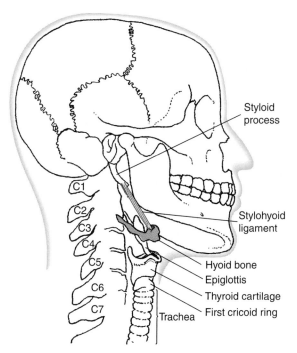

Figure 13-9. The hyoid bone is suspended from the styloid process of the temporal bone by the stylohyoid ligament. Right side view.

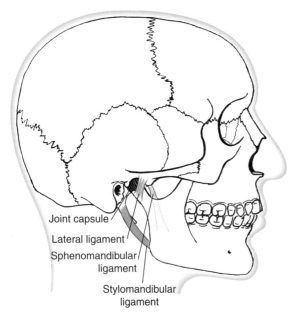

Figure 13-10.   The ligaments that suspend and/or limit excessive motion of the mandible. Right lateral view. Sphenomandibular ligament (distal attachment on medial side) is shown with dotted lines.

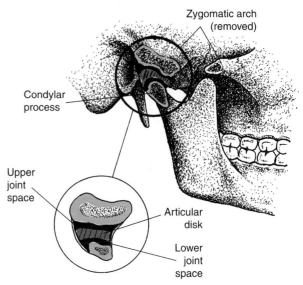

Figure 13-12.   Lateral view of the right TMJ with zygomatic arch removed and condylar process cut. This shows the relationship of the mandibular condyle, disk, and articular fossa in a closed-jaw position. The articular disk divides the joint space into upper and lower spaces.

medial pterygoid muscles and has a role in limiting excessive anterior motion.

The **stylohyoid ligament** attaches from the styloid process of the temporal bone to the hyoid bone (see Fig. 13-9). Its function is to hold the hyoid bone in place.

The **joint capsule** envelops the TMJ by attaching superiorly to the articular tubercle and borders of the

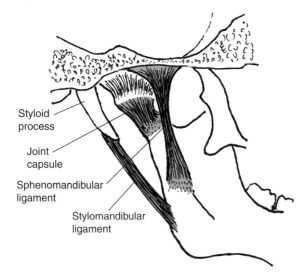

Figure 13-11.   Medial (inside) view of left TMJ shows joint capsule and ligaments. Lateral ligament is not visible from this view.

fossa of the temporal bone. Inferiorly, it attaches to the neck of the condyle of the mandible (see Figs. 13-10 and 13-11).

The **articular disk** of the TMJ is similar to the articular disk of the sternoclavicular joint. It is connected circumferentially to the capsule and tendon of the lateral pterygoid (Fig. 13-12). It also divides the joint space into two separate compartments: a larger upper joint space and a smaller lower joint space. The superior surface is both concave and convex to accommodate the shape of the fossa. The inferior surface is concave, accommodating the convex surface of the condyle and allowing the joint to remain congruent (compatible) throughout the motion. The disk's shape and attachments also allow it to rotate in an anterior/posterior direction on the condyle. Because the articular disk is more firmly attached to the mandible than the temporal bone, it allows the disk to move forward with the condyle of the mandible when the mouth opens. It returns posteriorly when the mouth closes.

Mechanics of Movement

Depression of the mandible (opening the jaw) involves two motions (Fig. 13-13). The first part is accomplished by anterior rotation of the mandibular condyle on the disk. The second part of the motion involves a

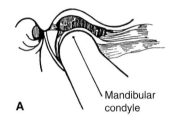

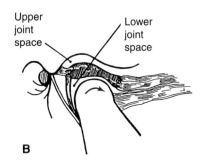

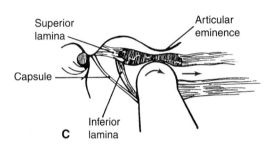

Figure 13-13.   Joint motion during mandibular depression (mouth opening). *(A)* Condyle sitting in articular fossa. *(B)* The condyle first rotates in the mandibular fossa, and *(C)* condyle then glides downward and forward over the articular eminence (tuberosity). (From Perry, JF, Rohe, DA, and Garcia, OA: The Kinesiology Workbook, ed 2. FA Davis, Philadelphia, 1996, p 168, with permission.)

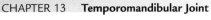

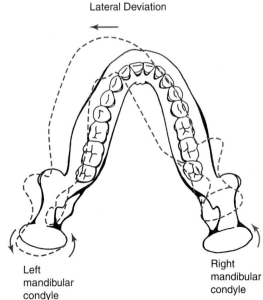

Figure 13-14.   Mandibular motion during lateral deviation to the left side—superior view. (Adapted from Perry, JF, Rohe, DA, and Garcia, OA: The Kinesiology Workbook, ed 2. FA Davis Company, Philadelphia, 1996, p 175, with permission.)

and the right condyle will slide forward (Fig. 13-14). This rotation occurs around a vertical axis.

Muscles of the TMJ

The TMJ is involved in activities such as talking, chewing, biting, swallowing, and yawning. Several muscles come into play, often in a synergistic manner. The muscles primarily involved are listed below. Unless stated otherwise, the action is considered a bilateral action that is occurring at each joint (right and left) simultaneously.

Temporalis	Medial pterygoid
Masseter	Lateral pterygoid

Other muscles involved in TMJ movements are:

Suprahyoid muscles	Infrahyoid muscles
Mylohyoid	Sternohyoid
Geniohyoid	Sternothyroid
Stylohoid	Thyrohyoid
Digastric	Omohyoid

The **temporalis** is a rather broad and fan-shaped muscle that lies in the temporal fossa (see Figs. 13-8 and 13-15). Because of its fan shape, the more anterior fibers run almost vertically, the middle fibers are at a diagonal, and the posterior fibers are nearly horizontal. From the temporal fossa, the fibers come together to form a

sliding of the disk and condyle forward and downward under the articular tubercle. Elevation of the mandible (closing the jaw) is the reverse action. It involves sliding the disk and condyle posteriorly and superiorly, which rotates the condyle posteriorly on the disk. These movements occur in the sagittal plane.

Protrusion and retrusion involve anterior/posterior movement in the horizontal plane. There is no rotation. All parts of the mandible move forward and backward the same amount. The mandibular condyle and disk move as one unit against the articular fossa of the temporal bone.

Lateral movement also occurs in the horizontal plane. It involves one condyle rotating in the articular fossa while the other condyle slides forward. To move the mandible toward the left, the left condyle will spin

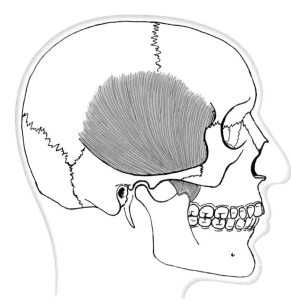

Figure 13-15. Temporalis muscle.

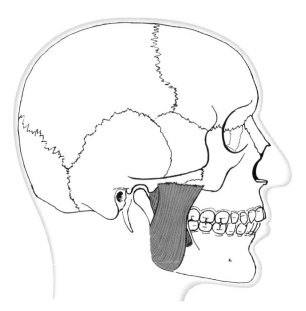

Figure 13-16. Masseter muscle.

tendon that passes deep to the zygomatic arch to insert on the coronoid process and anterior border of the ramus of the mandible. Its primary function is to elevate the mandible. Because of the horizontal direction of the posterior fibers, they also retract the jaw. In side-to-side movements, the temporalis contracts on one side, moving the mandible to the same side (ipsilaterally).

Temporalis Muscle

O	Temporal fossa
I	Coronoid process and ramus of mandible
A	Bilaterally: elevation, retrusion (posterior fibers) Unilaterally: ipsilateral lateral deviation
N	Trigeminal nerve (cranial nerve V)

The powerful **masseter** is a thick, almost quadrilateral-shaped muscle that produces the fullness of the posterior part of the cheek between the mandibular angle and zygomatic arch (Fig. 13-16). It is made up of two parts: the larger, superficial part, and the smaller, deep portion. The superficial part arises from the zygomatic process of the maxilla and inferior border of the zygomatic arch of the temporal bone. The deep part comes from the inferior and medial borders of the zygomatic arch. The two parts run inferiorly and posteriorly, coming together to attach on the angle of the ramus and coronoid process of the mandible. Both parts act as one muscle to elevate the mandible (close the jaw). Acting unilaterally, the masseter is an ipsilateral (same side) lateral deviator.

Masseter Muscle

O	Zygomatic arch of temporal bone and zygomatic process of maxilla
I	Angle of the ramus and coronoid process of mandible
A	Bilaterally: elevation Unilaterally: ipsilateral lateral deviation
N	Trigeminal nerve (cranial nerve V)

Although it is less powerful, the **medial pterygoid** is very similar to the masseter muscle. It is located on the medial side (inside) of the mandibular ramus (Fig. 13-17); the more superficial masseter is on the lateral side (outside). It arises from the medial side of the lateral pterygoid plate of the sphenoid bone and the tuberosity of the maxilla. It runs inferiorly, laterally, and posteriorly to attach on the medial side of the ramus and angle of the mandible (Fig. 13-18). Its actions are mandibular elevation, protrusion, and contralateral (opposite side) lateral deviation.

Medial Pterygoid Muscle

O	Lateral pterygoid plate of the sphenoid bone and tuberosity of the maxilla
I	Ramus and angle of the mandible
A	Bilaterally: elevation, protrusion Unilaterally: contralateral lateral deviation
N	Trigeminal nerve (cranial nerve V)

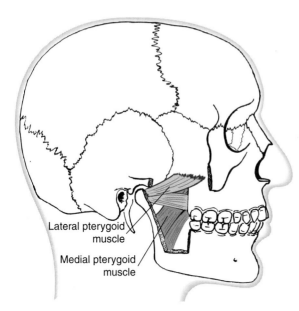

Figure 13-17. Lateral and medial pterygoid muscles. The mandible and zygomatic arch are cut to show inside the mandible.

The **lateral pterygoid** muscle is short, thick, and somewhat cone-shaped. It has two heads: superior and inferior. The superior part comes off the lateral surface of the greater wing of the sphenoid bone. The inferior, more horizontal part comes off the lateral surface of the lateral pterygoid plate. Both parts run nearly horizontal in a posterior and lateral direction. They attach

on the neck of the mandibular condyle, the articular disk, and the capsule (see Figs. 13-17 and 13-18). This muscle depresses, protrudes, and laterally deviates the mandible to the opposite side (contralateral).

Lateral Pterygoid Muscle

O	Lateral pterygoid plate and greater wing of the sphenoid
I	Mandibular condyle and articular disk
A	Bilaterally: depression, protrusion Unilaterally: contralateral lateral deviation
N	Trigeminal nerve (cranial nerve V)

The **suprahyoid muscles,** as their name implies, are a group of muscles located above the hyoid bone. They connect the hyoid bone to the skull, primarily to the mandible. Individually, these muscles are known as the mylohyoid, geniohyoid, stylohyoid, and digastric muscles. Although their primary function is to elevate the hyoid, they can assist in mandibular depression when the infrahyoid muscles stabilize the hyoid bone. Therefore, these muscles will be described here in terms of their importance to the TMJ only.

The **mylohyoid** is a broad muscle running from the interior (inside) medial part of the mandible to the superior border of the hyoid bone (Figs. 13-19 and 13-20). The **geniohyoid** is a narrow muscle located superior to the mylohyoid (Fig. 13-19). It attaches to the mental spine on the inside midline of the mandible and runs down to the hyoid. The **digastric** muscle has two bellies connected in the middle by a tendon (Figs. 13-20 and 13-21). The anterior belly goes from the internal inferior surface of the mandible near the midline posteriorly and inferiorly, where it attaches to the tendinous inscription at the hyoid bone. The tendon is

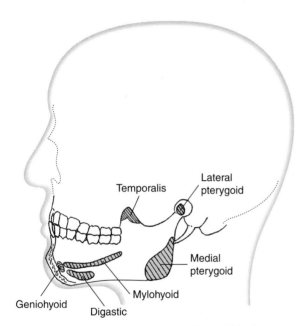

Figure 13-18. Medial (inside) view of mandible showing muscle attachments.

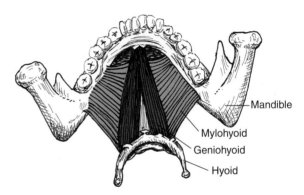

Figure 13-19. Muscles of the floor of the mouth. Posterior, superior view (looking down toward the front inside of the mandible).

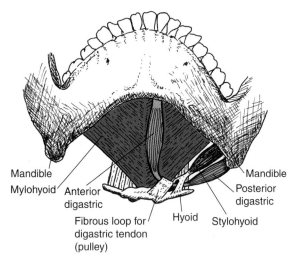

Mandible

Mylohyoid   Anterior
digastric

Mandible

Posterior
digastric

Fibrous loop for
digastric tendon
(pulley)

Hyoid   Stylohyoid

Figure 13-20. Muscles of the floor of the mouth. Anterior, inferior view (looking up under chin from the front). Geniohyoid muscle is not visible from this view.

held in place by a fibrous sling attached to the hyoid bone. From this point the posterior belly runs posterior and superior to attach to the mastoid process of the temporal bone. This pulleylike tendon is an example of how a muscle changes its line of pull. The **stylohyoid** is almost parallel to the digastric muscle. It attaches to the styloid process of the temporal bone and goes to the hyoid bone (see Fig. 13-20).

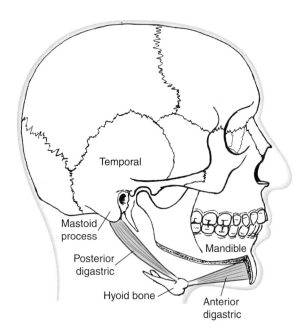

Temporal

Mastoid
process

Posterior
digastric

Hyoid bone

Mandible

Anterior
digastric

Figure 13-21. The digastric muscle. Right lateral view with the mandible cut away to show anterior attachment.

Mylohyoid Muscle

O	Interior medial mandible
I	Hyoid
A	Assists in depressing mandible
N	Branch of trigeminal nerve (cranial nerve V)

Geniohyoid Muscle

O	Mental spine of mandible
I	Hyoid
A	Assists in depressing mandible
N	Branch of C1 via hypoglossal nerve (cranial nerve XII)

Stylohyoid Muscle

O	Styloid process of temporal bone
I	Hyoid
A	Assists in depressing mandible
N	Branch of facial nerve (cranial nerve VII)

Digastric Muscle

O	Anterior: internal inferior mandible Posterior: mastoid process
I	Via pulleylike tendon to hyoid
A	Assists in depressing mandible
N	Branch of trigeminal nerve (cranial nerve V) and branch of facial nerve (cranial nerve VII)

The **infrahyoid muscles,** as their name implies, are located below the hyoid bone and serve to depress it (Fig. 13-22). Individually, these muscles are known as the sternohyoid, sternothyroid, thyrohyoid, and omohyoid muscles. In terms of their effect on the TMJ, they stabilize the hyoid bone, allowing the suprahyoid muscles to depress the mandible. These muscles will be described here in terms of their importance to the TMJ only.

The **sternohyoid** is a thin, narrow muscle that runs vertically next to the midline from the posterior aspect of the medial end of the clavicle, sternoclavicular ligament, and sternal manubrium. It is covered distally by the sternocleidomastoid. It, like all the infrahyoid muscles, attaches to the inferior border of the hyoid bone. The sternothyroid is shorter, wider, and lies deep to the sternohyoid. It runs vertically from the sternal manubrium and cartilage of the first rib to the thyroid cartilage. It indirectly pulls down on the hyoid bone by

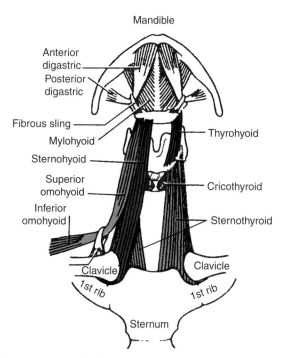

Figure 13-22.   Infrahyoid muscles. Anterior view showing inferior mandible, hyoid bone, thyroid cartilage, superior sternum, and medial end of clavicle. Left side shows more superficial muscle layer, and right side shows deeper muscles. (From Moore, K: Clinically Oriented Anatomy, ed. 2. Williams & Wilkins, Baltimore, 1985, p 1001, with permission.)

pulling down on the thyroid cartilage, which, in turn, is connected to the hyoid bone via the thyrohyoid muscle. The **thyrohyoid** is a short, rectangular muscle that acts much like a continuation of the sternothyroid muscle. It runs from the thyroid cartilage vertically to the inferior border of the hyoid bone. It serves to close the laryngeal opening, thus preventing food from going into the larynx during swallowing. In terms of the TMJ, it pulls down on the hyoid bone, stabilizing it so that the suprahyoid muscles can assist in depressing the jaw.

The **omohyoid** has two bellies connected by a tendon in between, much like the digastric muscle. The inferior belly comes off the superior border of the scapula and runs mostly horizontally. At the tendinous inscription, the muscle changes direction and the superior belly runs mostly vertically to the inferior border of the hyoid. The tendon is held in place by a fibrous sling attached to the clavicle that allows the muscle to make an almost right-angle turn. This is another example of an internal fixed pulley changing the line of pull of a muscle. This muscle also stabilizes the hyoid bone by pulling down on it.

Sternohyoid Muscle

O	Medial end of clavicle, sternoclavicular ligament, and manubrium of sternum
I	Inferior border of hyoid bone
A	Stabilize hyoid bone
N	Branch of hypoglossal nerve (cranial nerve XII) communicating with C1 to C3

Sternothyroid Muscle

O	Manubrium of sternum and cartilage of the first rib
I	Thyroid cartilage
A	Stabilize hyoid bone
N	Branch of hypoglossal nerve (cranial nerve XII) communicating with C1 to C3

Thyrohyoid Muscle

O	Thyroid cartilage
I	Inferior border of hyoid bone
A	Stabilize hyoid bone
N	Branch of hypoglossal nerve (cranial nerve XII) communicating with C1

Omohyoid Muscle

O	Superior border of the scapula
I	Inferior border of hyoid bone
A	Stabilize hyoid bone
N	Branch of hypoglossal (cranial nerve XII) communicating with C1 to C3

Summary of Muscle Action

The actions of the prime movers of the temporomandibular joint are summarized as:

Mandibular Action	Muscle
Elevation	Temporalis, masseter medial pterygoid
Depression	Lateral pterygoid
Protrusion	Lateral pterygoid, medial pterygoid
Retrusion	Temporalis (posterior)
Ipsilateral lateral deviation	Temporalis, masseter
Contralateral lateral deviation	Medial pterygoid, lateral pterygoid

Summary of Muscle Innervation

The innervation of the TMJ muscles comes from cranial nerve V, the trigeminal nerve. If the assisting muscles of the suprahyoid and infrahyoid group are included,

Table 13-1	Innervation of TMJ Muscles	
Muscle	Nerve	Cranial Nerve Number
Temporalis	Trigeminal	CN 5
Masseter	Trigeminal	CN 5
Lateral pterygoid	Trigeminal	CN 5
Medial pterygoid	Trigeminal	CN 5
Suprahyoid group		
Mylohyoid	Trigeminal	CN 5
Geniohyoid	C1, hypoglossal	CN 12
Stylohyoid	Facial	CN 7
Digastric	Trigeminal, facial	CN 5, 7
Infrahyoid group		
Sternohyoid	C1 to C3, hypoglossal	CN 12
Sternothyroid	C1 to C3, hypoglossal	CN 12
Thyrohyoid	C1, hypoglossal	CN 12
Omohyoid	C1 to C3, hypoglossal	CN 12

innervation additionally comes from cranial nerves VII and XII (the facial and hypoglossal nerves, respectively). The hypoglossal nerve communicates with the first three cervical nerves as well. Innervation of all TMJ muscles is summarized in Table 13-1.

Points to Remember

- The trigeminal nerve is the fifth cranial nerve, which has both sensory and motor components.

- The sensory component of the trigeminal nerves involves the facial area, while the motor component involves the chewing muscles.
- The facial nerve is the seventh cranial nerve which also has sensory and motor components.
- The sensory component of the facial nerve involve the tongue area, whereas the motor component involves the muscles of the face.

Review Questions

General Anatomy Questions

1. The zygomatic arch is made up of which two bones?
2. Synonymous terms for TMJ motions are:
   a. Opening the jaw
   b. Closing the jaw
   c. Moving the jaw posteriorly
   d. Moving the jaw anteriorly
   e. Moving the jaw toward the side
3. What two bones make up the temporomandibular joint?
4. What muscle can be palpated superior and anterior to the ear?
5. What muscle makes up the fullness of the posterior portion of the cheek?

6. What muscle works like a pulley?
7. The muscle in question No. 5 performs which pulley function?
8. If the fifth and seventh cranial nerves were damaged, which would impair function of the TMJ more?
9. Two motions occur during mandibular depression: (1) sliding the disk and condyle posteriorly and superiorly and (2) anterior rotation of the mandible on the disk. Which occurs first?
10. Lateral deviation of the mandible to the left involves both spinning and sliding motions. Describe how that happens.
11. What is another term for "Adam's apple"?

Functional Activity Questions

1. Forming the letter "O" with your lips requires what motion of the TMJ?

2. Biting off a tough piece of bread is usually done by placing it in one side of the mouth.
   a. The biting action requires what motion of the TMJ?
   b. Which side of the jaw experiences some distraction?
   c. Which side of the jaw experiences some compression?

3. Grinding your teeth could involve motions in the sagittal plane and frontal plane. What are these motions?

4. Clenching your teeth involves what TMJ motion and muscles?

Clinical Exercise Questions

1. Sit in a good posture position with your hands on each side of your jaw. Move your jaw from side to side against slight resistance.
   a. What is the joint motion?
   b. What type of contraction is occurring? (isometric, concentric, eccentric).
   c. Name the muscles responsible for moving the jaw to the right.

2. Sit in a good posture position with your thumb beneath your chin. Open your mouth against slight pressure. (Fig 13-23)
   a. What is the joint motion?
   b. What type of muscle contraction is occurring?
   c. Name the muscles responsible for moving the mouth.

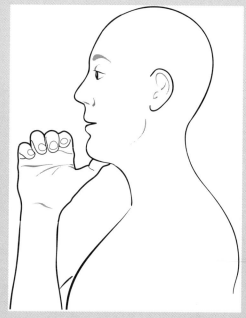

Figure 13-23.   Opening mouth against slight pressure.

3. Sit in a good posture position with your index and middle fingers on the anterior surface of your lower jaw in the midline. Without allowing your fingers to move, push against them with your lower jaw. Describe (a) the joint action, (b) the type of contraction (isometric, concentric, eccentric), and (c) the muscle(s) performing the action.
   a. What is the joint motion?
   b. What type of muscle contraction is occurring?
   c. Name the muscles responsible for moving the jaw to the right.

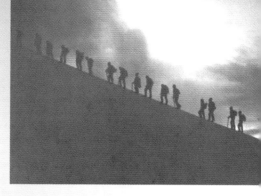

CHAPTER 14
Neck and Trunk

Vertebral Curves

Clarification of Terms

Joint Motions

Bones and Landmarks

Joints and Ligaments

Common Vertebral Column Pathologies

Muscles of the Neck and Trunk

Muscles of the Cervical Spine

Muscles of the Trunk

Summary of Muscle Actions

Summary of Muscle Innervation

Points to Remember

Review Questions

General Anatomy Questions

Functional Activity Questions

Clinical Exercise Questions

The vertebral column establishes and maintains the longitudinal axis of the body. Because it is a multijointed rod, the vertebral column's motions occur as the result of the combined motions of individual vertebrae.

The spinal column provides a pivot point for motion and support of the head at the cervical region. The weight of the head, shoulder girdle, upper extremities, and trunk are transmitted through the vertebral column. Because it encases the spinal cord, the vertebral column is able to provide protection to the cord. Not only does this multijointed rod provide movement, but the arrangement of these segments also provides effective shock absorption and transmission.

Sitting on this long, multijointed rod (vertebral column) is the skull. The skull is the bony structure of the head and can be divided into the bones of the cranium. The skull contains and protects the brain and the facial bones. Because the sensory organs for sight, hearing, taste, and vestibular responses are located within the cranium, it is important that the head be able to move freely. This occurs through movements at various levels of the cervical spine.

Vertebral Curves

The vertebrae are arranged in such a way as to form anterior-posterior (concave-convex) curves in the vertebral column, which can be seen from the side (Fig. 14-1). These curves provide the vertebral column with much more strength and resilience, approximately 10 times more than if it were a straight rod. The curves are summarized in Table 14-1.

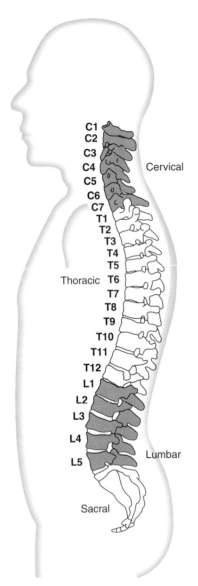

Figure 14-1. The anterior-posterior curves of the vertebral column.

Table 14-1	Vertebral Segments	
Segment	**Number**	**Anterior Curve**
Cervical	7	Convex
Thoracic	12	Concave
Lumbar	5	Convex
Sacral	5 (fused)	Concave

process of the vertebra below with the inferior articular process of the vertebra above (see Fig 14-5).

Joint Motions

The vertebral column as a whole is considered to be triaxial. Therefore, it has movement in all three planes (Fig. 14-2). **Flexion, extension,** and **hyperex-**

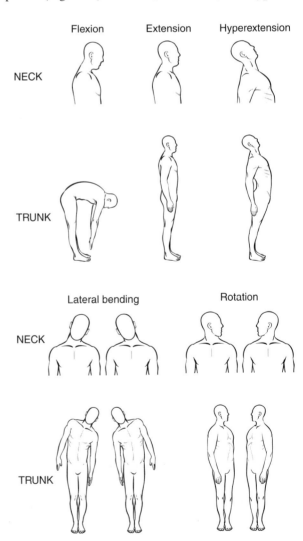

Figure 14-2. Motions of the neck and trunk.

Clarification of Terms

The term "spine" can be used in more than one way. The spinal cord, sometimes called the *spine,* is made of nervous tissue. The *spine, spinal column,* and *vertebral column* are synonymous terms referring to the bony components housing the spinal cord. This chapter discusses the spine as a bony structure.

Another term that needs clarifying is *facet.* A **facet** is a small, smooth, flat surface on a bone. Facets, as will be discussed, are found on thoracic vertebrae at the point of contact with a rib (see Fig 14-9). A **facet joint** is the articulation between the superior articular

tension occur in the sagittal plane around a frontal axis. **Lateral bending,** also called *side bending* or *lateral flexion,* occurs in the frontal plane around a sagittal axis. **Rotation** occurs in the transverse plane around a vertical axis, except between the skull and the atlas (C1). Alignment of the facet joints will greatly determine the amount of rotation and other motions possible.

The cervical spine allows movement and positioning of the head, and requires additional explanation. The articulation between the head and C1 (atlas) is often called the **atlanto-occipital joint.** The main motion here is **flexion** and **extension,** as when nodding your head in agreement. There is some lateral bending, although, most of this motion occurs between C1 and C2 at the atlantoaxial joint. Most rotation of the head on the neck, as in shaking your head in disagreement, occurs at these joints. The muscles having the most control over the head moving on the neck are the prevertebral muscles anteriorly and the suboccipital muscles posteriorly. Obviously, to have the ability to move the head on the neck, a muscle must have an attachment on the head and the cervical region. Tucking your chin in involves the head flexing on C1, as well as neck extension (C2–C7). This combined motion is sometimes referred to as *axial extension* or **cervical retraction.** Conversely, extending the head on C1 and flexing the neck (C2–C7) would be **cervical protraction.** Relaxed forward head posture, or looking at a computer screen through bifocals tends to accentuate cervical protraction. "Standing up straight" emphasizes cervical retraction.

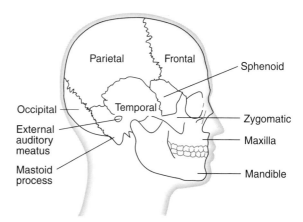

A

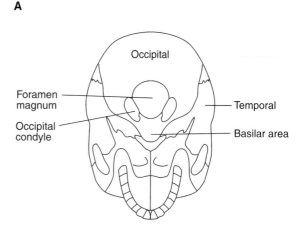

B

Figure 14-3. The bones of the skull as viewed from *(A)* lateral view and *(B)* the base of the skull, as seen from below.

Bones and Landmarks

The skull is made up of 21 separate bones and is considered the skeleton of the head (Fig. 14-3). Only those bones directly connected with the vertebral column will be discussed. They are as follows:

Occipital bone
Also called the occiput, it forms the posterior inferior part of the cranium.

Occipital protuberance
The small prominence in the center of the occiput.

Nuchal line
The ridge running horizontally along the back of the head from the occipital protuberance toward the mastoid processes.

Basilar area
Refers to the base, or inferior, portion of the occiput.

Foramen magnum
Opening in the occipital bone through which the spinal cord enters the cranium.

Occipital condyles
Located laterally to the foramen magnum on the occiput; provides articulation with the atlas (C1).

Temporal bone
Forms part of the base and lateral inferior sides of the cranium.

Mastoid process
Bony prominence behind the ear to which the sternocleidomastoid muscle attaches.

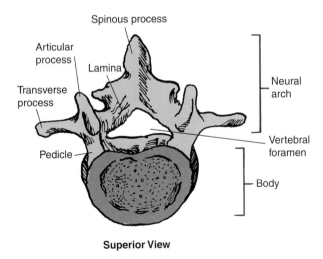

Superior View

Figure 14-4. The body landmarks of the anterior and posterior portions of a typical vertebra.

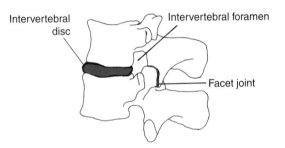

Figure 14-5. Lateral view of two vertebrae showing the intervertebral foramen and the facet joint. Both are formed by parts from each vertebra. The vertebrae are separated anteriorly by the intervertebral disk.

Vertebrae differ in size and shape but generally have the same layout (Figs. 14-4 and 14-5). The typical parts of a vertebra are as follows:

Body
Being primarily a cylindrical mass of cancellous bone, it is the anterior portion of the vertebra and the major weight-bearing structure. It is not present in the atlas (C1).

Between C3 and S1, bodies become progressively larger, bearing progressively more weight.

Neural arch
Also called the *vertebral arch,* it is the posterior portion of the vertebra with many different parts.

Vertebral foramen
Opening formed by the joining of the body and neural arch through which the spinal cord passes.

Pedicle
Portion of the neural arch just posterior to the body and anterior to the lamina.

Lamina
Posterior portion of the neural arch that unites from each side in the midline.

Transverse process
Formed at the union of the lamina and pedicle, the lateral projections of the arch to which muscles and ligaments attach.

Vertebral notches
Depressions located on the superior and inferior surfaces of the pedicle, and are so named (see Fig. 14-10).

Intervertebral foramen
Opening formed by the superior vertebral notch of foramen, the vertebra below, and the inferior vertebral notch of the vertebra above.

Articular process
Projecting superiorly and inferiorly off the posterior surface of each lamina, and so named.

Superior articular processes face posteriorly or medially, whereas inferior processes face anteriorly or laterally (see Fig. 14-10).

Spinous process
The most posterior projection on the neural arch; located at the junction of the two laminae. It serves as a point of attachment for many muscles and ligaments, and can be palpated throughout the length of the vertebral column.

Between each vertebra is an **intervertebral disk** that articulates with adjacent bodies (Figs. 14-5 and 14-6). There are 23 disks. Their main function is to absorb and transmit shock and maintain flexibility of the vertebral column. The disks make up approximately 25 percent of the total length of the vertebral column.

Annulus fibrosus
The outer portion of the disk consisting of several concentrically arranged fibrocartilaginous rings that serve to contain the nucleus pulposus.

Nucleus pulposus
Pulpy gelatinous substance with a high water content in the center of the disk. At birth, it is approximately 80 percent water, decreasing to less than 70 percent at 60 years of age. This is partially why an individual loses height with advanced age.

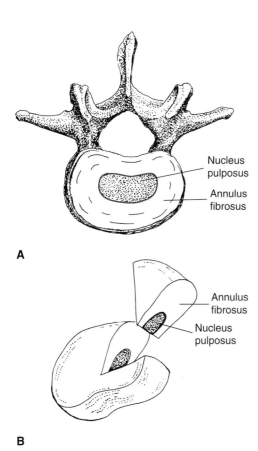

A

B

Figure 14-6. The two parts of the intervertebral disk. Viewed from above, the nucleus pulposus cannot be seen as it is covered by the annulus fibrosus. Its approximate location is show within the dotted lines. The longitudinal section view shows the relationship between the annulus fibrosus and nucleus pulposus.

There are a few vertebrae with distinguishing characteristics that must be identified. They are as follows:

Atlas (C1)
The first cervical vertebra upon which the cranium rests (Fig. 14-7). It is named after the Titan in Greek mythology who held up the Earth because it supports the globe of the head. The atlas is ring-shaped and has no body or spinous process.

Anterior arch
The anterior portion of C1.

Axis (C2)
The second cervical vertebra (Fig. 14-8) is so named because it forms the pivot upon which the atlas (C1), supporting the head, rotates.

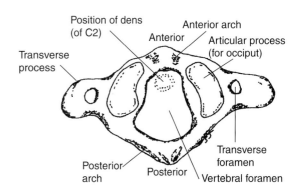

Figure 14-7. The parts of the first cervical vertebra (C1), also called the atlas. Superior view.

Dens
Also called the *odontoid process;* large vertical projection located anteriorly on the axis. Cervical rotation occurs through its articulation with the atlas.

C7
Also known as *vertebra prominens* because of its long and prominent spinous process. It resembles a thoracic vertebra and can be easily palpated with the neck in flexion.

Transverse foramen
Holes or openings in the transverse process of the cervical vertebra through which the vertebral artery passes (see Fig. 14-7).

Facet
Also called *costal facets,* they are located superiorly and inferiorly on the sides of the bodies and on the transverse processes of thoracic vertebrae

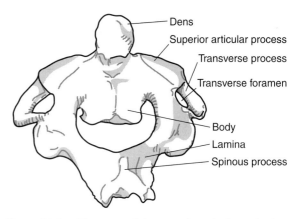

Figure 14-8. The parts of the second cervical vertebral (C2), also called the axis.

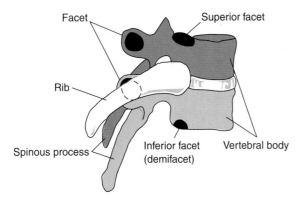

Figure 14-9. Costal facets (rib attachments) of the thoracic vertebrae

(Fig. 14-9). It is here that the ribs articulate with the vertebrae.

Demifacet

(In Latin *demi* means "half.") A partial, or half facet; located laterally on the superior and inferior edges of the vertebral body where ribs articulate with thoracic vertebrae. Depending on rib placement on the body, a facet or demifacet may be found on these edges.

Although the three different vertebrae have all the same parts, there are differences. These differences are illustrated in Figure 14-10 and summarized in Table 14-2.

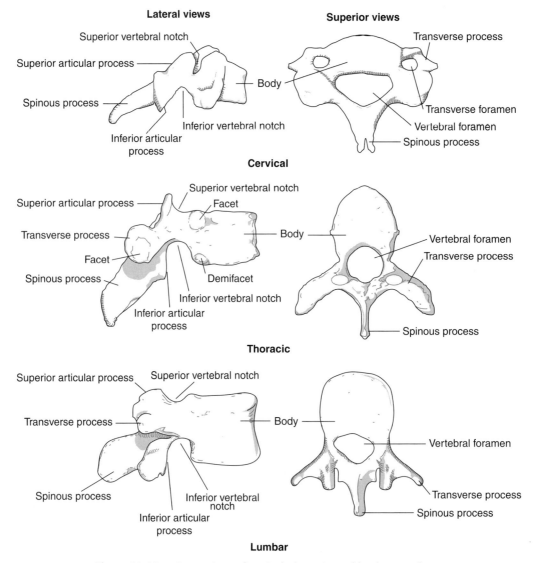

Figure 14-10. Comparison of cervical, thoracic, and lumbar vertebrae.

Table 14-2	Parts of the Vertebra		
	Cervical	**Thoracic**	**Lumbar**
Size	Smallest	Intermediate	Largest
Body shape	Small oval	Heart-shaped, with facets that connect with ribs	Large oval
Vertebral foramen	Large, triangular	Smallest	Intermediate
Transverse process	Foramen for vertebral artery; laterally	Facets that connect with ribs; long, thick, point posteriorly and laterally	No foramen or articulation
Spinous process	Short, stout, bifid	Long, slender, point inferiorly	Thick, point posteriorly
Superior articular process	Face medially	Face posteriorly and laterally	Face posteriorly
Vertebral notches	Equal depth	Deeper inferior notches	Deeper inferior notches

Joints and Ligaments

The cervical spine begins with two very different articulations. The **atlanto-occipital joint** is formed by the condyles of the occiput articulating with the superior articular processes of the atlas. This union is strong and supports the weight of the head. The anterior atlanto-occipital membrane is an extension of the anterior longitudinal ligament, which is somewhat thin superiorly. The tectorial membrane is a continuation of the posterior longitudinal ligament. It serves as a sling to support the spinal cord as it enters the vertebral column. The posterior atlantoaxial ligament serves to secure the weight of the head on the neck. Each of the condyloid joints formed at the union of the occipital condyles and the superior articular processes of the atlas are synovial joints with a synovial membrane enclosed in an articular capsule.

The articulations between the atlas and the axis are known as the **atlantoaxial joints,** of which there are three. The **median atlantoaxial joint** consists of a synovial articulation between the odontoid process (dens) of the axis and the anterior arch of the atlas anteriorly and the transverse ligament posteriorly. There are two synovial cavities present, one on each side of the dens. Each is enclosed in an articular capsule. The anterior atlantoaxial ligament and the posterior atlantoaxial ligament are continuations of the anterior and posterior longitudinal ligaments, which traverse the length of the vertebral column. The two **lateral atlantoaxial joints** are between articular processes of the two vertebrae (Fig. 14-11).

The articulations between C2 through S1 are all basically the same. The strong, weight-bearing articula-

tions occur anteriorly on the vertebra between vertebral bodies. The posterior portion of the vertebrae have two articulations (one on each side), called **facet joints** (also *apophyseal* or *zygapophyseal joints*) (see Fig. 14-5).

The facet joints are formed by the articulation between the superior articular processes of the vertebra below with the inferior articular processes of the vertebra above. Each facet joint is a synovial joint housing a synovial membrane and enclosed in an articular capsular ligament. Each vertebra has two superior articular processes and two inferior articular processes. Therefore, each vertebra is involved with two facet joints. These facet joints, by the direction they face, determine, to a great extent, the type and amount of motion possible (Fig. 14-12) at that part of the vertebral column.

In the lumbar area, the processes are located in the sagittal plane, whereas in the thoracic area they are in the frontal plane. Therefore, most flexion and exten-

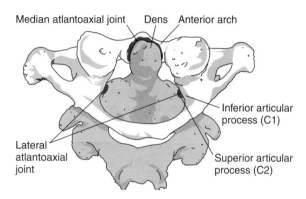

Median atlantoaxial joint   Dens   Anterior arch

Inferior articular process (C1)

Lateral atlantoaxial joint

Superior articular process (C2)

Figure 14-11.   The relationship of C1 sitting on top of C2 showing the three atlantoaxial joints. Posterior view.

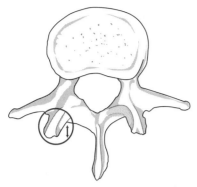

Lumbar orientation is in the sagittal plane

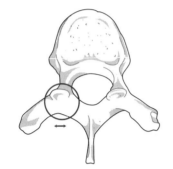

Thoracic orientation is in the frontal plane

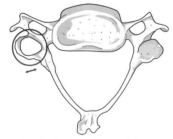

Cervical orientation is triplanar

Figure 14-12.   A comparison of the orientation of the superior articular process on the cervical, thoracic, and lumbar vertebrae.

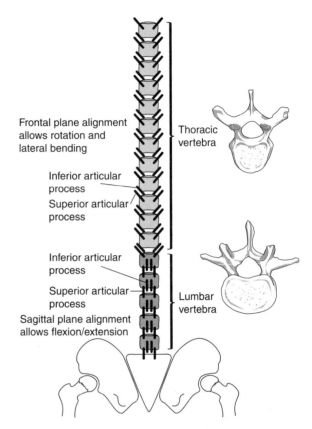

Figure 14-13.   The direction in which facet joints (in circles) are aligned will determine the type of motions allowed.

sion of the vertebral column occurs in the lumbar spine, and most rotation and lateral bending occurs in the thoracic spine. The attachment of ribs to the vertebra also contributes to the lack of flexion and extension in the thoracic spine. Because the processes are located diagonally between the sagittal and frontal planes, the cervical spine has a great deal of all three types of motion (Fig. 14-13).

Many ligaments hold these vertebrae together (Fig. 14-14). The **anterior longitudinal ligament** runs down the vertebral column on the anterior surface of the bodies and tends to prevent excessive hyperextension. It is thin superiorly and thick inferiorly where it

fuses to the sacrum. It is found in the thoracic and lumbar regions just deep to the aorta. The **posterior longitudinal ligament** runs along the vertebral bodies posteriorly inside the vertebral foramen. Its purpose is to prevent excessive flexion. It is thick superiorly where it helps support the skull. It is thin inferiorly, which contributes to instability and increased disk injury in the lumbar region. The **supraspinal ligament** extends from the seventh cervical vertebra distally to the sacrum posteriorly along the tips of the spinous processes. The interspinal ligament runs between successive spinous processes. The very thick ligamentum nuchae (nuchal ligament) takes the place of the supraspinal and **interspinal ligaments** in the cervical region (Fig. 14-15). The **ligamentum flavum** connects adjacent laminae anteriorly.

The lumbar spine is the region of the human body most often injured. It absorbs the majority of our body weight and any weight we carry. The center of gravity is located anterior to the second sacral vertebra. Most movement of the lumbar spine occurs between L4 and L5 and L5 and S1, and most disk herniations occur at these two levels.

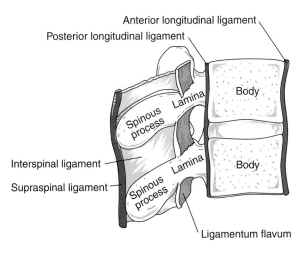

Sagittal Section View

A

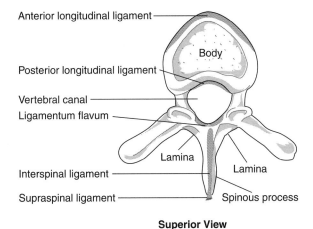

Superior View

B

Figure 14-14. The vertebral ligaments. *(A)* Sagittal section view showing the ligaments inside and outside the vertebral canal. *(B)* Superior view showing the attachments of the ligaments on the vertebra.

The thoracic spine has much less motion than the cervical and lumbar regions due to its attachments to the rib cage. The shape of the vertebral bodies and the length of the spinous processes also limit thoracic motion.

The cervical spine is also freely movable. Unlike the lumbar spine, weight distribution is not its job. The cervical region supports the head, allows freedom of motion of the head on the neck, allows for the nervous tissue to enter the vertebral canal, and also allows for entrance and exit of the major blood vessels in the skull.

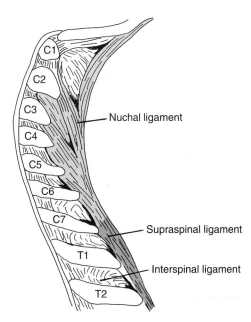

Figure 14-15. The nuchal ligament (ligamentum nuchae) becomes the supraspinal ligament in the cervical region.

Common Vertebral Column Pathologies

Thoracic outlet syndrome is a general term referring to compression of the neurovascular structures (brachial plexus and subclavian artery and vein) that run from the neck to the axilla. The thoracic outlet is located between the first rib, clavicle, and scalene muscles. The brachial plexus and subclavian artery pass between the anterior and middle scalene muscles, the first rib, and the clavicle. A variety of signs and symptoms can occur depending on the structures involved. **Torticollis** (from the Latin *tortus,* meaning twisted and *collum,* meaning neck) is a deformity of the neck in which the person's head is laterally bent to one side and rotated toward the other side. It is also known as "wry" (twisted) neck. **Cervical sprains** occur when the head suddenly and violently hyperextends and then flexes. *"Whiplash"* is the layman's term for this condition. **Sciatica** is pain that tends to run down the posterior thigh and leg. It is caused when there is pressure on the sciatic nerve, which, in most cases, is symptomatic of an underlying pathology.

The vertebral column has a normal anterior-posterior curvature. In the cervical and lumbar regions, these are concave posterior curves. In the thoracic and sacral regions, they are concave anterior curves (see Fig. 14-1). **Lordosis** is an abnormally increased curve of the lumbar spine. The layman's term is *swayback.* **Flat back** is an abnormally decreased lumbar curve. **Kyphosis** is an abnormally increased thoracic curve. Any amount of lateral curve is a pathological condition known as **scoliosis.**

Spondylosis (spinal osteoarthritis), is a degenerative disorder of the vertebral structure and function. It may result from bony spurs, thickening of ligaments, and a decrease in disk height due to a decrease in water content of the nucleus pulposus. Loss of water content is part of the normal aging process. All of these problems may lead to nerve root and spinal cord compression. **Spinal stenosis** is a narrowing of the vertebral canal housing the spinal cord. It is also possible to have stenosis of the intervertebral foramen through which the nerve roots pass. **Herniated disks** occur when there is a weakness or degeneration of the annulus fibrosus (outer layer). This allows a portion of the nucleus pulposus to bulge, or herniate through the annulus. It becomes symptomatic when the herniation puts pressure on the spinal cord, or more commonly, the nerve root. L4 and L5 are the most common sites for disk lesions, and the fourth and fifth lumbar nerve roots are the most commonly affected nerve roots. **Anklyosing spondylitis** is an chronic inflammation of the vertebral column and sacroiliac joints leading to fusion. It is a progressive rheumatic disease, and over time, can lead to a total loss of spinal mobility.

Spondylolysis is a vertebral defect in the pars interarticularis (the part of the lamina between the superior and inferior articular processes). This defect is most commonly seen in L5, and less commonly in L4. **Spondylolisthesis** is usually the result of a fracture, or giving way, of the defect in the pars interarticularis. The result is that one vertebra slips forward in relation to an adjacent vertebra, usually L5 slipping anterior on S1.

Osteoporosis, meaning porous bone, is a disease in which bone is removed faster than it can be laid down. This results in a decrease in bone mass and density, making the bone more prone to fracture. Common sites for fracture are the hip, thoracic vertebral column, and wrist.

Compression fractures typically result in collapse of the anterior (body) portion of the vertebrae. They are usually caused by trauma in the lumbar region, and by osteoporosis in the thoracic region. This type of fracture does not commonly cause spinal cord damage and paralysis because the fracture is usually stable. A stable fracture does not have progressive displacement or dislocation. Unstable fractures, or **fractures with dislocation,** usually result in spinal cord injury and paralysis. A fracture involving C2, commonly called a **hangman's fracture,** typically occurs when there is a forceful, sudden hyperextension of the head. Striking the head against the windshield in a motor vehicle accident often provides the necessary mechanism. This is usually a stable fracture, but without proper care and handling, it could become unstable. Spinal cord paralysis at this level usually results in death because respiration stops.

Muscles of the Neck and Trunk

Muscles of the neck and trunk are numerous and can be divided generally into anterior and posterior muscles as shown in Table 14-3. The quadratus lumborum muscle is the one exception. It is located in the midline and is neither an anterior nor posterior muscle. The clinical significance of the anterior or posterior location is function. As with most other joints, anterior muscles will have a flexion function and posterior muscles will extend. Only those muscles that are clinically important from an exercise standpoint will be discussed here. Others will be summarized in charts and illustrations.

Table 14-3	Vertebral Muscles		
	Neck		**Trunk**
Anterior	Sternocleidomastoid		Rectus abdominis
	Scalenes (3)		External oblique
	Prevertebral group (4)		Internal oblique
			Transverse abdominis
Posterior	Erector spinae group (3)		Erector spinae group (3)
	Splenius capitis		Transversospinalis group (3)
	Splenius cervicis		Interspinales
	Suboccipital group (4)		Intertransversarii
Lateral			Quadratus lumborum

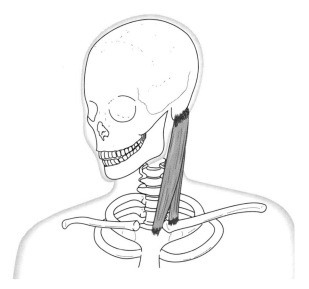

Figure 14-16. The sternocleidomastoid muscle.

Muscles of the Cervical Spine

Generally speaking, muscles located anterior to the vertebral column are neck flexors. The largest flexor, the **sternocleidomastoid muscle,** is a long, superficial, straplike muscle originating as two heads from the medial aspect of the clavicle and superior end of the sternum (Fig. 14-16). It runs superiorly and posteriorly to insert on the mastoid process of the temporal bone. When it contracts bilaterally, it flexes the neck, and when it contracts unilaterally, it laterally bends and rotates the head to the opposite side. What "rotating to the opposite side" means is that, for example, when the right sternocleidomastoid muscle contracts, your neck would rotate so that you would be looking over your left shoulder. Because it attaches on the head, it can have an affect on head motion. Looking at the muscle's line of pull from the side, one can see that in addition to flexing the neck, the sternocleidomastoid can also hyperextend the head. This would accentuate the "forward head" position common in faulty posture. To neutralize this action, one should always "tuck the chin" before doing such activities as sit-ups.

Sternocleidomastoid Muscle

O	Sternum and clavicle
I	Mastoid process
A	Bilaterally: flexes neck, hyperextends head Unilaterally: laterally bends the neck; rotates head to the opposite side
N	Accessory nerve (cranial nerve XI); second and third cervical nerves

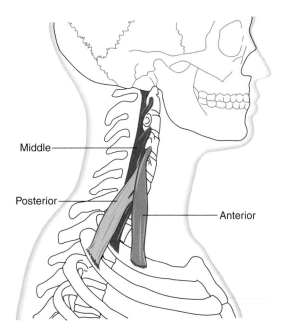

Figure 14-17. The three parts of the scalene muscles.

Deep to the sternocleidomastoid muscle lie the three **scalene muscles** (Fig. 14-17). The **anterior scalene muscle** originates on the transverse processes of C3 through C6 and inserts into the superior surface of the first rib. The **middle scalene muscle** originates on the transverse processes of C2 through C7 and inserts into the superior surface of the first rib also. The **posterior scalene muscle,** the smallest and deepest, originates from C5 through C7, and inserts into the second rib. Because they all perform the same action and are located close to each other, it is not necessary to differentiate between them. Located laterally at the neck, they are very effective in laterally bending the cervical spine. Because they are close to the axis, they are only assistive in flexion.

Scalene Muscles

O	Transverse processes of the cervical vertebrae
I	First and second ribs
A	Bilaterally: assists in neck flexion Unilaterally: neck lateral bending
N	Lower cervical nerve

There is an anterior group of muscles often referred to as the **prevertebral muscles.** They are located deep and run along the anterior portion of the cervical vertebrae (Fig. 14-18). These muscles have a role in flexing either the neck or head. Because of their small size in relation to other neck flexors, their greatest role, perhaps, is

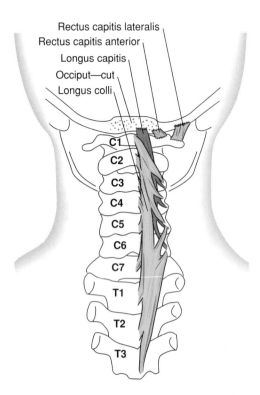

Figure 14-18.   The prevertebral muscles. Anterior view. Note that the anterior skull has been cut away to view the attachments on the occiput.

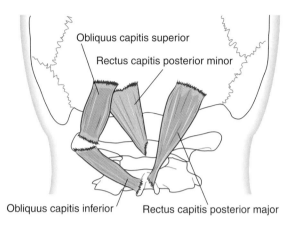

Figure 14-19.   Suboccipital muscles. Posterior view.

The **suboccipital muscles** are clustered together below the base of the skull and move only the head (Fig. 14-19). The muscles work together to extend the head with a rocking motion of the occipital condyles on the atlas, or to rotate by pivoting the skull and atlas around the odontoid process of the axis. These muscles are summarized in Table 14-6.

The postvertebral muscles are located posteriorly along the vertebral column and are considered the superior portions of the deep back muscles, known as the **erector spinae group,** which will be discussed later in more detail with the other trunk muscles. These muscles provide postural control over the gravitational pull of the head into flexion, and they act as extensors to bring the head back from the flexed position.

Erector Spinae Muscles

See the section on the trunk for muscle summary.

The most superficial of the neck extensors are the **splenius capitis** and **splenius cervicis muscles.** As their names imply, they attach to the head and cervical spine with the splenius capitis muscle being the more superficial of the two. They both attach from the spinous processes of the lower cervical and upper thoracic vertebrae, and run superiorly and laterally to the lateral

maintaining postural control and "tucking" the chin. Table 14-4 summarizes their locations and actions.

Several small muscles in the neck serve as anchors for the hyoid bone and the tongue. Except for the platysma, these muscles are illustrated in Figures 13-18 through 13-22. The hyoid bone is unique in that it has no bony articulation. It functions as a primary support for the tongue and its numerous muscles. The influence of these muscles on motions of the cervical spine is assistive at best. The muscles approach the base of the skull from all directions. Table 14-5 summarizes the actions of these muscles.

Table 14-4	Prevertebral Muscles		
Muscle	**Origin**	**Insertion**	**Action**
Longus colli	Bodies and transverse processes of C3–T2	Transverse processes and bodies of C1–C6	Flex neck
Longus capitis	Transverse processes of C3–C6	Occipital bone	Flex head
Rectus capitis anterior	Atlas	Occipital bone	Flex head
Rectus capitis lateralis	Transverse process of atlas	Occipital bone	Laterally bend head

Table 14-5	Muscles of the Mouth and Hyoid Bone	
Group	**Muscle**	**Action**
Superficial cervical	Platysma	Draws lower lip down and out, tensing skin over neck
Suprahyoid	Digastric	Raises hyoid bone and/or tongue
	Stylohyoid	
	Mylohyoid	
	Geniohyoid	
Infrahyoid	Sternohyoid	Lowers hyoid bone
	Sternothyroid	
	Thyrohyoid	
	Omohyoid	

occiput (capitis) and transverse processes of the upper cervical vertebrae (cervicis) (Fig. 14-20). When the muscles on only one side contract, they rotate and laterally bend the head and neck to the same side. When both sides contract, however, they extend the head and neck.

Splenius Capitis Muscles

O	Lower half of nuchal ligament; spinous processes of C7 through T3
I	Lateral occipital bone; mastoid process
A	Bilaterally: extend head and neck Unilaterally: rotate and laterally bend the head to same side
N	Middle and lower cervical nerves

Splenius Cervicis Muscles

O	Spinous processes of T3 through T6
I	Transverse processes of C1 through C3
A	Bilaterally: extend neck Unilaterally: rotate and laterally bend the neck to same side
N	Middle and lower cervical nerves

It should be noted that the upper trapezius and levator scapula can assist the splenius capitis and cervicis

under certain conditions. If the scapula is fixed, they can function in a reversal of muscle action. Instead of moving the scapula on the head and neck, the head and neck move on the scapula.

Muscles of the Trunk

Spanning the anterior trunk in the midline is the **rectus abdominis** muscle. The two sides are separated from each other by the linea alba. The rectus abdominis muscle arises from the crest of the pubis and inserts into the costal cartilages of the fifth, sixth, and seventh ribs. There are several tendinous inscriptions dividing the muscle horizontally into several small units (Figs. 14-21 and 14-22). Located in the anterior midline, the rectus abdominis muscle is a strong trunk flexor and, along with the other anterior trunk muscles, compresses the abdominal contents.

Note that when doing a sit-up, the trunk is moving on the hips. The hip flexor muscles, in a reversal of muscle action, are also involved in performing a sit-up if the ankles or legs are held down. Therefore, if the objective is to strengthen the abdominals (not the hip flexors), the hips and knees should be flexed and the ankles should not be held down. Flexing the hips and knees will shorten the hip flexors, making them less efficient. The hip flexors cannot work in a reversal of

Table 14-6	Suboccipital Muscles	
Muscle	**Location**	**Head Motion**
Obliquus capitis superior	Posterior	Extension
Obliquus capitis inferior	Posterior	Extension, lateral bending, rotation to the same side
Rectus capitis posterior minor	Posterior	Extension
Rectus capitis posterior major	Posterior	Extension, lateral bending, rotation to the same side

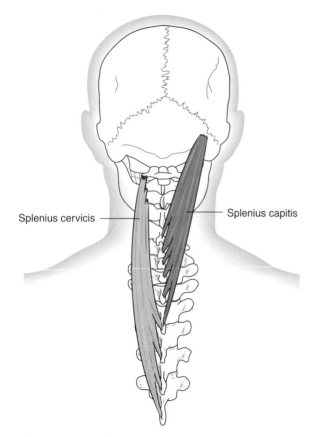

Splenius cervicis

Splenius capitis

Figure 14-20. The splenius capitis and cervicis muscles.

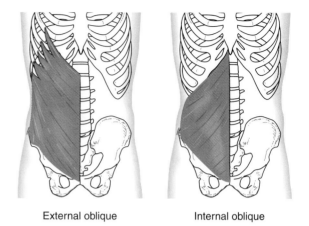

External oblique

Internal oblique

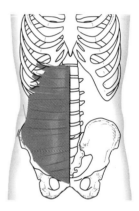

Transverse abdominis

Figure 14-22. The three layers of abdominal muscles. The external oblique is superficial, the internal oblique lies underneath it, and the transverse abdominis is the deepest layer.

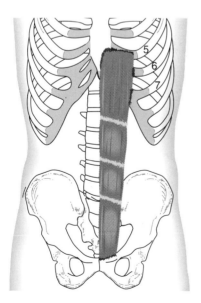

Figure 14-21. The rectus abdominis muscle. Note that the muscle is shown only on the left side.

muscle action role when the distal segment (feet or legs) is not stabilized (held down).

Rectus Abdominis Muscles

O	Pubis
I	Xiphoid process and costal cartilages of fifth, sixth, and seventh ribs
A	Trunk flexion; compression of abdomen
N	Seventh through twelfth intercostal nerves

The **external oblique muscle** is a large, broad (see Fig. 14-22), flat muscle lying superficially on the anterolateral abdomen. It originates laterally on the lower eight ribs, runs inferiorly and medially to insert into the iliac crest and, via the abdominal aponeurosis, into the linea alba at the midline. The direction of the fibers on both sides form the shape of a "V." When both sides contract, they flex the trunk and compress the abdominal contents. When one side contracts, it laterally bends and rotates the trunk to the opposite side. This means that the right external oblique muscle would rotate the right side of the trunk toward the midline. Visualize the right shoulder moving toward the left.

Located deep to the external oblique muscle and running at right angles to the external oblique muscle is the **internal oblique muscle.** It originates from the inguinal ligament, iliac crest, and thoracolumbar fascia. It then runs superiorly and medially to insert into the last three ribs and, via the abdominal aponeurosis, into the linea alba (see Fig. 14-22). The direction of the fibers on both sides form the shape of an inverted "V." Like the external oblique muscle, when both sides contract, they flex and compress the abdominal contents. When one side contracts, it laterally bends the trunk. However, the internal oblique muscle has the opposite action in rotation by rotating the trunk to the same side. This means that the right internal oblique muscle would rotate the right side of the trunk away from the midline. Visualize the right shoulder moving toward the right. Therefore, the right external oblique and left internal oblique are agonists in rotating the trunk to the left. During the same action, the left external and right internal obliques are antagonists.

External Oblique Muscle

O	Lower eight ribs laterally
I	Iliac crest and linea alba
A	Bilaterally: trunk flexion; compression of abdomen Unilaterally: lateral bending; rotation to opposite side
N	Eighth through 12th intercostal, iliohypogastric, and ilioinguinal nerves

Internal Oblique Muscle

O	Inguinal ligament, iliac crest, thoracolumbar fascia
I	Tenth, eleventh, and twelfth ribs; abdominal aponeurosis
A	Bilaterally: trunk flexion; compression of abdomen Unilaterally: lateral bending; rotation to same side
N	Eighth through 12th intercostal, iliohypogastric, and ilioinguinal nerves

The deepest of the abdominal muscles is the **transverse abdominis** muscle lying deep to the internal oblique muscle. It is named for the transverse, or horizontal, direction of its fibers. It originates from the lateral portion of the inguinal ligament, iliac crest, the thoracolumbar fascia, and the last six ribs. It spans the abdomen horizontally to insert into the abdominal aponeurosis and linea alba (see Fig. 14-22). Because of its horizontal line of pull, it plays no effective part in moving the trunk. However, it does work with the other abdominal muscles to compress and give support to the abdominal contents. This is important in such activities as coughing, sneezing, laughing, forced expiration, and "bearing down," such as during childbirth or while having a bowel movement.

Transverse Abdominis Muscle

O	Inguinal ligament, iliac crest, thoracolumbar fascia, and last six ribs
I	Abdominal aponeurosis and linea alba
A	Compression of abdomen
N	Seventh through 12th intercostal, iliohypogastric, and ilioinguinal nerves

There are many groups of muscles that extend, and, as summarized in Table 14-7, some general statements can be made regarding attachments and actions (Fig. 14-23). Generally speaking, muscles attaching from spinous process to spinous process have a vertical line of pull; thus, they extend. Because they are located in the midline, there is only one set of them Muscles that run from transverse process to transverse process have a vertical line of pull lateral to the midline; therefore, they laterally bend unilaterally and extend bilaterally. Muscles

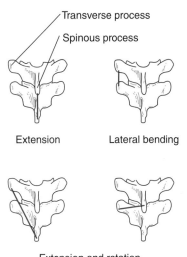

Figure 14-23. The line of pull determines muscle action as summarized for posterior trunk muscles.

Table 14-7	Posterior Trunk Muscles	
Attachments	**Action**	**Muscles**
Spinous processes	Extension	Spinalis (ES) Interspinales
Transverse processes	Extension, lateral bending	Longissimus (ES) Intertransversarii
Spinous to transverse process	Extension, rotation	Splenius cervicis
Transverse to spinous process	Extension, rotation	Semispinalis (T) Multifidus (T) Rotatores (T)
Transverse process to rib, or rib to rib	Extension, lateral bending	Iliocostalis (ES)

ES, erector spinae; T, transversospinalis.

attaching from rib to rib have the same line of pull as those attaching between transverse processes. Being more lateral, muscles attaching to ribs are even more effective at lateral bending. Muscles attaching from spinous process to transverse process or from transverse process to spinous process have an oblique line and, therefore, extend bilaterally and rotate unilaterally. Of these, shorter muscles are more effective at rotation, and longer muscles are more effective at extension.

The intermediate layer of back extensors is a group of muscles called the **erector spinae muscles,** sometimes called the *sacrospinalis muscle group*. This muscle group can be subdivided into three groups that tend to run parallel to the vertebral column connecting spinous processes, transverse processes, and ribs (Fig. 14-24). The most medial group is the **spinalis muscle group** that primarily attaches the nuchal ligament and spinous processes of the cervical and thoracic vertebrae. The portion of this group that attaches to the occiput also attaches to the transverse processes of the cervical vertebrae. Located in the midline, these muscles are prime movers in trunk extension.

The intermediate muscles, the **longissimus muscle group,** are located lateral to the spinalis muscle group, attaching the transverse processes from the occiput to the sacrum. These muscles have a vertical line of pull lateral to the midline and, therefore, laterally bend when contracting unilaterally and extend when contracting bilaterally. The **iliocostalis muscles** are the most lateral group and primarily attach to the ribs posteriorly. Superiorly, they attach to transverse processes, and inferiorly they attach to the sacrum and ilium. Because of their lateral position, these muscles are excellent at lateral bending. Acting bilaterally, they are effective extensors. These three groups of muscles generally tend to be referred to as the erector spinae muscle group and, therefore, will be summarized as a group. However, it

should be noted that the upper fibers of the spinalis and longissimus groups attach to the occiput, and therefore can extend the head on the neck.

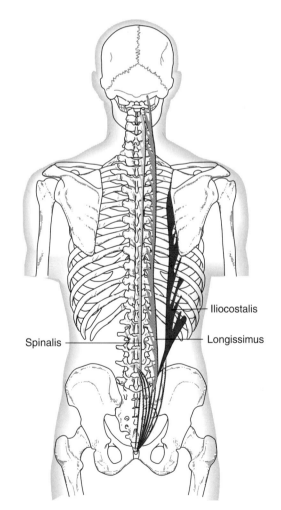

Figure 14-24.   The three parts of the erector spinae muscle group.

Erector Spinae Muscles

O	Spinous processes, transverse processes, and ribs from the occiput to the sacrum and ilium
I	Spinous processes, transverse processes, and ribs from the occiput to the sacrum and ilium
A	Bilaterally: extend
	Unilaterally: lateral bend
N	Spinal nerves

The deepest of the back extensor muscles is a group of three muscles called the **transversospinalis (transverse spinal) muscle group** (Fig. 14-25). They have an oblique line of pull, essentially attaching from a transverse process to the spinous process of a vertebra above and, therefore, are very effective at rotation. The *semispinalis muscles* tend to span five or more vertebrae; the *multifidus* muscles tend to span two to four vertebrae; and the *rotatores* muscles, the shortest and deepest of this group, span only one vertebra. These muscles rotate to the opposite side and extend the spine. The semispinalis is the most superficial muscle of this group. The multifidus lies underneath it, with the rotators being the deepest of these muscles.

Transversospinalis Muscles

O	Transverse processes
I	Spinous processes of vertebra above
A	Bilaterally: extend Unilaterally: rotate to opposite side
N	Spinal nerves

These next two muscles are located deep like the transversospinalis muscle group but have a vertical, not an oblique, line of pull and, therefore, must be considered separately. The names of the interspinales and intertransversarii muscles tell you about their attachments. The **interspinales muscles** attach from the spinous process below to the spinous process above throughout most of the vertebral column (Fig. 14-26). With this vertical line of pull in the midline, they are effective extensors. The **intertransversarii muscles** attach from the transverse process below to the transverse process above, also throughout most of the vertebral column (Fig. 14-27). They are effective at lateral bending.

Interspinales Muscles

O	Spinous process below
I	Spinous process above
A	Trunk extension
N	Spinal nerves

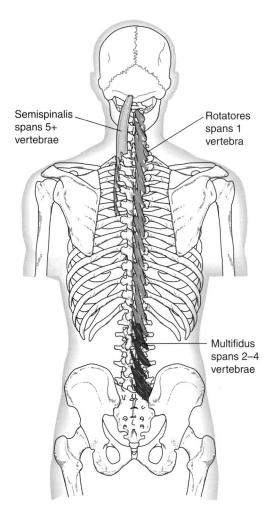

Semispinalis spans 5+ vertebrae

Rotatores spans 1 vertebra

Multifidus spans 2–4 vertebrae

Figure 14-25. The transversospinalis muscle group. For illustration purposes, muscles are shown in different parts of the vertebral column. In fact, all run the entire vertebral column in layers.

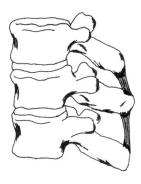

Figure 14-26. The interspinales muscles. Lateral view.

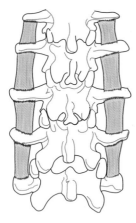

Figure 14-27. Intertransversarii muscles. Posterior view.

Intertransversarii Muscles

O	Transverse process below
I	Transverse process above
A	Trunk lateral bending
N	Spinal nerves

The **quadratus lumborum muscle** is a deep muscle that originates from the iliac crest and runs superiorly to insert into the last rib and transverse processes of all lumbar vertebrae (Fig. 14-28). Because it is located in the anterior-posterior midline, it does not have a function of flexion or extension; being vertical, it has no role in rotation. However, being lateral to the midline makes it effective at lateral bending. It has another function that occurs when its origin is pulled toward its insertion (reversal of muscle action). The action is called *hip hiking,* or *elevation,* of one side of the pelvis. This is an important function to anyone with a long leg cast or fused knee. It allows the foot to clear the floor without bending the knee.

Quadratus Lumborum Muscle

O	Iliac crest
I	Twelfth rib, transverse processes of all five lumbar vertebrae
A	Trunk lateral bending
N	Twelfth thoracic and first lumbar nerves

Summary of Muscle Actions

The muscle action of the prime movers of the neck and trunk are summarized as follows:

Action	Muscle
HEAD (Occiput on C1)	
Flexion	Prevertebral group
Extension	Suboccipital group
NECK	
Flexion	Sterneocleidomastoid
Extension	Splenius capitis, splenius cervicis, erector spinae
Lateral bending	Sternocleidomastoid, splenius capitis, splenius cervicis, scalenes, erector spinae
Rotation (same side)	Splenius capitis, splenius cervicis
Rotation opposite side	Sternocleidomastoid
TRUNK	
Flexion	Rectus abdominis, external oblique, internal oblique
Extension	Erector spinae, transversospinalis, interspinales
Lateral bending	Quadratus lumborum, erector spinae, internal oblique, external oblique, intertransversarii
Rotation same side	Internal oblique
Rotation opposite side	External oblique, transversospinalis
Compression of abdomen	Rectus abdominis, external oblique, internal oblique, transverse abdominis

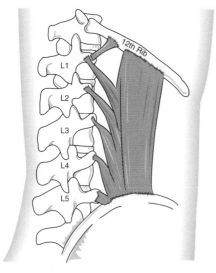

Figure 14-28. The quadratus lumborum muscle.

Summary of Muscle Innervation

The muscles of the neck and trunk do not receive innervation from branches or terminal nerves of a plexus for the most part. Because they tend to be groups that span several vertebral levels, their innervation tends to reflect that. Generally speaking, they receive innervation from spinal nerves at various levels. For example, a spinal cord injury at T12 will not cause paralysis of all erector spinae muscles but will cause paralysis of those located below that level.

Points to Remember

- When a muscle contracts, it knows no direction; it simply shortens.
- Usually when a muscle contracts, it moves its insertion (more movable end) toward its origin (more stable end).

- A muscle insertion is usually the distal end and the more movable end.
- A muscle origin is usually the proximal end and the more stable end.
- Reversal of muscle action occurs when the origin becomes more movable and moves toward the insertion, which has become more stable.
- Concentric contractions occur when the body part is moving against gravity.
- Eccentric contractions occur when the body part is moving in the same direction as the pull of gravity.
- Isometric contractions occur when a muscle contracts, but no significant joint motion occurs.
- The muscle group contracting isometrically is the same group as if the joint were contracting concentrically.

Review Questions

General Anatomy Questions

1. Describe neck and trunk motions in:
   a. The frontal plane around the sagittal axis
   b. The transverse plane around the vertical axis
   c. The sagittal plane around the frontal axis
2. You are handed a cervical, thoracic, and lumbar vertebra. What identifying features help you distinguish among them?
3. What structural features allow the thoracic vertebrae to rotate but not to flex?
4. What structural features allow the lumbar vertebrae to flex but not to rotate?
5. Name the ligament that extends over the spinous processes from the occiput to C7 and from C7 to the sacrum.
6. What is the name of the series of ligaments that connect the lamina above to the lamina below along the length of the vertebral column?
7. Name the ligaments that attach to the bodies of the vertebrae and run the length of the vertebral column.
8. Why doesn't the quadratus lumborum muscle play a role in trunk flexion, extension, or rotation?

9. Which posterior muscle groups are the most superficial?.
10. You ask your patient, who is in the supine position, to bring her left shoulder toward her right knee. What joint motion(s) and prime movers are involved?

Functional Activity Questions

Identify the main **cervical** positions in the following activities:

1. Sleeping on your stomach
2. Cradling the telephone between your ear and shoulder
3. Looking a the top of a tall building from the street below
4. Lying supine on a sofa with your head propped up on pillow or arm of sofa
5. Painting the ceiling

Identify the main **trunk** action in the following activities:

6. Preparing to hit a tennis ball with a backhand swing with the racket in your right hand (Fig. 14-29)

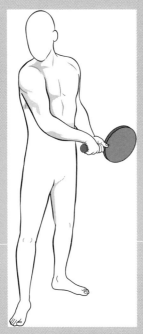

Figure 14-29.   Preparing to hit with tennis backswing.

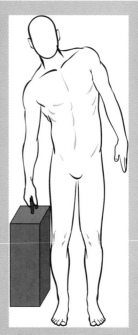

Figure 14-31.   Picking up suitcase.

7. Hitting the tennis ball with the backhand swing (Fig. 14-30)

8. Reaching down to pick up a suitcase beside you (Fig. 14-31)

9. The follow-through of punting a football

10. Doing a backward handstand

Clinical Exercise Questions

Head and Neck

1. Lie prone with your head and shoulders over the edge of the table and head down. Tuck your chin in and raise your head to anatomical position.
   a. What joint motion is occurring in the neck as you tuck in your chin?
   b. What joint motion is occurring in the neck as you raise your head?
   c. What type of contraction (isometric, concentric, eccentric) occurs as you raise your head?
   d. What type of contraction (isometric, concentric, eccentric) occurs as you hold your head in anatomical position while in this prone position.
   e. What are the prime movers that are working to raise your head?

2. Sitting or standing with your head and neck in anatomical position, press your right hand against the right side of your head. Try to move your head but resist any motion with your hand.
   a. What joint motion is occurring (or attempting to occur)?

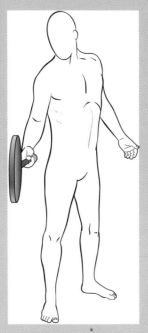

Figure 14-30.   Hitting with backswing.

b. What type of contraction (isometric, concentric, eccentric) is occurring?

c. What are the prime movers of this joint motion?

3. While lying supine, lean your head toward your right shoulder. Do not raise your right shoulder. Both stretching and strengthening are occurring here. In answering the questions below, be sure to indicate whether you are referring to the right or left side.

a. What joint motion is occurring (or attempting to occur)?

b. What muscle group is being stretched?

c. What are the prime movers of this joint motion?

d. What muscle group is being strengthened?

e. What are the prime movers of this joint motion?

4. Which muscle would be stretched if you leaned your head toward the right shoulder and rotated your head to the left?

5. From a supine position, tuck your chin and raise your head off the mat, hold for the count of 5, then return to the starting position.

a. Is the head flexing or extending on C1 as you tuck in your chin?

b. What type of contraction (isometric, concentric, eccentric) is occurring?

c. What is the muscle group involved in tucking your chin?

d. Is your neck flexing or extending as you raise your head?

e. What type of contraction is occurring as you raise your head?

f. What muscles are prime movers in this joint motion?

g. What type of contraction is occurring as you hold your head for the count?

h. What muscles are prime movers in this action?

i. Is neck flexion or extension occurring in the neck as you return to the starting position?

j. What type of contraction is occurring with this motion?

k. What muscle are involved with this action?

Trunk

1. Sit in a chair with your legs abducted. Drop your head and shoulders forward, bending at hips and trunk until your shoulders are between your knees.

a. Is trunk flexion or extension occurring in this activity?

b. Are the trunk flexors or extensors being stretched?

c. What muscles are being stretched?

2. Lie supine with your knees extended and your arms at your sides. First, press your lower back to the mat, and then curl your trunk. Lift your head and shoulders up (keeping your chin down) until your scapulae leave the floor.

a. Is trunk flexion or extension occurring in this activity?

b. What type of contraction (isometric, concentric, eccentric) is occurring?

c. What muscles are prime movers in this trunk motion?

3. Repeat the action of exercise No. 2, except this time have someone hold down your feet. In this exercise, the hip flexors are contracting.

a. Is the trunk motion still the same as in No.1?

b. Are the hips flexing or extending?

c. Is the hip muscle moving its origin toward its insertion or its insertion toward its origin?

d. What is the kinesiology term for a muscle that contracts in this direction?

e. What is the main one-joint hip muscle that is contracting in this motion?

f. Describe how holding the feet down allows certain hip muscles to contract.

4. Lie supine with your knees bent and feet flat. Put your right hand behind your head. Lift your right shoulder and scapula off the mat toward your left knee.

a. What two trunk motions are occurring (flexion, extension, right rotation, left rotation, right lateral bending, left lateral bending)?

b. What type of contraction (isometric, concentric, eccentric) is occurring?

c. What muscles are causing these trunk motions? Be sure to indicate which side the muscle is on that is contracting.

5. Lie prone with your face in the mat and your arms at your side. Tuck your chin in and raise your head and shoulders up off the mat. Be sure to keep your chin tucked and eyes looking down at the mat.

a. Is the head flexing or extending on C1 as you tuck in your chin?

b. What type of contraction (isometric, concentric, eccentric) is occurring as you tuck in your chin?

c. What type of contraction is occurring as you hold your chin tucked in?

d. What is the muscle group involved in tucking your chin?

e. Is your neck in flexion or extension as you raise your head and shoulders from the mat?

f. What type of contraction is occurring at the neck as you raise your shoulders from the mat?

g. What are the prime movers at the neck as you raise your shoulders from the mat?

h. Is your trunk flexing, extending, or hyperextending as your raise your shoulders from the mat?

i. What type of trunk muscle contraction is occurring as you raise your shoulders?

j. What muscles are causing the trunk motion that raises your shoulders?

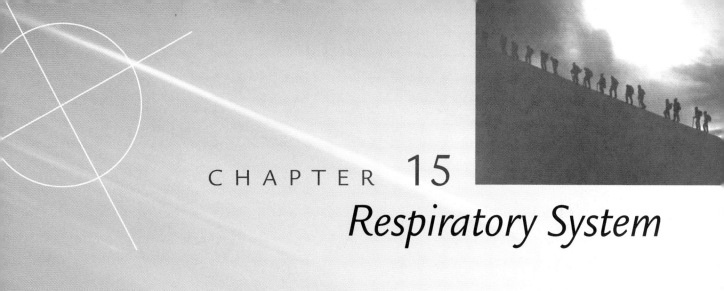

The Thoracic Cage

   Joints and Articulations

   Movements of the Thorax

Structures of Respiration

   Mechanics of Respiration

Phases of Respiration

Muscles of Respiration

   Diaphragm Muscle

   Intercostal Muscles

   Accessory Inspiratory Muscles

   Accessory Expiratory Muscles

   Diaphragmatic Versus Chest Breathing

   Summary of Innervation of the Muscles of Respiration

   Valsalva's Maneuver

   Common Respiratory Conditions or Pathologies

Review Questions

   General Anatomy Questions

   Functional Activity Questions

   Clinical Exercise Questions

Simply stated, the main function of the respiratory system is to supply oxygen to and eliminate carbon dioxide from the lungs. The respiratory organs are the conduits through which air gets into and out of the lungs. The thorax provides bony protection to the lungs, and assists in the air exchange. Although a brief description of the passage of air through the respiratory organs will be given, the main focus of this chapter will be the bony and muscular mechanisms that make air exchange possible.

The Thoracic Cage

The thorax consists of the sternum, the ribs and costal cartilages, and the thoracic vertebrae (Fig. 15-1). It is bounded anteriorly by the sternum, posteriorly by the bodies of the 12 thoracic vertebrae, superiorly by the clavicle, and inferiorly by the diaphragm. The thorax is wider from side to side than it is from front to back.

The **rib cage** serves to attach the vertebral column posteriorly to the sternum anteriorly. Due to these attachments, movement within the thoracic spine is very limited. The internal organs (heart, lungs) are housed and protected within the rib cage. There are 12 ribs on each side, for a total of 24. The upper seven are called **true ribs,** attaching directly to the sternum anteriorly. Ribs eight through ten are called **false ribs** because they attach indirectly to the sternum via the costal cartilage of the seventh rib. The 11th and 12th ribs are called **floating ribs** because they have no anterior attachment. Each rib corresponds to the thoracic vertebral articulations above and below its number.

The **sternum** is the long, flat bone in the midline of the anterior chest wall. Its shape resembles a dagger and consists of three parts: manubrium, body, and xiphoid process (see Fig. 15-1).

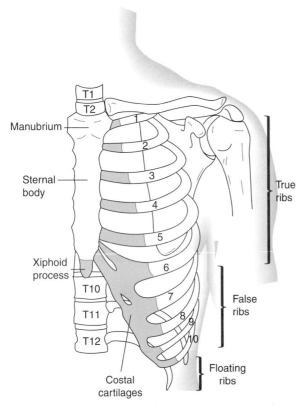

Figure 15-1.   The thoracic cage.

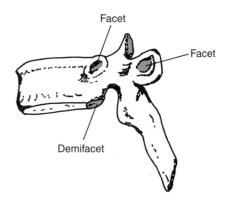

Figure 15-3.   The facets and demifacets on the thoracic vertebra. Lateral view.

is called the **facet** and is located laterally and posteriorly on the body near the beginning of the neural arch. Some ribs articulate partially with two bodies. These articulations are with the superior part of the vertebral body below and the inferior part of the vertebral body above. These facets are often called **demifacets** because they articulate with only about half of the rib. In other words, the rib articulates with a demifacet on the vertebra above plus a demifacet on the vertebra below. A facet that articulates with the tubercle and neck of the rib is located on the anterior tip of the transverse vertebra. These facets and demifacets are illustrated in Figure 15-3.

Movements of the Thorax

Like the costovertebral articulations, the articulations of the ribs and the sternum, with the costal cartilage in between, are nonaxial, diarthrodial, gliding joints. Because most of the ribs attach anteriorly and posteriorly, there is little movement, but **elevation** and **depression** of the rib cage do occur. These movements are associated with inspiration and expiration of the lungs, respectively

As you inhale, the rib cage moves up and out, increasing the medial-lateral diameter of the chest. Accordingly, as you exhale, the rib cage returns to its starting position by moving down and in, decreasing the medial-lateral chest diameter. This type of movement has been associated with the up and down movement of a *bucket handle* (Fig. 15-4A). When the handle is resting down against the side of the bucket, it is comparable to the lowered position of the rib cage during expiration. As the handle (lateral aspect of the ribs) moves up and away from the bucket (vertebral column and sternum), it is comparable to the increased mediolateral diameter of the rib cage during inspiration.

In addition to a change in medial-lateral diameter, there is a change in the anterior-posterior diameter of

The *manubrium* (Latin, meaning "handle") is the superior part; the *body* is the middle and longest part; and the *xiphoid process* (Greek, meaning "sword") is the inferior tip portion. The ribs, sternum, and vertebral bodies form the thorax.

Joints and Articulations

The ribs articulate with the vertebrae in mainly two areas: (1) the bodies of the vertebrae, and (2) the transverse processes. These joints are called **costovertebral joints** (Fig. 15-2). The articulating surface on the vertebral body

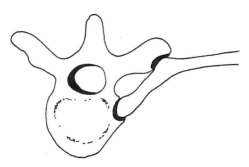

Figure 15-2.   Costovertebral joints.

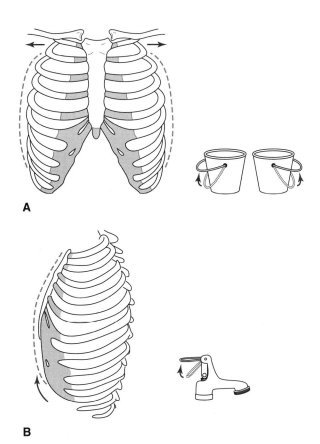

A

B

Figure 15-4. Comparison of thorax movements during breathing with movements of bucket and pump handles.

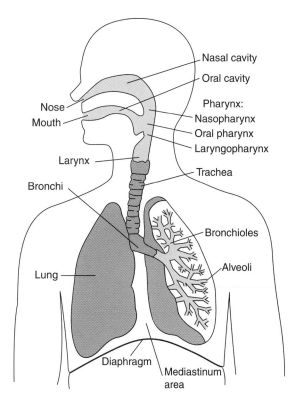

Figure 15-5. The respiratory structures are divided into the upper and lower airway tracts. Note that the left lung is cut in cross section to show terminal structures.

the chest. This is called the "pump-handle" effect (Fig. 15-4B). As you inhale, the sternum and ribs move upward and outward (forward), which increases the anterior-posterior diameter of the chest. This is comparable to the pump handle moving up. Conversely, as the ribs and sternum are lowered, the diameter of the anterior-posterior thorax decreases, resulting in expiration. This movement is comparable to the pump handle moving back down.

Structures of Respiration

Respiratory structures can be divided into upper and lower airway tracts (Fig. 15-5). The **upper respiratory tract** consists of the nose, oral cavity, pharynx, and larynx. The **lower respiratory tract** is made up of the trachea and bronchial tree. To allow the airways to remain open, all structures down to the smallest bronchi are made up of cartilaginous material. The **nose** is mostly made up of relatively soft cartilage and consists of the two nostrils, also called *nasal nares*. Only the upper part, or bridge, is bony. The two nostrils lead into the

nasal cavity. The nasal septum, formed by the vomer and part of the ethmoid bones, separates the nasal cavity into two fairly equal chambers. The ethmoid, sphenoid, and a small part of the frontal bone form the roof of the nasal cavity, whereas the palatine and part of the maxillae bones form the floor. These bones also make up the hard palate of the mouth. The functions of the nasal cavity are to warm, filter, and moisten the air you breathe in.

If you breathe through your mouth, air enters the **oral cavity** over the lips and tongue, and into the pharynx. The roof of the mouth is made up of the bony hard palate and the fibrous soft palate. The uvula is the soft tissue structure that hangs down in the middle of the back of the mouth and is part of the soft palate. The function of the soft palate is to close off the opening between the nasal and oral pharynx during such activities as swallowing, blowing, and certain speech sounds. This forces food and liquids down into the throat during swallowing and air out through the mouth when blowing and speaking.

Once air passes through the nasal cavity, it enters the pharynx through the nasopharynx. The **pharynx,** or throat, has three parts: the nasal pharynx, which has primarily a respiratory function; the oral pharynx, which receives food from the mouth; and the laryngopharynx. This last part is located between the base of the tongue and the entrance to the esophagus. Next, air passes into the **larynx,** or voice box. The larynx is located between the pharynx and the trachea and anterior to C4 through C6 vertebrae. Anteriorly, it is fairly easy to locate by the laryngeal prominence, or *Adam's apple,* which tends to be more prominent in men than women. The larynx is made up of cartilages, ligaments, muscles, and vocal cords. It function is to (1) act as a passageway for air between the pharynx and trachea, (2) prevent food or liquid from passing into the trachea, and (3) generate speech sounds. The epiglottis, which is one of the cartilaginous structures of the larynx, closes over the vocal cords during swallowing to allow food and/or liquids to pass into the esophagus and not into the trachea during swallowing, thus preventing food or drink from being aspirated into the lungs. The glottis is the opening between the vocal cords and the area where sound is produced. It is also an important part of the cough mechanism, which is important for keeping the airways clear.

Passing out of the larynx, air then enters the **trachea,** commonly called the windpipe. It is located anterior to the esophagus and C6 through T4 vertebrae. To keep the airway open, the trachea is made up of C-shaped cartilage, on all sides except posteriorly. It divides into right and left **main stem bronchi.** The right bronchus is shorter and wider and subdivides into three **lobar bronchi** (upper, middle, and lower) with one going to each lobe of the lung. The longer, narrower left bronchus subdivides into two lobar bronchi (upper and lower). As the bronchi continue to divide, they become progressively smaller, narrower, and more numerous. The trachea, bronchi, and their subdivisions are sometimes referred to as the "*bronchial tree.*" The smallest bronchi, less than 1 mm in diameter, are called **bronchioles.** It is at this point where the airway becomes noncartilaginous. The **alveolus** is at the very end of the bronchial tree subdivision. These saclike alveoli are in clusters around the terminal bronchioles. Exchange of oxygen and carbon dioxide is made at the alveoli.

When the trachea divides into the right and left bronchi, they each enter a lung. The **lungs** are somewhat triangular shaped, being wider and concave at the bottom. This concave shape fits with the convex dome shape of the diaphragm located below. The right lung has an upper, middle, and lower lobe, whereas the left lung has an upper and lower lobe. There is a double-walled sac encasing each lung called the **pleura** The

outer wall lines the chest wall and covers the diaphragm, and the inner wall adheres to the lung. Between the two walls is the **pleural cavity.** Between the two lungs is the **mediastinum.** This cavity contains several structures including the heart, esophagus, and several vital blood vessels and nerves.

Mechanics of Respiration

The lungs are passive in the process of breathing. The pleural cavities around the lungs are closed, whereas the inside of the lungs are in communication with the outside atmosphere and subject to its pressure. It is important to remember that air flows from higher pressure to lower pressure until pressure is equalized. During inspiration, the thoracic cavity is made larger, causing the pressure within the thorax to decrease, forcing air into the lungs. This inspiration action can be simulated by the pulling apart of the handles of a bellows (Fig. 15-6A). When the handles are pulled apart, the bellows become larger as air rushes into the bellows. The reverse happens during expiration. The thoracic cavity returns to its smaller size, pressure in the thorax increases, and air is forced out of the lungs. This action is simulated by pushing the handles of the bellows together, making them smaller and forcing air out of the bellows (Fig. 15-6B).

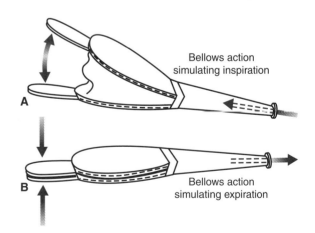

Figure 15-6. *(A)* Simulation of inspiration. As the handles of the bellows are pulled apart, air is brought into the bellows. As the ribs elevate and the diaphragm moves down, the thoracic cavity gets larger and air is pulled into the lungs. *(B)* Simulation of expiration. As the handles of the bellows are pushed together, air is pushed out of the bellows. Similarly, as the ribs move downward and the diaphragm moves upward, the thoracic cavity gets smaller and air is pushed out of the lungs.

Phases of Respiration

Inspiration is commonly broken down into three phases of increasing effort: quiet, deep, and forced. **Quiet inspiration** occurs when an individual is resting or sitting quietly. The diaphragm and external intercostal muscles are the prime movers. As **deep inspiration** occurs the actions of quiet inspiration are increased. A person needs more oxygen and is, therefore, breathing harder. Muscles that can pull the ribs up are being called into action. **Forced inspiration** occurs when an individual is working very hard, needs a great deal of oxygen, and is in a state of "air hunger." Not only are the muscles of quiet and deep inspiration working, but so are muscles that stabilize and/or elevate the shoulder girdle, thus directly, or indirectly, elevating the ribs.

Expiration is divided into two phases: quiet and forced. **Quiet expiration** is mostly a passive action. It occurs through relaxation of the external intercostal muscles, the elastic recoil of the thoracic wall and tissue of the lungs and bronchi, and gravity pulling the rib cage down from its elevated position. Essentially, no muscle action is occurring. **Forced expiration** brings in muscles that can pull down on the rib and muscles that can compress the abdomen, forcing the diaphragm upward.

Muscles of Respiration

Respiration is the result of changes in thoracic volume, hence thoracic pressure. There are two ways of changing thoracic volume: (1) move the ribs, and (2) lower the diaphragm. To accomplish either of these, muscles are required. The muscles of primary importance during respiration are the diaphragm and the intercostal muscles. The role of accessory muscles, which come into play during forced respiration, can be determined by noting whether a muscle's action will pull the ribs up (inspiration) or pull them down (expiration). There has been a great deal of controversy over which muscles are active during which phases of respiration. In recent years, more refined electromyographic (EMG) instruments and techniques may have helped to clarify the roles of various muscles. Because there have been numerous studies conducted, many of which disagree, the waters are still cloudy.

Diaphragm Muscle

The thoracic cavity is separated from the abdominal cavity by the diaphragm muscle, a large sheetlike, dome-shaped muscle (Fig. 15-7). It has a somewhat circular

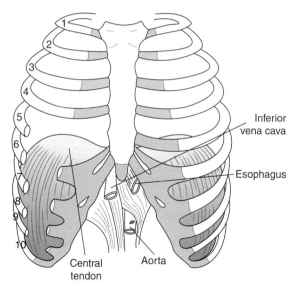

Figure 15-7.   The diaphragm muscle.

origin on the xiphoid process anteriorly, the lower six ribs laterally, and the upper lumbar vertebra posteriorly. Its insertion is rather unique. Because the muscle is somewhat circular, it inserts into itself at the broad central tendon. There are three openings in the diaphragm muscle to allow passage of the esophagus, the aorta, and the inferior vena cava. Because the insertion (central tendon) is located higher than the origin, the diaphragm muscle descends when it contracts (Fig. 15-8). This

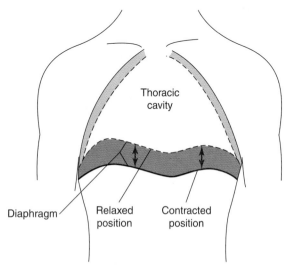

Figure 15-8.   Movement of the diaphragm. When the diaphragm contracts, it descends, making the thoracic cavity larger. As in the bellows example, this allows air to be pulled into the lungs. When it relaxes, it moves upward, decreasing the size of the thoracic cavity and forcing air out of the lungs.

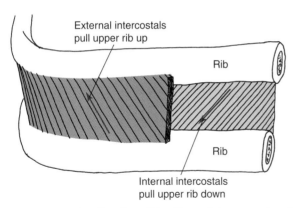

Figure 15-9. The direction of the fibers of the external and internal intercostals muscles, anterior view.

makes the thoracic cavity larger and the abdominal cavity smaller, causing inspiration. Very forced inspiration may lower the dome as much as 4 inches.

Diaphragm Muscle	
O	Xiphoid process, ribs, lumbar vertebrae
I	Central tendon
A	Inspiration
N	Phrenic nerve (C3, C4, C5)

Intercostal Muscles

The intercostal muscles are located between the ribs and run at right angles to each other (Fig. 15-9). The most superficial muscles are the **external intercostal muscles,** which run inferiorly and medially from the rib above to the rib below (Fig. 15-10). They elevate the

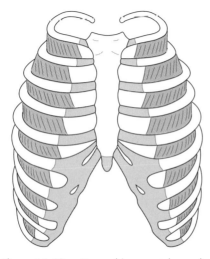

Figure 15-10. External intercostal muscles.

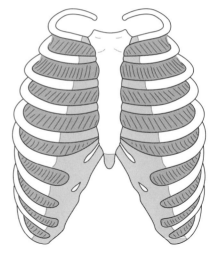

Figure 15-11. Internal intercostal muscles.

ribs by each muscle pulling up on and lifting the rib below. The fibers of the **internal intercostal muscles,** deep and at a 90-degree angle to the external intercostal muscles, perform the opposite action. They run superiorly and medially from the rib below to the rib above (Fig. 15-11). By pulling down on the rib above, they depress the ribs.

Anteriorly, the external intercostal muscles run in the same direction as the external oblique muscles of the abdomen, and the fibers on both sides are in the shape of a "V." As you would expect, the internal intercostal muscles, which run in the opposite direction, form the shape of an inverted "V."

If you view these two sets of muscles posteriorly, the direction of their fibers is just the opposite from their direction anteriorly. Posteriorly, the external intercostals are in the shape of an inverted "V," while the internal intercostals are now in the shape of a "V." To clearly understand how this change occurs, take a pencil and place it diagonally next to the sternum of a skeleton (or your partner). Next, move the pencil around the rib cage posteriorly toward the vertebral column without changing the *direction* of the pencil. Notice that the pencil (muscle fibers) direction posteriorly is opposite to what it was when in front. Although the fibers have not changed direction, the ribs have curved 180 degrees causing this apparent change in direction.

External Intercostal Muscles	
O	Rib above
I	Rib below
A	Elevate ribs
N	Intercostal nerve (T2 through T6)

Internal Intercostal Muscles

O	Rib below
I	Rib above
A	Depress ribs
N	Intercostal nerve (T2 through T6)

Accessory muscles of inspiration assist the diaphragm and external intercostals in pulling up on the rib cage. These muscles demonstrate reversal of muscle action by pulling from origin toward insertion, instead of insertion toward origin. For example, the sternocleidomastoid usually pulls from its insertion on the skull toward the sternum, causing the head to move. When acting in inspiration, the head and neck are stabilized by other muscles and the sternocleidomastoid now pulls from origin on the sternum toward insertion on the head (Fig. 15-12). Pulling in this direction will elevate the rib cage.

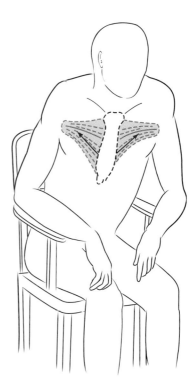

Figure 15-13.   The pectoralis major muscle assisting with inspiration in a reversal of muscle action by pulling the sternum toward the humerus, which is stabilized by resting the forearms on the arms of the chair (closed-chain action).

It is common to see athletes who have just completed a sprint put their hands on their hips while trying to "catch their breath." What they are doing is making breathing a closed-chain activity. With the arms braced, the pectoralis major can now pull the sternum toward the humerus, thus increasing the diameter of the rib cage. Individuals with chronic obstructive pulmonary disease commonly brace their arms against the arms of the chair to accomplish the same thing (Fig. 15-13).

The scalenes usually move the head and neck. However, when they act as accessory breathing muscles, they elevate the first and second ribs, assisting in inspiration.

Accessory expiratory muscles operate in much the same fashion, except that they pull down on the rib cage. For example, the rectus abdominis, which usually flexes the trunk, now pulls the sternum toward the pubis in a reversal of muscle action, which assists in expiration (see Fig. 15-12). The quadratus lumborum pulls the lower ribs toward the iliac crest in the same fashion.

Many of the accessory breathing muscles have already been discussed with the vertebral column or shoulder girdle. Those that have not been discussed

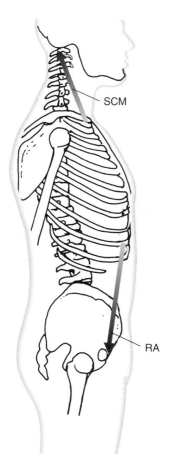

Figure 15-12.   Sternocleidomastoid (SCM) muscle pulling up and rectus abdominis (RA) pulling down.

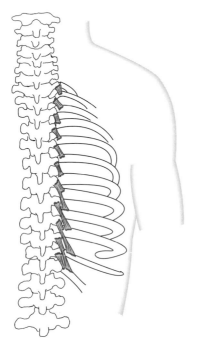

Figure 15-14.   The levator costarum muscles.

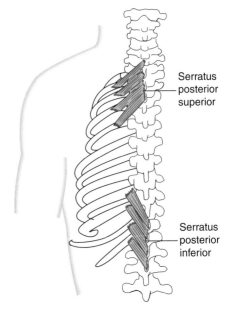

Figure 15-15.   The serratus posterior superior and inferior muscles.

here or in previous chapters are illustrated in Figures 15-14 and 15-15. They are as follows:

Accessory Inspiratory Muscles

Deep Inspiration Muscles
Sternocleidomastoid
Pectoralis major
Scalenes
Levator costarum (Fig. 15-14)
Serratus posterior superior (Fig. 15-15)

Forced Inspiration Muscles
Levator scapulae
Upper trapezius
Rhomboids
Pectoralis minor

Accessory Expiratory Muscles

Forced Expiration Muscles
Rectus abdominis
External oblique
Internal oblique
Transverse abdominis
Quadratus lumborum
Serratus posterior inferior (see Fig. 15-15)

Table 15-1 summarizes the phases of respiration.

Diaphragmatic Versus Chest Breathing

Diaphragmatic breathing is the most efficient method of breathing and requires the least amount of energy. Normally, when the diaphragm contracts, it lowers, causing the abdomen to move out, the lungs to expand, and air to flow into the lungs. When the diaphragm relaxes, it raises, the abdomen moves in, and the lungs recoil, and air flows out of the lungs. When sitting or standing, the gravitational pull on the abdominal viscera also tends to lower the diaphragm. However, when lying, gravity's effect on the abdominal viscera tends to push the diaphragm up into the thoracic cavity. This requires the diaphragm to work harder. This gravitational effect provides the rationale for elevating the head of the bed of an individual with respiratory difficulty. This elevated position will allow easier breathing.

There are certain habits, conditions, or pathologies that don't allow the diaphragm to work effectively. In this case, the upper chest and rib cage must play a major role. **Chest breathing** requires greater effort and is much less efficient than diaphragmatic breathing. As described earlier, during inspiration the rib cage moves up and out (both in a medial-lateral direction and in an anterior-posterior direction), the lungs expand, and air flows into the lungs. During expiration, the rib cage relaxes, the lung recoil, and air flows out of the lungs. With chest breathing, a much smaller volume of air is drawn into the lungs. With shorter

Table 15-1	Phases of Respiration

INSPIRATION: elevation (raising) of ribs and increase in size of thoracic cavity via descent of the diaphragm muscle and expansion of the thoracic wall

Phase	Muscles
Quiet inspiration	Diaphragm
	External intercostals
Deep inspiration	Muscles of quiet inspiration *plus:*
	Sternocleidomastoid
	Scalenes
	Pectoralis major
	Levator costarum
	Serratus posterior superior
Forced inspiration	Muscles of quiet and deep inspiration *plus:*
	Levator scapula
	Upper trapezius
	Rhomboids
	Pectoralis minor

EXPIRATION: depression (lowering) of ribs and decrease in size of the thoracic cavity

Phase	Muscles
Quiet expiration	Relaxation of external intercostals
	Elastic recoil of thoracic wall, lungs, and bronchi
	Gravity
	(Internal intercostals)
Forced expiration	Internal intercostals *plus:*
	Rectus abdominis
	External oblique
	Internal oblique
	Quadratus lumborum
	Transverse abdominis
	Serratus posterior inferior

breaths, the individual must breathe more rapidly. With this type of breathing, a person is more prone to hyperventilate and/or faint.

To be aware of the two methods of breathing, lie supine in a comfortable position with a pillow under your knees and head. Place one hand on your upper chest and the other hand on your stomach just below your ribs. Breathe in slowly through your nose with your mouth closed. With diaphragmatic breathing, you will notice that the hand on your stomach moves up and down as you breathe in and out. There should be little or no movement of the hand on your chest. With chest breathing, the opposite occurs. You will notice movement of the hand on your chest instead of the one on your stomach.

A century ago, it was considered fashionable for women to wear dresses with tightly laced-up girdles. Aesthetically, this made for a small waist, but functionally, it forced the internal organs up against the diaphragm, greatly restricting its effectiveness and forcing women to become chest breathers. No wonder the literature is full of accounts of women "swooning" or fainting. Today, we have the "designer jeans syndrome." Tight-fitting clothing, tight belts and waistbands restrict diaphragmatic breathing and force a person to chest breathe. Extremely obese people and women in the later stages of pregnancy cannot effectively contract diaphragm, therefore, they also tend to chest breathe.

Summary of Innervation of the Muscles of Respiration

Muscles of respiration, like other trunk muscles, receive innervation from spinal nerves at various levels primarily in the thoracic region. The notable exception is the diaphragm muscle that receives its innervation from the phrenic nerve. The phrenic nerve arises from the third, fourth, and fifth cervical nerves. The functional significance of this is that an individual with a spinal cord injury at C3 or above will not be able to breathe unassisted. They will be dependent on a respirator. Individuals with a cervical spinal cord injury below C3 will have impaired respiration but be able to breathe unassisted. Activities such as coughing, yelling, or taking deep breaths are limited. Not only are the intercostal muscles involved but other accessory breathing muscles as well. Activities requiring forced inspiration or expiration are affected to the degree that the accessory breathing muscles are involved.

Valsalva's Maneuver

Valsalva's maneuver occurs when people hold their breath and exhale. Several things can happen. Forcibly exhaling while keeping the mouth closed and nose pinched shut forces air into the eustachian tubes and increases pressure inside the eardrum. This is sometimes helpful in "clearing your ears," which may have become blocked from diving, or quickly descending in elevation.

Prolonged breath-holding and straining is forcible exhalation against the closed glottis. This causes an increase of intrathoracic pressure, which, in turn, traps blood in veins, preventing it from entering the heart. When the breath is released, the intrathoracic pressure drops and the trapped blood is quickly propelled through the heart, increasing heart rate (tachycardia) and blood pressure. Immediately, a reflex bradycardia (slowed heart rate) follows. This can either be an event with no consequences, or lead to cardiac arrest.

Young children having a temper tantrum will take several deep fast breaths, then usually stick their thumb in their mouth, and blow hard without releasing any air. This causes them to get dizzy and pass out. Adults, when exerting, may also take a deep breath, and blow hard or "bear down" without exhaling. Because this maneuver helps to create intra-abdominal pressure and strong contraction of the abdominal muscles that help to stabilize the spine and keep the trunk tight during a heavy lift, it may be purposefully done during exercise. It is also commonly done during birth delivery, moving up in bed, straining when urinating, defecating, vomiting, coughing, or sneezing.

A healthy heart can usually withstand these sudden and changing demands placed on the heart. However, in a weakened heart, it can, and occasionally does, lead to cardiac arrest. Therefore, during exercise, it is a good general rule to breathe out slowly during exertion to avoid breath holding.

Common Respiratory Conditions or Pathologies

An **upper respiratory infection (URI)** is any infection confined to the nose, throat, and larynx. The larynx marks the transition between the upper and lower airways. The common cold is perhaps the most frequent URI. Other URIs are influenza (flu), laryngitis, rhinitis (inflammation of the nasal mucosa), and hay fever.

Lower respiratory infections (LRIs) involve structures from the trachea to the alveoli. **Pneumonia** is perhaps the most common. It is an inflammation of the alveoli caused by bacterial or viral infection. It can affect an entire lobe (lobar pneumonia), or be scattered throughout the entire lung (bronchopneumonia). This form is more common in the very young and very old. "Walking pneumonia" is so named because, in most cases, the disease is not severe enough to confine the patient to bed or to be hospitalized. Bronchitis, emphysema, and asthma are other common LRIs. **Bronchitis** involves the bronchi and the many subdivisions. With **emphysema,** the walls of the alveoli become distended and lose their elasticity due to chronic bronchial obstruction. **Asthma** symptoms are usually due to a spasm of the bronchial walls. This will make it very difficult for the individual to exhale.

Hyperventilation exists commonly during rapid breathing when more carbon dioxide is removed from the system than is metabolically being produced. Breathing into a paper bag to "rebreathe" carbon dioxide is a common treatment. A **stitch** is a temporary condition common in runners. It is a localized sharp pain usually felt just below the rib cage, commonly caused by a cramp in the diaphragm. **Hiccups** are involuntary spasms of the diaphragm accompanied by rapid closure of the glottis producing short, sharp, inspiratory sounds.

A quite painful condition called **pleurisy** is an inflammation of the pleura. A *collapsed lung* or **pneumothorax** occurs by introducing air or otherwise destroying the vacuum of the pleural cavity, thereby reducing ventilation capacity.

Rib separation refers to a dislocation between the rib and its costal cartilage. A **rib dislocation** is the displacement of the costal cartilage from the sternum. A **flail chest** occurs when four or more ribs are fractured in two places (comminuted). This causes that part of the chest wall to collapse instead of expand during inspiration. Conversely, the chest wall will also expand during expiration.

Review Questions

General Anatomy Questions

1. What bony structures make up the thorax?
2. Costovertebral articulations involve what bony structures?
3. What type of movement is allowed at the costovertebral articulations?
4. How do movements of the thorax affect inspiration and expiration? Of the diaphragm?
5. What is the muscle origin of all accessory inspiratory muscles in relation to the rib cage?
6. The line of pull of the external intercostal muscles forms a "V" shape in front similar to the external obliques. However, in the back, they have the opposite line of pull. Why?
7. The diaphragm has only one bony attachment. How is the other end attached? How does the muscle work?

8. When you talk, are you doing so during inspiration, expiration, or both?

9. How do the accessory muscles assist with breathing?

10. Movement of the rib cage is often compared mechanically to what, while movement of the thoracic cavity (lung expansion/deflation) is often compared to what?

11. What is the functional significance between a person with a C3 spinal cord injury versus a person with a C5 level injury?

Functional Activity Questions

Identify the phase(s) of respiration occurring during the following activities:

1. Blowing up a balloon
2. Holding your breath for the count of 15
3. Sneezing
4. Whistling a tune
5. Sitting quietly

Clinical Exercise Questions

1. Lie supine in a comfortable position with a pillow under your knees and head. Place your right hand on your upper chest and your left hand on your stomach just below your ribs. Breathe in slowly through your nose with your mouth closed.
   a. What type of breathing is occurring if your <u>right</u> hand is moving up and down?
   b. What type of breathing is occurring if your <u>left</u> hand is moving?

2. Lying in the same position, place one hand on your stomach and the other covering your mouth. Cough. What muscles are you feeling contract?

3. Place one hand on your chest and the other on the anterior lateral side of your neck. Sniff strongly (as if you had a drippy nose).
   a. What movement occurred at your chest?
   b. Did you feel any muscle contraction at your neck?
   c. What phase of respiration occurs when sniffing, and what neck muscles in a reversal of muscle action caused the sniffing?

4. Sit in a chair with your elbows supported on the arms of the chair. Place your right hand on your left chest with your fingers pointing up toward the left shoulder. Take a deep breath.
   a. What rib movement occurred and in what phase of respiration did it occur?
   b. What accessory breathing muscle is working?
   c. What type of chain activity is occurring?

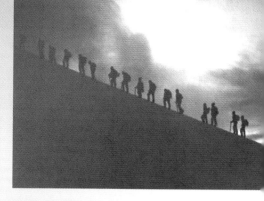

CHAPTER 16

Pelvic Girdle

Structure and Function

False and True Pelvis

   Sacroiliac Joint

   Pubic Symphysis

   Lumbosacral Joint

Pelvic Girdle Motions

   Muscle Control

Review Questions

   General Anatomy Questions

   Functional Activity Questions

   Clinical Exercise Questions

Structure and Function

Four bones make up the **pelvic girdle:** the sacrum, coccyx, and the two hip bones, comprising the ilium, ischium, and pubis. The joints or articulations in the pelvic girdle include the right and left **sacroiliac joints** posterolaterally, the **symphysis pubis** anteriorly, and the **lumbosacral joint** superiorly (Fig. 16-1).

The pelvic girdle, also referred to as the **pelvis,** performs several functions. Perhaps most important to movement and posture is that it supports the weight of the body through the vertebral column and passes that force on to the hip bones. Conversely, it receives the ground forces generated when the foot contacts the ground and transmits them upward toward the vertebral column. During walking, the pelvic girdle moves as a unit in all three planes to allow for relatively smooth motion. In addition, it supports and protects the pelvic viscera, provides attachment for muscles, and makes up the bony portion of the birth canal in females.

False and True Pelvis

There are several terms commonly used when referring to the birth canal. Therefore, it is appropriate to briefly describe a few of these terms and identify some of the differences between the male and female bony pelvis.

The **false pelvis,** also called the *greater* or *major pelvis,* is the bony area between the iliac crests and superior to the pelvic inlet. The **pelvic inlet** can be described by drawing a line between the sacral promontory posteriorly and the superior border of the symphysis pubis anteriorly (Fig. 16-2). There are no pelvic organs within the false pelvis.

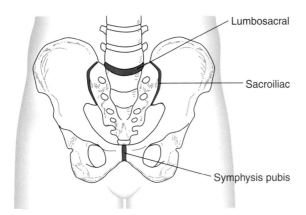

Figure 16-1. Joints of the pelvic girdle.

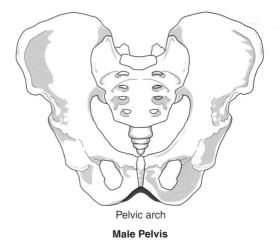

Male Pelvis

A

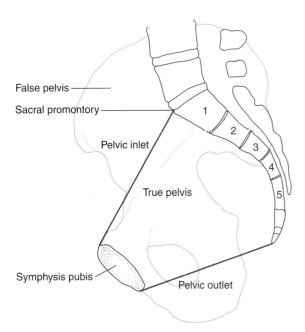

The **true pelvis,** also called the *lesser* or *minor pelvis,* lies between the pelvic inlet and the pelvic outlet. The **pelvic outlet** can be described by drawing a line from the tip of the coccyx to the inferior surface of the pubic symphysis (see Fig. 16-2). The true pelvis area makes up the **pelvic cavity.** It contains portions of GI tract, urinary tract, and some reproductive organs. In females, it forms the *birth canal.*

Several comparisons can be made between the male and female pelvis (Fig. 16-3). The superior open-

Female Pelvis

B

Figure 16-3. Comparison of the male and female pelvis, anterior view. *(A)* Male pelvis. *(B)* Female pelvis.

Figure 16-2. Pelvic inlet and outlet, sagittal section. The bony area between them is called the true pelvis, which makes up the pelvic cavity. The bony area above the pelvic inlet is called the false pelvis.

ing into the pelvic cavity is more oval in females and more heart-shaped in males. The pelvic cavity is shorter and less funnel-shaped in females. The sacrum is shorter, and less curved. The walls are not as vertical. The acetabula and ischial tuberosities are farther apart. These features make the area within the female pelvic cavity greater than the longer, funnel-shaped, cavity of the male pelvis. It can also be noted that the pelvic arch is wider and more rounded in females. These arches can be visually represented by the arch of the extended thumb and index finger in females, and the extended index and middle finger in males.

Sacroiliac Joint

Joint Structure and Motions

The **sacroiliac joint,** commonly referred to as the **SI joint,** is a synovial, nonaxial joint between the sacrum and the ilium. It is described as a plane joint; however its articular surfaces are very irregular. It is this irregularity that helps to lock the two surfaces together.

The function of the sacroiliac joint is to transmit weight from the upper body through the vertebral column to the hip bones. It is designed for great stability and has very little mobility. Like other synovial joints, its articular surface is lined with hyaline cartilage. Synovial membrane lines the nonarticular portions of the joint. It has a fibrous capsule reinforced by ligaments.

SI Joint Motion

The actual type and amount of movement occurring at the SI joint is the subject of considerable controversy. However, it is generally accepted that the motions that do occur at the SI joint are nutation and counternutation (Fig. 16-4).

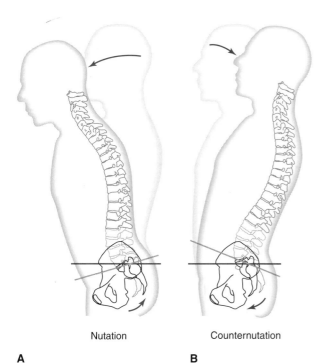

| Nutation | Counternutation |

A   **B**

Figure 16-4. Sacroiliac joint motions: *(A)* nutation occurs when the sacral promontory moves anteriorly and inferiorly while the tip of the coccyx moves in the opposite direction; *(B)* counternutation occurs when the sacral promontory moves posteriorly and superiorly while the tip of the coccyx moves in the opposite direction.

Nutation, sometimes referred to as sacral *flexion,* occurs when the base of the sacrum (on the superior end) moves anteriorly and inferiorly. This causes the inferior portion of the sacrum and the coccyx to move posteriorly. The pelvic outlet becomes larger. The pelvic outlet can be described by drawing a line from the tip of the coccyx to the bottom surface of the pubic symphysis.

Counternutation, sometimes called *sacral extension,* refers to the opposite motion. The base of the sacrum moves posteriorly and superiorly causing the tip of the coccyx to move anteriorly. The pelvic inlet becomes larger. The pelvic inlet can be described by drawing a line from the base of the sacrum across to the top of the symphysis pubis.

The amount of motion that occurs in nutation and counternutation is minimal, and can only occur in association with other joint motions. Nutation occurs with trunk flexion or hip extension. Conversely, counternutation occurs with trunk extension or hip flexion. These motions are also important during childbirth. In the early stages, when the baby moves through the pelvic inlet, the anterior-posterior diameter here needs to be larger. Therefore, the SI joints are in counternutation. In the latter stages, when the baby passes through the pelvic outlet, it is important that this A-P diameter has increased. Putting the SI joints in nutation increases the A-P diameter.

Bones and Landmarks

The two bones of the SI joint are the sacrum and the superior portion of the hip bone, the ilium. The **sacrum** is wedge-shaped and consists of five fused sacral vertebrae. It is located between the two hip bones and makes up the posterior border of the bony pelvis. Its anterior surface, often called the pelvic surface, is concave (Fig. 16-5). Because it is tilted, the sacrum articulates with the fifth lumbar vertebra at an angle. This angle is referred to as the lumbosacral angle. The significant landmarks are as follows (Fig. 16-6):

Base
Superior surface of S1.

Promontory
Ridge projecting along the anterior edge of the body of S1.

Superior articular process
Located posteriorly on the base, it articulates with the inferior articular process of L5.

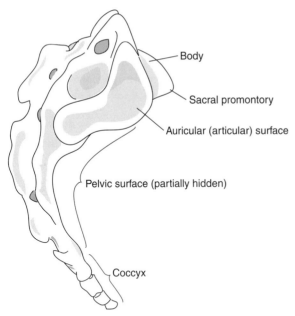

Figure 16-5.   Sacrum, lateral view.

Ala
Lateral flared wings that are actually fused transverse processes.

Foramina
Located on the anterior (pelvic) and dorsal surfaces are four pair of foramina. They serve as the exit for the anterior and posterior divisions of the sacral nerves. The anterior foramina are larger.

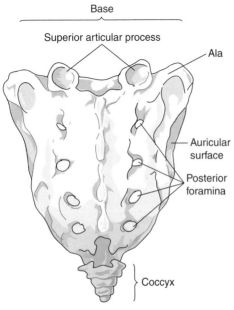

Figure 16-6.   Sacrum, posterior view.

Auricular surface
Named because its shape is similar to the external ear (*auricular* is Latin for "earlike"). It is located on the lateral surface of the sacrum and articulates with the ilium. The irregular surface assists in locking the two surfaces together, providing greater stability.

Pelvic surface
Concave anterior surface.

The **ilium** will be described in more detail in the hip joint chapter. It makes up the superior part of the hip bone. Landmarks relevant to the sacroiliac joint are as follows (Fig. 16-7):

Tuberosity
Large roughened area between the posterior portion of the iliac crest and the auricular surface. It serves as an attachment for the interosseous ligament.

Auricular surface
Named for its earlike shape, it is the articular surface of the ilium with the sacrum. It is located inferior and anterior to the iliac tuberosity.

Iliac crest
Superior ridge of the ilium, the bony area felt when you place your hands on your hips.

Posterior superior iliac spine
Often abbreviated PSIS, it is the posterior projection of the iliac crest and serves as an attachment for the posterior sacroiliac ligaments.

Posterior inferior iliac spine
Often abbreviated PIIS; it lies inferior to the PSIS and serves as an attachment for the sacrotuberous ligament.

Greater sciatic notch
Formed by the ilium superiorly and the ilium and ischium inferiorly.

Greater sciatic foramen
Formed from the greater sciatic notch by ligamentous attachments. The sacrotuberous ligament forms the posterior medial border of the foramen and the sacrospinous ligament forms the inferior border (see Figs. 16-8 and 16-9). The sciatic nerve passes through this opening.

The **ischium** will also be described in more detail in Chapter 17 on the hip joint. The portions of the ischium pertaining to the sacroiliac joint are (see Fig. 16-7):

Body
Makes up all of the ischium superior to the tuberosity.

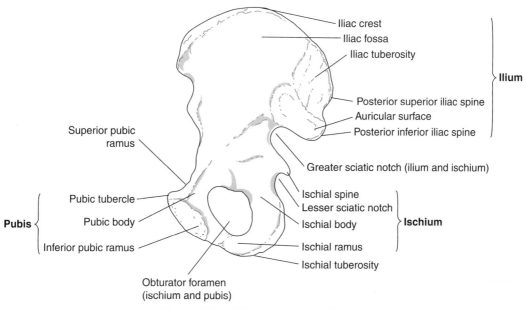

Figure 16-7. Right hip bone, medial view.

Lesser sciatic notch

Smaller concavity located on the posterior body between the greater sciatic notch and the ischial tuberosity.

Spine

Located on the posterior body and between the greater sciatic and lesser sciatic notches. It provides attachment for the sacrospinous ligament.

Tuberosity

The blunt, rough projection on the inferior part of the body. It is a weight-bearing surface when you are sitting.

Ligaments

Because the sacroiliac joint is meant to take a great deal of stress while providing great stability, it is a joint heavily endowed with ligaments. The **anterior sacroiliac ligament** is a broad, flat ligament on the anterior (pelvic) surface connecting the ala and pelvic surface of the sacrum to the auricular surface of the ilium (Fig. 16-8). It holds the anterior portion of the joint together. The **interosseous sacroiliac ligament** is the deepest, shortest, and strongest of the sacroiliac ligaments (Fig. 16-9). It fills the roughened area immediately above and behind the auricular surfaces and anterior sacroiliac ligament. It connects the tuberosities of the ilium to the sacrum.

The posterior sacroiliac ligament comprises two parts (Fig. 16-10). The **short posterior sacroiliac ligament** runs more oblique between the ilium and the upper portion of the sacrum on the dorsal surface. It prevents forward movement of the sacrum. The **long posterior**

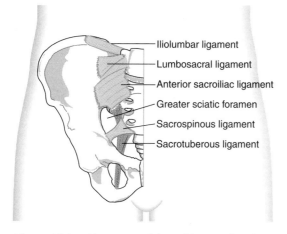

Figure 16-8. Ligaments of the pelvis, anterior view.

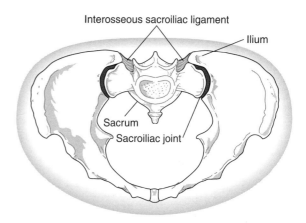

Figure 16-9. Cross section of the sacroiliac joints.

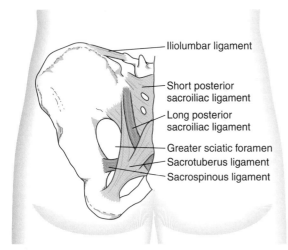

Figure 16-10. Ligament of the pelvis, posterior view.

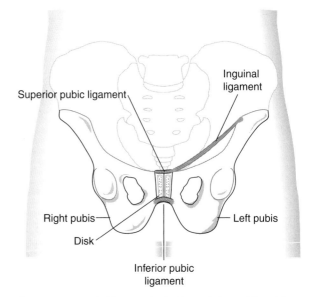

Figure 16-11. Pubic symphysis, frontal view with pubic bone cut away.

sacroiliac ligament runs more vertically between the posterior superior iliac spine and the lower portion of the sacrum. It prevents downward movement of the sacrum.

Three accessory ligaments further reinforce the sacroiliac joint and are seen in Figures 16-8 and 16-10. The **sacrotuberous ligament** is a very strong, triangular-shaped ligament running from between the PSIS and PIIS of the ilium, from the posterior and lateral side of the sacrum inferior to the auricular surface, and from the coccyx. These fibers come together to attach on the ischial tuberosity. It serves as an attachment for the gluteus maximus, and prevents forward rotation of the sacrum. The **sacrospinous ligament** is also triangular-shaped and lies deep to the sacrotuberous ligament. It has a broad attachment from the lower lateral sacrum and coccyx on the posterior side. It then narrows to attach to the spine of the ischium. These two ligaments convert the greater sciatic notch into a foramen through which passes the sciatic nerve. The **iliolumbar ligament** connects the transverse process of L5 with the ala of the sacrum. It is described in more detail under the lumbosacral joint.

Pubic Symphysis

The pubic symphysis joint is located in the midline of the body (Fig. 16-11). The right and left pubic bones are joined anteriorly forming the pubic symphysis. A fibrocartilage disk lies between the two bones. Because it is an amphiarthrodial joint, there is little movement. However, in women during childbirth, it becomes much more moveable.

The pubic symphysis is held together primarily by two ligaments (Fig. 16-11). The **superior pubic liga-**

ment attaches to the pubic tubercles on each side of the body and strengthens the superior and anterior portions of the joint. The **inferior pubic ligament** attaches between the two inferior pubic rami. It strengthens the inferior portion of the joint.

Landmarks

The **pubis** will be described in greater detail under the hip joint. The landmarks relevant to the pubic symphysis are (see Fig. 16-7):

Body
Main portion of the pubic bone, it has a superior and inferior projection (ramus).

Superior ramus
Superior projection of the pubic body.

Inferior ramus
Inferior projection of the pubic body that provides attachment for the inferior pubic ligament.

Tubercle
Projects anteriorly on the superior ramus near the midline and provides attachment for superior pubic ligament.

Lumbosacral Joint

Joint Structure and Ligaments

The lumbosacral joint is made up of the fifth lumbar vertebra and the first sacral vertebra. The articulation between these vertebrae is the same as that for all other

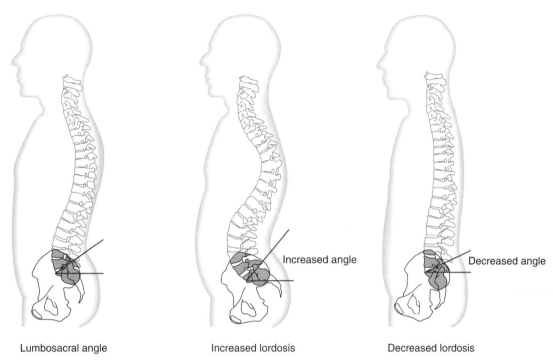

Lumbosacral angle   Increased lordosis   Decreased lordosis

Figure 16-12.   The lumbosacral angle is determined by drawing one line parallel to the ground and another line along the base of the sacrum. The angle increases or decreases as lumbar lordosis increases or decreases, respectively.

vertebrae. The bodies of these two bones are separated by an intervertebral disk and are held together at the bodies by the anterior and posterior longitudinal ligaments. The vertebrae articulate at the articular processes (inferior articular process of L5 and superior articular process of S1). The ligaments holding together this portion of the joint are the supraspinal, interspinal, and ligamentum flava. All of these ligaments are described in Chapter 14.

There are two additional ligaments that specifically hold the lumbosacral joint together (see Fig. 16-8). The **iliolumbar ligament** attaches on the transverse process of L5 and runs laterally to the inner lip of the posterior portion of the iliac crest. This ligament limits the rotation of L5 on S1, and assists the articular processes in preventing L5 from moving anteriorly on S1. The **lumbosacral ligament** also attaches on the transverse process of L5. It runs inferiorly and laterally to attach on the ala of the sacrum. Here its fibers intermingle with the fibers of the anterior sacroiliac ligament.

Lumbosacral Angle

Lumbosacral angle (Fig. 16-12) is determined by drawing one line parallel to the ground and another line along the base of the sacrum. This angle will increase as the pelvis tilts anteriorly and decrease as the pelvis tilts

posteriorly. The optimal lumbosacral angle is approximately 30 degrees. As the lumbar lordosis increases, the angle increases. This causes the shearing stresses of L5 on S1 to increase. Forward movement of L5 on S1 is prevented by ligamentous support, the shape and fit of the inferior articular process of L5 inside and behind the superior articular process of S1. Conversely, as the lumbar lordosis decreases, lumbosacral angle decreases.

Pelvic Girdle Motions

The joints directly involved in movement of the pelvic girdle include the two hip joints and the lumbar joints, particularly the lumbosacral articulation between L5 and S1. The pelvic motions occur in all three planes. When standing in the upright position, the pelvis should be level; in the sagittal plane, the anterior superior iliac spine (ASIS) and pubic symphysis should be in the same vertical plane. **Anterior tilt** occurs when the pelvis tilts forward, moving the ASIS anterior to the pubic symphysis. **Posterior tilt** occurs when the pelvis tilts backward, moving the ASIS posterior to the pubic symphysis. These motions are shown in Figure 16-13.

For the body to remain upright when the pelvis tilts forward, movement in the opposite direction must occur in the joints above and below the pelvis. Therefore,

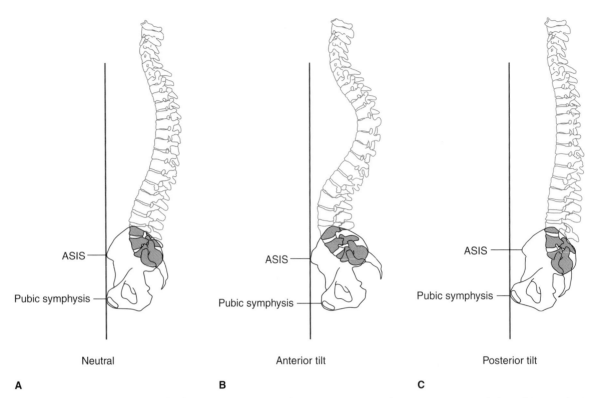

ASIS ——

Pubic symphysis ——

Neutral

A

ASIS ——

Pubic symphysis ——

Anterior tilt

B

ASIS ——

Pubic symphysis ——

Posterior tilt

C

Figure 16-13. Pelvic movement in the sagittal plane. *(A)* The anterior superior iliac spine (ASIS) and the pubic symphysis should be in the same vertical plane. *(B)* Anterior tilt occurs when the pelvis tilts forward, moving the ASIS anterior to the pubic symphysis. *(C)* Posterior tilt occurs when the pelvis tilts backward, moving the ASIS posterior to the pubic symphysis.

when the pelvis tilts anteriorly, the lumbar portion of the vertebral column goes into hyperextension while the hip joints flex. Thus, when a person with a hip flexion contracture stands in the upright position, the pelvis will tilt anteriorly while the lumbar region becomes hyperextended. Conversely, a person with tight hamstrings may stand with the pelvis tilted posteriorly and lumbar curve flattened.

In the frontal plane, the iliac crests should be level (Fig. 16-14). Placing your thumbs on the ASISs and determining if your thumbs are at the same level can assess this. **Lateral tilt** occurs when the two iliac crests are not level. Because the pelvis moves as a unit, one side moves up as the other side moves down (Fig. 16-15). Therefore, a point of reference must be used. *The side that is unsupported will be the point of reference.* Another way of identifying the reference point is to identify the *side of the pelvis farthest from the joint axis.* For example, in right unilateral stance, the joint axis would be the right hip. The side of the pelvis farthest away would be the left side. During walking, the pelvis is level when both legs are in contact with the ground. However, when one leg leaves the ground (swing phase), it becomes

unsupported and the pelvis on that side drops slightly. It is impossible to drop the pelvis on the weight-bearing side. Therefore, the point of reference for lateral tilt will be the unsupported, or less supported, side, or the

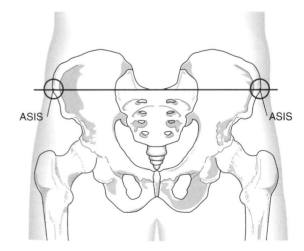

ASIS   ASIS

Figure 16-14. Pelvic movement in the frontal plane. When standing upright on both feet, the iliac crests and the ASISs should be level.

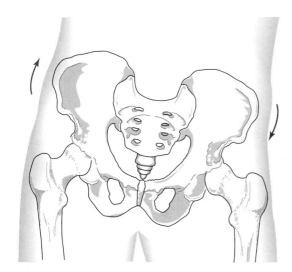

Figure 16-15. Lateral tilt. One side of pelvis moves up while the other side moves down.

side farthest from the weight-bearing joint axis. Figure 16-16 illustrates a left lateral tilt. The person bears weight on the right leg while lifting the left leg from the ground. The left side of the pelvis becomes unsupported and drops, or laterally tilts to the left.

To keep the body balanced, joints directly above and below will shift in the opposite direction. Notice in

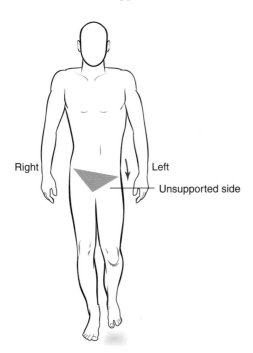

Figure 16-16. Left lateral tilt. When one leg leaves the ground, the pelvis on that side becomes unsupported. This causes the pelvis on that side to drop slightly. Therefore, lateral tilt is named by the unsupported side.

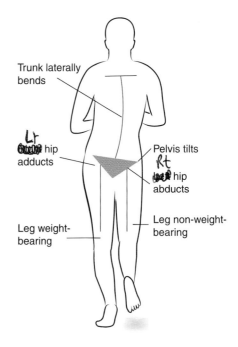

Posterior View

Figure 16-17. Other joint motions affected by pelvic tilting. As the pelvis tilts to the right, the vertebral column laterally bends to the left. The left hip (weight-bearing side) adducts and the right hip (non–weight-bearing) abducts.

Figure 16-17 that, as the pelvis tilts (drops) to the right, the vertebral column laterally bends to the left. While the weight-bearing hip joint (left) adducts, the unsupported hip (right) becomes more abducted.

Although this discussion has centered on one side of the pelvis dropping below the level of the other side, it is possible to raise the pelvis on the unsupported side. This is commonly called "*hip hiking.*" When walking with a long leg cast or brace, this motion assists the foot in clearing the floor during the swing phase. Shifting from one ischial tuberosity to the other also involves raising the pelvis on one side. This is useful in allowing some pressure relief during sitting.

Pelvic rotation occurs in the transverse plane around a vertical axis when one side of the pelvis moves forward or backward in relation to the other side. Looking down on the pelvis, the significant landmarks again are the ASISs. In the anatomical (neutral) position (Fig. 16-18A), both ASISs should be in the same plane. With forward rotation of the pelvis, as in the example in Figure 16-18B, the left leg is weight-bearing and the right leg is swinging forward. Once again, *the unsupported side is the point of reference.* This causes the right side of the pelvis to rotate forward

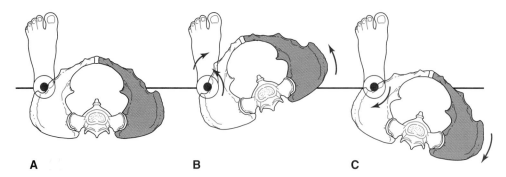

A   **B**   **C**

Figure 16-18.   Pelvic rotation in the transverse plane, superior view. *(A)* In the anatomical (neutral) position, both ASISs are in the same plane. *(B)* With forward rotation, the pelvis on the right moves forward. This causes the left pelvis to rotate around the femoral head, resulting in hip medial rotation. *(C)* With backward rotation, the pelvis on the right moves backward. This causes the left pelvis to rotate on the femoral head resulting, in hip lateral rotation.

moving the right ASIS forward of the left ASIS. If the right leg were to swing backward, as in Figure 16-18C, the pelvis would rotate backward. Stated another way, if you bear weight on your left leg and swing your right leg backward, the right side of your pelvis rotates backward.

This pelvic rotation is occurring because the pelvis is moving on the weight-bearing hip joint. If there is right forward rotation of the pelvis, there is left hip medial rotation (Fig 16-18B). It should be remembered that this hip medial rotation is occurring because the pelvis is moving on the femoral head, instead of the more common other way around. With right backward rotation of the pelvis, there is left hip lateral rotation (Fig 16-18C). The combinations of joint motions occurring during walking will be described in greater detail in Chapter 21. However, a summary of some of the associated joint motions can be found in Table 16-1.

Muscle Control

The pelvis is moved and controlled by groups of muscles acting as force couples. As the pelvis tilts in the anterior/posterior direction, it is the opposing muscle groups that provide the movement and control (Fig. 16-19). To tilt the pelvis anteriorly, the lumbar trunk extensors, primarily the erector spinae, pull up posteriorly while the hip flexors pull down anteriorly. Conversely, to tilt the pelvis posteriorly, the abdominals pull up anteriorly while the gluteus maximus and hamstrings pull down posteriorly (Fig. 16-20). In both cases, the opposite muscle groups are acting as a force couple, causing the pelvis to tilt.

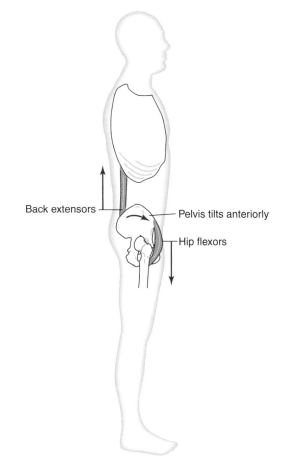

Back extensors —

— Pelvis tilts anteriorly

— Hip flexors

Figure 16-19.   Force couple causing anterior pelvic tilt. The trunk extensors pulling up (posteriorly) and the hip flexors anterior pulling down (anteriorly) cause the pelvis to tilt anteriorly.

Table 16-1	Associated Motions of the Pelvic Girdle, Vertebral Column, and Hip Joints	
Pelvic Girdle	**Vertebral Column**	**Hip**
Anterior tilt	Hyperextension	Flexion
Posterior tilt	Flexion	Extension
Lateral tilt (unsupported side)	Lateral bending (to supported side)	Adduction—weight-bearing side Abduction—non-weight-bearing side
Rotation (forward)	Rotation—to opposite side	Medial rotation—weight-bearing side
Rotation (backward)	Rotation—to opposite side	Lateral rotation—weight-bearing side

The force of gravity, without any muscle action, can tilt the pelvis laterally when that leg becomes unsupported. However, to control or limit the amount of lateral tilting, opposite muscle groups work as a force couple as well. Using the example in Figure 16-21, in a reversal of muscle function action, the left trunk lateral benders, primarily the erector spinae and quadratus lumborum, pull up on the left side of the pelvis, while the right hip abductors (gluteus medius and minimus) pull down on the right side to keep the pelvis fairly level.

All of these same muscle groups can work together to provide stability by preventing the pelvis from moving. Pelvic and trunk control are necessary to provide the stable foundation upon which the head and extremities can move.

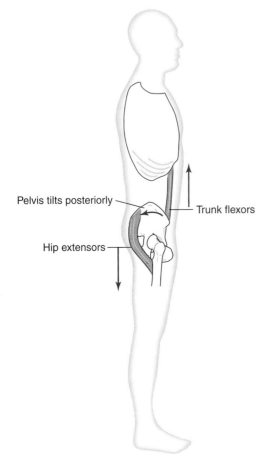

Figure 16-20.   Force couple causing posterior pelvic tilt. The trunk flexors pulling up (anteriorly) and the hip extensors pulling down (posteriorly) cause the pelvis to tilt posteriorly.

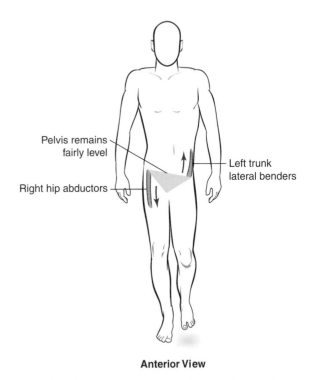

Anterior View

Figure 16-21.   Force couple keeps the pelvis level in the frontal plane. In a reversal of muscle action, the left trunk lateral benders pull up while the right hip abductors pull down. This keeps the pelvis fairly level as opposed to letting the pelvis drop on the unsupported side.

Review Questions

General Anatomy Questions

1. What pelvic girdle motions occur in the following?
   a. The sagittal plane around the frontal axis
   b. The frontal plane around the sagittal axis
   c. The transverse plane around the vertical axis

2. Concentric contraction of the right quadratus lumborum would cause the pelvis to laterally tilt to which side?

3. Motion occurs at the lumbosacral joint when the pelvis tilts anteriorly and posteriorly and at what other distal joint?

4. What associated hip motion occurs when the pelvis tilts:
   a. Anteriorly
   b. Posteriorly
   c. Laterally

5. What associated hip motion occurs when the left pelvis rotates:
   a. Forward
   b. Backward

6. What associated lumbar motion occurs when the pelvis tilts:
   a. Anteriorly
   b. Posteriorly
   c. Laterally

7. If a person maintained a posture in which the pelvis were tilted excessively in an anterior position, what muscle groups would tend to be tight?

Functional Activity Questions

Identify the position of the pelvis in the following activities:

1. Lying supine, bring your right leg up to your chest.

2. Kneeling on your hands and knees, let your trunk sag downward.

3. Kneeling on your hands and knees, arch your back.

4. Standing with your left foot on a telephone book and your right foot on the floor with weight on both feet. Identify the position of right and left hips in terms of abducted or adducted positions (Fig. 16-22).

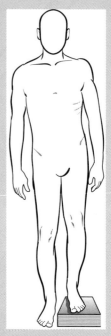

Figure 16-22.   Standing with one foot on a telephone book and the other foot on the floor.

Clinical Exercise Questions

1. Lying supine with the knees flexed and soles of the feet flat on the mat. Place your hand in the small of your back (lumbar curve). Push your back against your hand. Identify the main trunk, pelvic, and hip motions occurring. What are the muscles contributing to this force couple action?
   Motions:
   Muscles:

2. Standing in anatomical position, lift your left foot off the ground, keeping your hip and knee extended.
   Identify the main pelvic and hip motions occurring. What are the muscles contributing to this force couple action?
   Motions:
   Muscles:

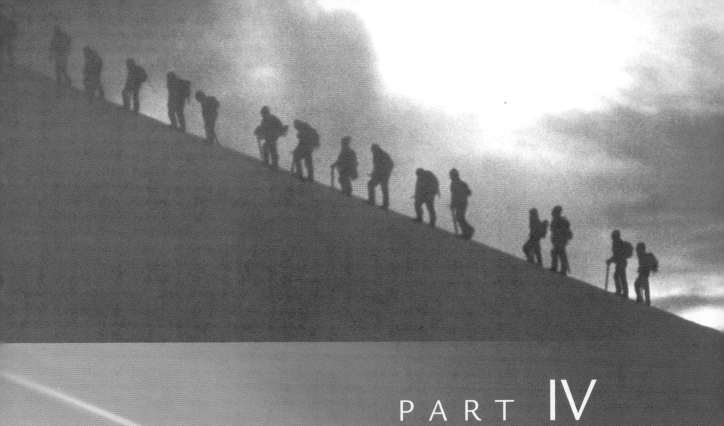

PART IV

Clinical Kinesiology and Anatomy of the Lower Extremities

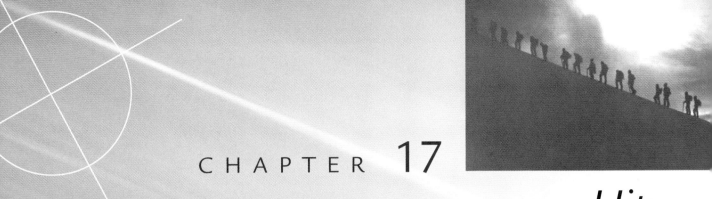

CHAPTER 17

Hip

Joint Structure and Motions

Bones and Landmarks

Ligaments and Other Structures

    Common Hip Pathologies

Muscles of the Hip

    Summary of Muscle Action

    Summary of Muscle Innervation

Review Questions

    General Anatomy Questions

    Functional Activity Questions

    Clinical Exercise Questions

The lower extremity includes the pelvis, thigh, leg, and foot (Fig. 17-1). Bones of the pelvis are the two hip bones (os coxae bones), the sacrum, and the coccyx. The hip bone consists of three bones (ilium, ischium, and pubis) fused together. The thigh contains the femur and patella. The leg includes the tibia and fibula, and the foot includes seven tarsal bones, five metatarsals, and 14 phalanges. Table 17-1 summarizes these bones.

Joint Structure and Motions

The **hip** is the most proximal of the lower extremity joints. It is very important in weight-bearing and walking activities. Like the shoulder, it is a ball-and-socket joint. The rounded or convex-shaped femoral head fits into and articulates with the concave-shaped acetabulum (Fig. 17-2). Unlike the shoulder, the hip is a very stable joint and therefore sacrifices some range of motion. Conversely, the shoulder allows a great deal of motion but is not as stable.

Being a triaxial joint, the hip has motion in all three planes (Fig. 17-3). Flexion, extension, and hyperextension occur in the sagittal plane with approximately 120 degrees of flexion and 15 degrees of hyperextension. Extension is the return from flexion. Abduction and adduction occur in the frontal plane with about 45 degrees of abduction. Adduction is usually thought of as the return to anatomical position, although there is approximately an additional 25 degrees possible beyond the anatomical position. In the transverse plane, medial and lateral rotation are sometimes referred to as *internal* and *external rotation,* respectively. There are approximately 45 degrees of rotation possible in each direction from the anatomical position.

The two hip bones are connected to each other anteriorly and to the sacrum posteriorly. The sacrum is also

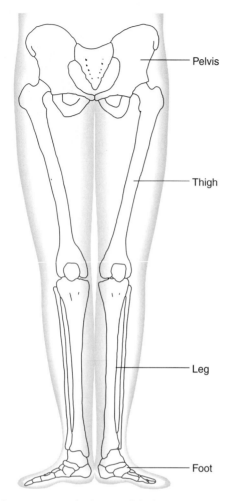

Figure 17-1.   The bones of the lower extremities.

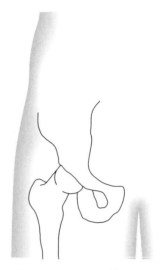

Figure 17-2.   The hip joint.

connected distally to the coccyx. These four bones (two hip bones, sacrum, and coccyx) are collectively known as the pelvis, or pelvic girdle (Fig. 17-4). Note that the pelvis does not include the femur.

Bones and Landmarks

As mentioned, the hip joint is made up of the hip bone and the femur. The hip bone, also known as the *os coxae,*

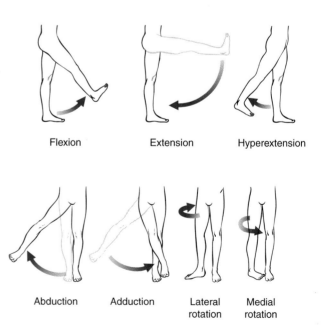

Figure 17-3.   Motions of the hip.

Table 17-1	Bones of the Lower Extremity	
Region	**Bones**	**Individual Bones**
Pelvis	Os coxae	Ilium, ischium, pubis
	Sacrum	
	Coccyx	
Thigh	Femur	
	Patella	
Leg	Tibia	
	Fibula	
Foot	Tarsals (7)	Calcaneus, talus, cuboid, navicular, cuneiform (3)
	Metatarsals (5)	First through fifth
	Phalanges (14)	Proximal (5), middle (4), distal (5)

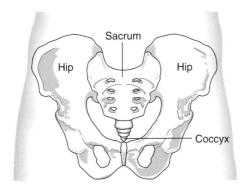

Figure 17-4. The bones of the pelvis.

is irregularly shaped and actually made up of three bones (Fig. 17-5). These bones fuse together as one by adulthood. The three bones are the ilium, ischium, and pubis.

The fan-shaped **ilium** makes up the superior portion of the hip bone. Its significant landmarks are as follows (Fig. 17-6):

Iliac fossa
Large, smooth, concave area on the internal surface to which the iliac portion of the iliopsoas muscle attaches.

Iliac crest
Bony part that your hands rest on when you put your hands on your hips. Its borders are the anterior superior iliac spine (ASIS) anteriorly and the posterior superior iliac spine (PSIS) posteriorly.

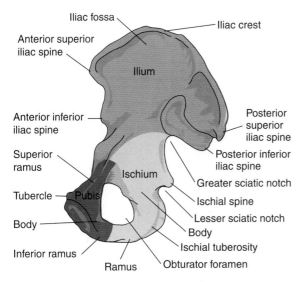

Figure 17-5. Right hip bone, medial view, consists of the ilium, ischium, and pubis. The greater sciatic notch, acetabulum, and obturator foramen are formed by different combinations of these bones.

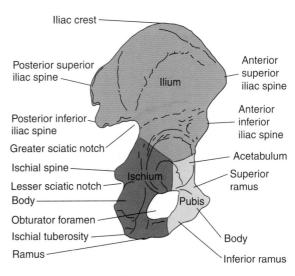

Figure 17-6. Right hip bone, lateral view.

Anterior superior iliac spine
Abbreviated ASIS; the projection on the anterior end of the iliac crest. The tensor fascia lata, sartorius, and inguinal ligament attach here.

Anterior inferior iliac spine
Abbreviated AIIS. The projection is just inferior to the ASIS to which the rectus femoris muscle attaches.

Posterior superior iliac spine
Abbreviated PSIS. It is the posterior projection on the iliac crest.

Posterior inferior iliac spine
Abbreviated PIIS; located just below the PSIS.

The **ischium** is the posterior inferior portion of the hip bone. Its significant landmarks are as follows (see Fig. 17-6):

Body
Makes up about two-fifths of the acetabulum.

Ramus
Extends medially from the body to connect with the inferior ramus of the pubis. The adductor magnus, obturator externus, and obturator internus muscles attach here.

Ischial tuberosity
Rough, blunt projection of the inferior part of the body, which is weight-bearing when you are sitting. It provides attachment for the hamstring and adductor magnus muscles.

Spine

Located on the posterior portion of the body between the greater and lesser sciatic notchs. It provides attachment for the sacrospinous ligament.

The **pubis** forms the anterior inferior portion of the hip. It can be divided into three parts, the body and its two rami (see Fig. 17-5):

Body

Externally forms about one-fifth of the acetabulum and internally provides attachment for the obturator internus muscle.

Superior ramus

Lies superior between the acetabulum and the body and provides attachment for the pectineus muscle.

Inferior ramus

Lies posterior, inferior, and lateral to the body. Provides attachment for the adductor magnus and brevis and gracilis muscles.

Symphysis pubis

A cartilaginous joint connecting the bodies of the two pubic bones at the anterior midline.

Pubic tubercle

Projects anteriorly on the superior ramus near the symphysis pubis and provides attachment for the inguinal ligament.

The following are made up of combinations of the hip bones (see Fig. 17-5):

Acetabulum

A deep, cup-shaped cavity that articulates with the femur. It is made up of nearly equal portions of the ilium, ischium, and pubis.

Obturator foramen

A large opening made up of the bodies and rami of the ischium and pubis and through which pass blood vessels and nerves.

Greater sciatic notch

Large notch just below the PIIS that is actually made into a foramen by the sacrospinous ligament. The sciatic nerve, piriformis muscle, and other structures pass through this opening.

The **femur** is the longest, strongest, and heaviest bone in the body. A person's height can roughly be estimated to be four times the length of the femur (Moore, 1985). It articulates with the hip bones to form the hip joint and has the following significant landmarks (Fig. 17-7):

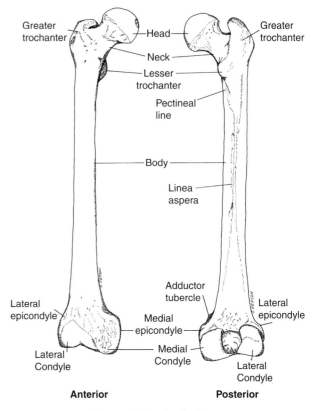

Figure 17-7.   Right femur.

Head

The rounded portion covered with articular cartilage articulating with the acetabulum.

Neck

The narrower portion located between the head and the trochanters.

Greater trochanter

Large projection located laterally between the neck and the body of the femur, providing attachment for the gluteus medius and minimus, and most deep rotator muscles.

Lesser trochanter

A smaller projection located medially and posteriorly just distal to the greater trochanter, providing attachment for the iliopsoas muscle.

Body

The long cylindrical portion between the bone ends; also called the *shaft*. It is bowed slightly anteriorly.

Medial condyle

Distal medial end.

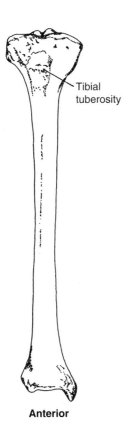

Figure 17-8.   Right tibia, anterior view.

Lateral condyle
Distal lateral end.

Lateral epicondyle
Projection proximal to the lateral condyle.

Medial epicondyle
Projection proximal to the medial condyle.

Adductor tubercle
Small projection proximal to the medial epicondyle to which a portion of the adductor magnus muscle attaches.

Linea aspera
Prominent longitudinal ridge or crest running most of the posterior length.

Pectineal line
Runs from below the lesser trochanter diagonally toward the linea aspera. It provides attachment for the adductor brevis.

Patellar surface
Between the medial and lateral condyle anteriorly. It articulates with the posterior surface of the patella.

The **tibia** will be discussed in more detail in Chapter 18. It is important to identify one landmark now (Fig. 17-8):

Tibial tuberosity
Large projection at the proximal end in the midline. It provides attachment for the patellar tendon.

Ligaments and Other Structures

Like all synovial joints, the hip has a fibrous joint capsule. It is strong, thick, and covers the hip joint in a cylindrical fashion. It attaches proximally around the lip of the acetabulum and distally to the neck of the femur (Fig. 17-9). It forms a cylindrical sleeve that encloses the joint and most of the femoral neck.

Three ligaments reinforce the capsule. They are the iliofemoral, ischiofemoral, and pubofemoral ligaments (Fig. 17-10). The most important of these ligaments is the **iliofemoral ligament.** It reinforces the capsule anteriorly by attaching proximally to the anterior inferior iliac spine and crossing the joint anteriorly. It splits into two parts distally to attach to the intertrochanteric line of the femur. Because it resembles an inverted "Y," it is often referred to as the *Y ligament.* It is also known as the *ligament of Bigelow.* Its main function is to limit hyperextension.

The **pubofemoral ligament** spans the hip joint medially and inferiorly, attaching from the medial part of the acetabular rim and superior ramus of the pubis, running down and back to attach on the neck of the femur. Like the iliofemoral ligament, it also limits hyperextension. In addition, it limits abduction.

The **ischiofemoral ligament** covers the capsule posteriorly. It attaches on the ischial portion of the acetabulum, crosses the joint in a lateral and superior

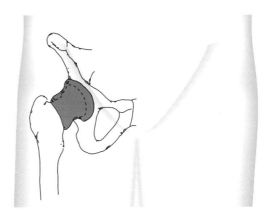

Figure 17-9.   The hip joint capsule.

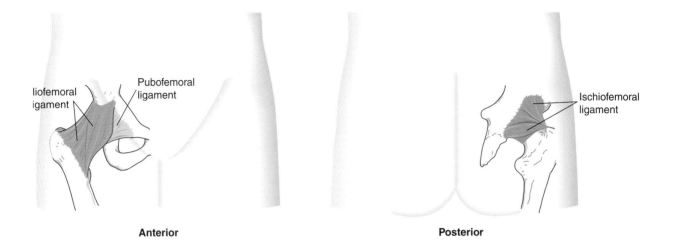

Figure 17-10. The hip joint capsule is reinforced by three ligaments: the iliofemoral, pubofemoral, and ischiofemoral.

direction, and attaches on the femoral neck. Its fibers limit hyperextension and also medial rotation.

These three ligaments all attach along the rim of the acetabulum and cross the hip joint in a spiral fashion to attach on the femoral neck. The combined effect of this spiral attachment is to limit motion in one direction (hyperextension) while allowing full motion (flexion) in the other direction. Therefore, these ligaments are slack in flexion and become taut as the hip moves into hyperextension. By thrusting the hips forward so

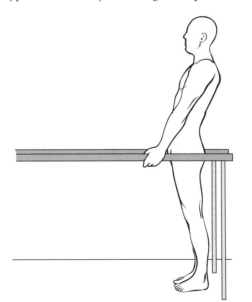

Figure 17-11. The spiral attachment of the hip ligaments tends to limit hyperextension. An individual with paraplegia can therefore stand in the upright position by thrusting the hips forward of the shoulders and knees.

that they are in front of the shoulders and knees, it is possible to stand in the upright position without using any muscles by, essentially, resting on the iliofemoral ligament. This is the basis for the standing posture of an individual with spinal cord paralysis (Fig. 17-11).

The **ligamentum teres** is a small intracapsular ligament of debatable importance (Fig. 17-12). It attaches proximally in the acetabulum and distally in the fovea of the femoral head. Some sources indicate that it becomes taut during adduction or during lateral rotation, when the hip is semiflexed. However, given its size, it is doubtful that it adds significantly to the strength of the joint. Its other feature is that it contains a blood vessel that supplies the head of the femur. However, by itself, this vessel is unable to supply enough blood to the head to keep it viable.

The depth of the acetabulum is increased by the fibrocartilaginous **acetabular labrum,** which is located around the rim. The free end of the labrum surrounds the femoral head and assists in holding the head in the acetabulum.

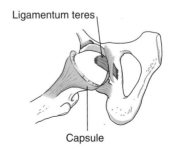

Figure 17-12. The ligamentum teres. Oblique view with femur laterally rotated and capsule cut away.

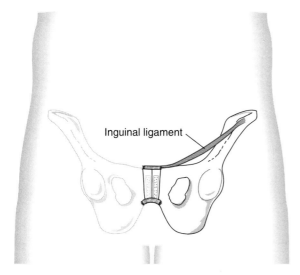

Figure 17-13.   The inguinal ligament.

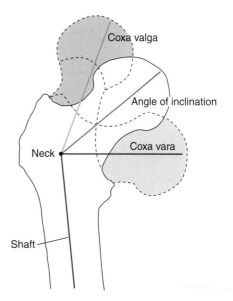

Figure 17-14.   Angle of inclination is normally about 125 degrees, coxa valga is an angle greater than 125 degrees, and coxa vara is an angle less than 125 degrees.

Although the **inguinal ligament** has no function at the hip joint, it should be identified because of its presence. It runs from the anterior superior iliac spine to the pubic tubercle and is the landmark that separates the anterior abdominal wall from the thigh (Fig. 17-13). When the external iliac artery and vein pass under the inguinal ligament, their names change to the *femoral artery* and *vein.*

The **iliotibial band** or **tract** is the very long, tendinous portion of the tensor fascia latae muscle (see Fig. 17-28). It attaches to the anterior portion of the iliac crest and runs superficially down the lateral side of the thigh to attach to the tibia. Both the gluteus maximus and tensor fascia latae muscles have fibers attaching to it.

Common Hip Pathologies

The hip joint is the site of many orthopedic conditions occurring throughout life that can have an affect on lower extremity alignment. **Congential hip dislocation** or **dysplasia** is the result of an unusually shallow acetabulum causing the femoral head to slide upward. The joint capsule remains intact, though stretched. **Legg-Calvé-Perthes disease** or **coxa plana** is a condition in which the femoral head undergoes necrosis. It is usually seen in children between the ages of 5 and 10 years. The course of the disease may take about 2 to 4 years for the head to die, revascularize, and then remodel. **Slipped capital femoral epiphysis** is seen in children during the growth spurt years. The proximal epiphysis slips from its normal position on the femoral head.

The angle between the shaft and the neck of the femur in the *frontal plane* is referred to as the **angle of inclination,** which is normally at 125 degrees. This angle can vary greatly as the result of many factors, such as congenital, trauma, or disease. Coxa valga is characterized by a neck-shaft angle greater than 125 degrees (Fig. 17-14). Because this angle is "straighter," it tends to make the limb longer, thus placing the hip in an adducted position during weight-bearing. **Coxa vara** is a deformity in which the neck-shaft angle is less than the normal of 125 degrees. Because it is "more bent," it tends to make the involved limb shorter, dropping the pelvis on that side during weight-bearing.

The angle between the shaft and the neck of the femur in the *transverse plane* is called the **angle of torsion,** which normally has the head and neck rotated outward from the shaft approximately 15 to 25 degrees (Fig. 17-15). Looking down on the femur, as in Figure 17-15, one would see the femoral head and neck superimposed on the shaft. The shaft is best shown here by a line through the femoral condyles, which are attached to the shaft distally. As the shaft rotates, so do the condyles. An increase in this angle is called **anteversion,** and forces the hip joint into a more medially rotated position. This would cause a person to walk in a more "toed-in" position. A decrease in the angle of torsion is called **retroversion.** This position would force the hip joint into a more laterally rotated position, causing the person to walk more "toed out."

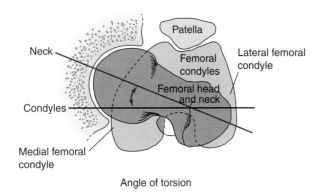

A

Angle of torsion

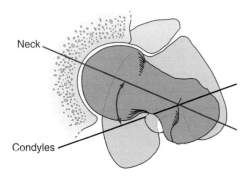

Anteversion is an increased angle and results in toed-in gait

B

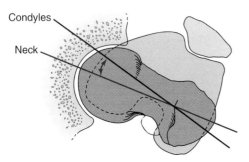

Retroversion is a decreased angle and results in toed-out gait

C

Figure 17-15. Superior view. Angle of torsion normally has the head and neck rotated outward from the shaft approximately 15 to 25 degrees. An increase in this angle is called anteversion, and a decrease in this angle is called retroversion.

Osteoarthritis is a degeneration of the articular cartilage of the joint. It may be the result of trauma or wear and tear, and is typically seen later in life. It is commonly treated with a total joint replacement. **Hip** **fractures** tend to be of two types: intertrochanteric and femoral neck. These are very common among the elderly, usually resulting from falls. High impact trauma, such as motor vehicle accidents, may cause hip fractures in younger individuals.

Iliotibial band syndrome is an overuse injury causing lateral knee pain. It is commonly seen in runners and bicyclists. Repeated friction of the band sliding over the lateral femoral epicondyle during knee motion caused by such conditions as muscle tightness, worn down shoes, or running on uneven surfaces is believed to create the syndrome. Because many muscles insert at the greater trochanter, there are many bursae providing a friction-reducing cushion between the muscles and bone. **Trochanteric bursitis** is the result of either acute trauma or overuse. It can be seen in runners or bicyclists, someone with a leg length discrepancy, or other factors putting repeated stress on the greater trochanter. A **hamstring strain,** also called **"pulled hamstring,"** is probably the most common muscle problem in the body. Unfortunately, it is often recurrent. It may result from an overload of the muscle or trying to move the muscle too fast. Therefore, this is a common injury among sprinters and in sports that require bursts of speed or rapid acceleration, such as soccer, track and field, football, and rugby. Hamstring strains can occur at one of the attachment sites or at any point along the length of the muscle.

Hip pointer is a misnomer because it doesn't occur at the hip, but at the pelvis. It is a severe bruise caused by direct contact to the iliac crest of the pelvis. It is most commonly associated with football but can be seen in almost any contact sport. Spearing the hip/pelvis with a helmet while tackling may be the most common cause.

Muscles of the Hip

There are many similarities between the shoulder and hip joints. Like the shoulder, the hip has a group of one-joint muscles that provide most of the control and a group of longer, two-joint muscles that provide the range of motion. These muscles can also be grouped according to their location and somewhat by their function. For example, the anterior muscles tend to be flexors, lateral muscles tend to be abductors, posterior muscles tend to be extensors, and medial muscles tend to be adductors. Table 17-2 classifies the hip muscles by location and function.

The **iliopsoas muscle** is actually two muscles with separate proximal attachments and a common distal attachment (Fig. 17-16). The iliacus muscle

Table 17-2	Muscles of the Hip		
Muscle Group	**One-Joint Muscles**		**Two-Joint Muscles**
Anterior	Iliopsoas		Rectus femoris
			Sartorius
Medial	Pectineus		Gracilis
	Adductor magnus		
	Adductor longus		
	Adductor brevis		
Posterior	Gluteus maximus		Semimembranosus
	Deep rotators (6)		Semitendinosus
			Biceps femoris
Lateral	Gluteus medius		Tensor fascia latae
	Gluteus minimus		

portion arises from the iliac fossa, and the psoas major muscle portion comes from the transverse processes, bodies, and intervertebral disks of the T12 through L5 vertebrae. These muscles blend together to attach on the lesser trochanter of the femur. The iliopsoas muscle is a prime mover in hip flexion. The psoas muscle portion, because of its attachment on the vertebra, contributes to trunk flexion when the femur is stabilized.

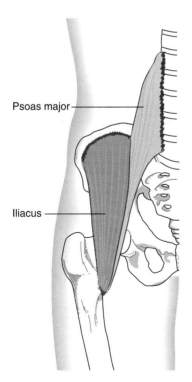

Psoas major

Iliacus

Figure 17-16. The iliopsoas muscle is made up of the psoas major and iliacus.

Iliopsoas Muscle

O	Iliac fossa, anterior and lateral surfaces of T12 through L5
I	Lesser trochanter
A	Hip flexion
N	Iliacus portion: Femoral nerve (L2, L3) Psoas major portion: L2 and L3

The **rectus femoris muscle** is part of the quadriceps muscle group and the only one of that group to cross the hip (Fig. 17-17). Its proximal attachment is on the AIIS. It runs almost straight down the thigh to be joined by the three vasti muscles to blend into the quadriceps muscle tendon (also called the patellar tendon). This tendon encases the patella, crosses the knee joint, and attaches to the tibial tuberosity. The rectus femoris muscle is a prime mover in hip flexion and knee extension.

Rectus Femoris Muscle

O	Anterior inferior iliac spine
I	Tibial tuberosity
A	Hip flexion, knee extension
N	Femoral nerve (L2, L3, L4)

The **sartorius muscle** is the longest muscle in the body (Fig. 17-18). This long, straplike muscle arises from the anterior superior iliac spine. It runs diagonally across the thigh from lateral to medial and proximal to distal to cross the medial knee joint posteriorly. Because of its line of pull, it is capable of flexing, abducting, and laterally rotating the hip and flexing the knee. However, it is not considered a prime mover in any one of these motions. It is most efficient when doing all four of these motions at the same time. An example of this motion is when you cross your legs by putting one foot on the opposite knee.

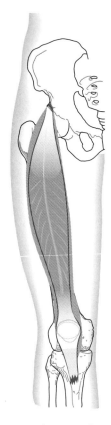

Figure 17-17. The rectus femoris muscle.

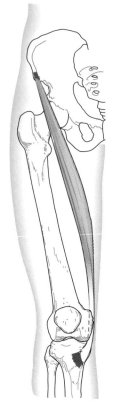

Figure 17-18. The sartorius muscle.

Sartorius Muscle

O	Anterior superior iliac spine
I	Proximal medial aspect of tibia
A	Combination of hip flexion, abduction, lateral rotation and knee flexion
N	Femoral nerve (L2, L3)

Located medial to the iliopsoas muscle and lateral to the adductor longus muscle is the **pectineus muscle.** Its origin is on the superior ramus of the pubis, and its insertion is on the pectineal line of the femur (Fig. 17-19). Because it spans the hip anteriorly as well as medially, it provides hip flexion and adduction.

Pectineus Muscle

O	Superior ramus of pubis
I	Pectineal line of femur
A	Hip flexion and adduction
N	Femoral nerve (L2, L3, L4)

There are three other one-joint hip adductors, all with the same first name (Fig. 17-20). The **adductor longus muscle,** the most superficial of the three, originates from the anterior surface of the pubis near the tubercle and inserts on the middle third of the linea aspera of the femur. Because it is superficial, its tendon can easily be felt in the anterior-medial groin. Being able to palpate this tendon is important when checking for correct fit of the quadrilateral socket of an above-knee prosthesis. It is a prime mover in hip adduction.

Adductor Longus Muscle

O	Pubis
I	Middle third of the linea aspera
A	Hip adduction
N	Obturator nerve (L3, L4)

The **adductor brevis muscle** implies by its name that it is shorter. It lies deep to the adductor longus muscle, but superficial to the adductor magnus muscle. It arises from the inferior ramus of the pubis and inserts on the pectineal line and proximal linea aspera above the adductor longus muscle. It is a prime mover in hip adduction.

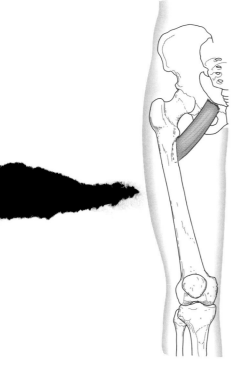

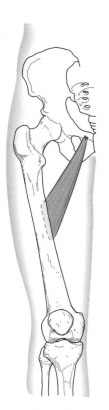

Adductor Brevis Muscle

O	Pubis
I	Pectineal line and proximal linea aspera
A	Hip adduction
N	Obturator nerve (L3, L4)

The largest, most massive, and deepest of the adductors is the **adductor magnus muscle.** It arises from the ischial tuberosity and ramus of the ischium and inferior ramus of the pubis. It makes up most of the bulk on the medial thigh. It inserts along the entire linea aspera and adductor tubercle. There is an interruption, or hiatus, in the distal attachment between the linea aspera and adductor tubercle. The femoral artery and vein pass through this opening. After these structures have passed through to the posterior surface, their names become the *popliteal artery* and *vein.* Because of its size, the adductor magnus muscle is a very strong hip adductor.

Adductor Magnus Muscle

O	Ischium and pubis
I	Entire linea aspera and adductor tubercle
A	Hip adduction
N	Obturator and sciatic nerve (L3, L4)

Figure 17-19. The pectineus muscle. Note that the distal attachment is on the posterior femur.

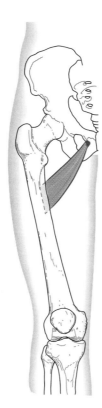

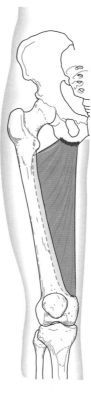

Adductor longus

Adductor brevis

Adductor magnus

Figure 17-20. The three adductor muscles. Note that the distal attachments are on the posterior femur.

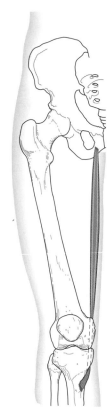

Figure 17-21. The gracilis muscle. Note that it passes behind the knee but attaches anteriorly.

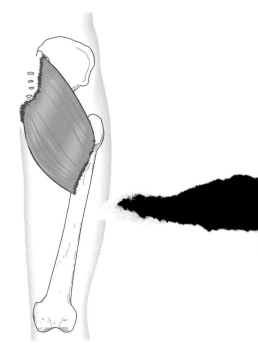

Figure 17-22. The gluteus maximus muscle.

The only hip adductor that is a two-joint muscle is the **gracilis muscle** (Fig. 17-21). It arises from the symphysis and inferior ramus of the pubis and descends the thigh medially and superficially. It crosses the knee joint posteriorly and curves around the medial condyle to attach distally on the antero-medial surface of the proximal tibia. It is assistive in knee flexion.

Gracilis Muscle

O	Pubis
I	Anterior medial surface of proximal end of tibia
A	Hip adduction
N	Obturator nerve (L2, L3)

The **gluteus maximus muscle** can be described as a large, one-joint, quadrilateral-shaped, thick muscle located superficially on the posterior buttock (Fig. 17-22). It arises from the general area of the posterior sacrum, coccyx, and ilium, and runs in a diagonal direction distally and laterally to the posterior femur inferior to the greater trochanter. Some fibers also attach to the iliotibial band. Because it spans the hip posteriorly in this diagonal direction, it is very strong in hip extension, hyperextension, and lateral rotation.

Gluteus Maximus Muscle

O	Posterior sacrum and ilium
I	Posterior femur distal to greater trochanter and to iliotibial band
A	Hip extension, hyperextension, lateral rotation
N	Inferior gluteal nerve (L5, S1, S2)

There are six small, deep, mostly posterior muscles that span the hip joint in a horizontal direction, and they all laterally rotate the hip. Because they all work together to produce the same motion, their individual attachments are not functionally important. Therefore, they can be grouped together as the **deep rotator muscles** (Fig. 17-23). The piriformis is, however, the best known of this group, perhaps because of its close relationship to the sciatic nerve. Table 17-3 summarizes their attachments and innervation.

Table 17-3	Deep Rotator Muscles		
Muscle	**Proximal Attachment**	**Distal Attachment**	**Innervation**
Obturator externus	Rami of pubis and ischium	Trochanteric fossa	Obturator nerve
Obturator internus	Rami of pubis and ischium	Greater trochanter	Nerve to obturator internus
Quadratus femoris	Ischial tuberosity	Intertrochanteric crest	Nerve to quadratus femoris
Piriformis	Sacrum	Greater trochanter	S1, S2 segments
Gemellus superior	Ischium	Greater trochanter	Nerve to obturator internus
Gemellus inferior	Ischial tuberosity	Greater trochanter	Nerve to quadratus femoris

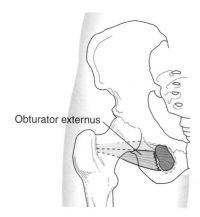

Anterior

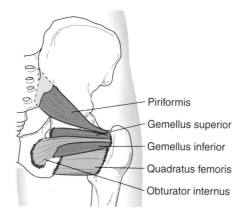

Posterior

Figure 17-23. The deep rotator muscles.

Deep Rotator Muscles

O	Posterior sacrum, ischium, pubis
I	Greater trochanter area
A	Hip lateral rotation
N	Numerous, see Table 17-3

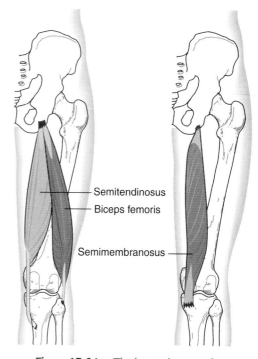

Figure 17-24. The hamstring muscles.

Three muscles that are known collectively as the **hamstring muscles** cover the posterior thigh. They consist of the semitendinosus, the semimembranosus, and the biceps femoris muscles (Fig. 17-24). They have a common site of origin on the ischial tuberosity.

The **semimembranosus muscle** runs down the medial side of the thigh deep to the semitendinosus muscle and inserts on the posterior surface of the medial condyle of the tibia. The **semitendinosus muscle** has a much longer and narrower distal tendon that after spanning the knee joint posteriorly, moves anteriorly to attach to the anteromedial surface of the tibia with the gracilis and sartorius muscles. The **biceps femoris muscle** has two heads and runs down the thigh laterally on the posterior side. The long head arises with the other two muscles on the ischial tuberosity, but the short head arises from the lateral lip of the linea aspera. Both heads join together, spanning the knee posteriorly to attach laterally on the head of the fibula and by a small slip to the lateral condyle of the tibia. Because they span the knee posteriorly, they flex the knee. The long head, because it spans the hip posteriorly, also extends the hip.

Semimembranosus Muscle

O	Ischial tuberosity
I	Posterior surface of medial condyle of tibia
A	Extend hip and flex knee
N	Sciatic nerve (L5, S1, S2)

Semitendinosus Muscle

O	Ischial tuberosity
I	Anteromedial surface of proximal tibia
A	Extend hip and flex knee
N	Sciatic nerve (L5, S1, S2)

Biceps Femoris Muscle

O	Long head: ischial tuberosity Short head: lateral lip of linea aspera
I	Fibular head
A	Long head: extend hip and flex knee Short head: flex knee
N	Long head: sciatic nerve (S1, S2, S3) Short head: common peroneal nerve (L5, S1, S2)

The other two gluteal muscles are more laterally located. The **gluteus medius muscle** is triangular-shaped, much like the deltoid muscle of the shoulder (Fig. 17-25). It attaches proximally to the outer surface of the ilium and distally to the lateral surface of the greater trochanter. Because it spans the hip laterally, it is able to abduct the hip. Its anterior fibers are able to assist the gluteus minimus muscle in medially rotating the hip.

Gluteus Medius Muscle

O	Outer surface of the ilium
I	Lateral surface of the greater trochanter
A	Hip abduction
N	Superior gluteal nerve (L4, L5, S1)

Proximally, the **gluteus minimus muscle** lies deep and inferior to the gluteus medius muscle on the lateral ilium (Fig. 17-26). The distal attachment is on the

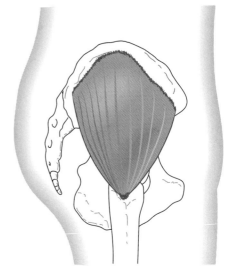

Figure 17-25.   The gluteus medius muscle.

anterior aspect of the greater trochanter. This gives the gluteus minimus muscle a somewhat diagonal line of pull, making it able to medially rotate the hip. Because it spans the hip laterally, it also abducts the hip.

Gluteus Minimus Muscle

O	Lateral ilium
I	Anterior surface of the greater trochanter
A	Hip abduction, medial rotation
N	Superior gluteal nerve (L4, L5, S1)

Attaching to the ilium and the femur and spanning the hip laterally, these two gluteal muscles have another

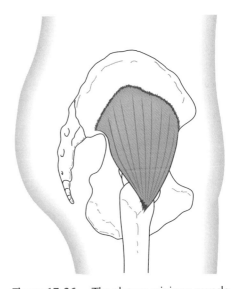

Figure 17-26.   The gluteus minimus muscle.

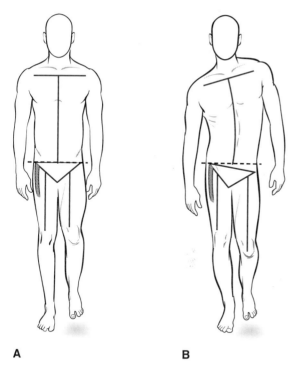

A   **B**

Figure 17-27. *(A)* In reversal of muscle function, the right hip abductors contract to keep the pelvis steady when the left leg is lifted. *(B)* When right hip abductors are weak, the left side of the pelvis drops.

very important function. When you stand on one leg, the distal segment (femur) becomes more stable than the proximal segment (pelvis); therefore, the origin moves toward the insertion. Another term for this change is **reversal of muscle function.** If these muscles did not contract when you stood on one leg, the opposite side of your pelvis would drop (Fig. 17-27). Therefore, the gluteus medius and minimus muscles contract to keep the pelvis fairly level and prevent the opposite side of the pelvis from dropping very much when you stand on one leg. This occurs every time you pick up one leg, as when walking. Weakness or loss of these muscles results in a "Trendelenberg gait." For example, if your right hip abductors are weak, your left pelvis will drop significantly when you stand on your right leg and lift your left leg off the ground.

The **tensor fascia latae muscle** is a very short muscle with a very long tendinous attachment (Fig. 17-28). It arises from the ASIS, crosses the hip laterally and slightly anteriorly, then attaches to the long fascial band called the *iliotibial band,* which proceeds down the lateral thigh and attaches into the tibia. It is a hip abductor but, because of its slight anterior position, it

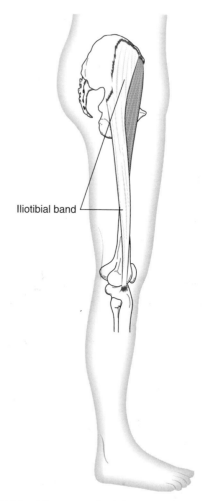

Iliotibial band

Figure 17-28. The tensor fascia latae muscle. The very long, tendinous portion of this muscle is known as the iliotibial band.

is perhaps strongest when performing a combination of flexion and abduction. Stated another way, it is most efficient when abducting in a slightly anterior direction.

Tensor Fascia Latae Muscle

O	Anterior superior iliac spine
I	Lateral condyle of tibia
A	Combined hip flexion and abduction
N	Superior gluteal nerve (L4, L5)

Summary of Muscle Action

The actions of the prime movers of the hip joint are summarized as follows:

Action	Muscle
Combination of flexion and abduction	Tensor fascia latae
Combination of flexion, abduction, and lateral rotation	Sartorius
Flexion	Rectus femoris, iliopsoas, pectineus
Extension	Gluteus maximus, semitendinosus, semimembranosus, biceps femoris (long head)
Hyperextension	Gluteus maximus
Abduction	Gluteus medius, gluteus minimus
Adduction	Pectineus, adductor longus, adductor brevis, adductor magnus, gracilis
Medial rotation	Gluteus minimis
Lateral rotation	Gluteus maximus, deep rotators

Summary of Muscle Innervation

Generally speaking, the femoral nerve innervates muscles on the anterior surface of the hip and thigh region (hip flexors). The obturator nerve innervates hip adductors on the medial side. The hip abductors on the lateral side are supplied by the superior gluteal nerve. The hamstring muscles, which are hip extensors and located posteriorly, receive innervation from the sciatic nerve.

There are, of course, exceptions to all generalizations. The gluteus maximus, a posterior muscle, receives innervation from the inferior gluteal nerve. The deep rotators do not fit neatly into any sort of generalization; therefore, they are included in the summary of hip joint muscle innervation in Table 17-4 individually instead of as a group. Table 17-5 summarizes the segmental innervation. As has been stated in previous chapters, there is variation among sources regarding some segmental innervation. The deep rotators are included here as a group.

Table 17-4 Innervation of the Muscles of the Hip

Muscle	Nerve	Spinal Segment
Iliopsoas: psoas part	Anterior rami	L2, L3
Iliacus part	Femoral	L2, L3
Rectus femoris	Femoral	L2, L3, L4
Sartorius	Femoral	L2, L3
Pectineus	Femoral	L2, L3
Gracilis	Obturator	L2, L3
Adductor longus	Obturator	L2, L3, L4
Adductor brevis	Obturator	L2, L3, L4
Adductor magnus	Obturator	L3, L4
Gluteus maximus	Inferior gluteal	L5, S1, S2
Gluteus medius	Superior gluteal	L5, S1, S2
Gluteus minimis	Superior gluteal	L5, S1, S2
Tensor fascia latae	Superior gluteal	L4, L5
Semitendinosus	Sciatic	L5, S1, S2
Semimembranosus	Sciatic	L5, S1, S2
Biceps femoris		
Long	Sciatic	L5, S1, S2
Short	Common peroneal	L5, S1, S2
Obturator externus	Obturator	L3, L4
Obturator internus	Nerve to the obturator internus	L5, S1
Gemellus superios	Nerve to the obturator internus	L5, S1
Quadratus femoris	Nerve to the quadratus femoris	L5, S1
Gemellus inferior	Nerve to the quadratus femoris	L5, S1
Piriformis	Anterior rami	S1, S2

Table 17-5	Segmental Innervation of Hip Muscles						
Spinal Cord Level	L2	L3	L4	L5	S1	S2	S3
Illiopsoas	X	X					
Sartorius	X	X					
Gracillis	X	X					
Rectus femoris	X	X	X				
Pectineus	X	X	X				
Adductor longus		X	X				
Adductor brevis		X	X				
Adductor magnus		X	X				
Tensor fascia latae			X	X			
Gluteus medius			X	X	X		
Gluteus minimus			X	X	X		
Semitendinosus				X	X	X	
Semimembranosus				X	X	X	
Biceps femoris				X	X	X	X
Deep rotators		X	X	X	X	X	

Review Questions

General Anatomy Questions

1. List the bones that make up the:
   a. Pelvis
   b. Hip bone
   c. Hip joint
   d. Acetabulum
   e. Obturator foramen
   f. Greater sciatic notch

2. If you were handed an unattached hip bone, what landmarks would you use to determine if it were a right or left hip bone?

3. How would you determine if an unattached femur is a right or left one?

4. Describe the hip joint:
   a. Number of axes:
   b. Shape of joint:
   c. Type of motion allowed:

5. What hip motions occur in:
   a. the transverse plane around the vertical axis?
   b. the sagittal plane around the frontal axis?
   c. the frontal plane around the sagittal axis?

6. What is referred to as the *Y ligament?* Why?

7. Why is the hip joint not prone to dislocation?

8. What is the direction of the line of attachment of the ligaments of the hip—vertical, horizontal, or spiral? What does this line of attachment allow for?

9. Which two-joint hip joint muscles attach below the knee?

10. Which hip joint muscles are not prime movers in any single action but are effective in a combination of movements? List the movements.

11. What muscle(s) keeps your pelvis from dropping on one side when you lift one foot off the floor? Describe what happens.

Functional Activity Questions

1. A right-handed tennis player strikes a ball with a forehand swing. The left hip is moving into what positions (Fig. 17-29)?

2. a. How is hip flexion affected by sitting on a low surface versus a higher one, for example, a regular versus a raised toilet seat?

   b. What accompanying hip motions or positions may occur if a person has her feet apart, knees

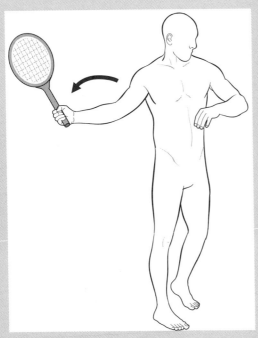

Figure 17-29.   Position of tennis player when hitting a forehand swing.

together, puts her hands on her knees, and pushes down to assist when standing (Fig. 17-30)?

3. Standing in anatomical position and keeping your pelvis fairly level, shift your weight to your right foot.
   a. What hip joint motion has occurred at your right hip?
   b. What muscle group initiates this action?

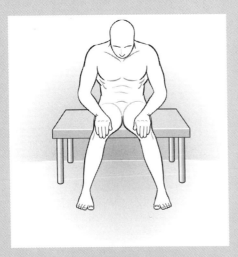

Figure 17-30.   Position of hips when beginning to stand.

4. While weight-bearing on the left leg, note the motions of your right hip as you swing your right leg in the following activities:
   a. Walking
   b. Stepping up onto a curb
   c. Getting into a car
   d. Getting on a boy's bicycle (bar between handlebars and seat)

5. Lie supine on a table with knees bent and your feet flat. Note the position of your pelvis and determine if you can put your hand in the small of your back.
   a. If you cannot, what is the position of your pelvis?
   b. If you can, what then is the position of your pelvis and lumbar spine?

6. Next, slowly slide your feet down the table until your hips and knees are extended. Again, note the position of your pelvis and determine if you can put your hand in the small of your back. Repeat this again keeping your right knee and hip flexed with foot flat, while you move your left foot down until your left hip and knee are extended.
   a. What is accomplished at the pelvis by keeping your right hip and knee flexed?
   b. What can be said about left hip muscle length if you cannot rest your left thigh completely on the table? In other words, why wouldn't you be able to extend your left hip?
   c. What is the one-joint hip muscle attaching on the pelvis and lumbar spine that may be responsible?
   d. What difference does the position of the pelvis have on anterior hip muscle length?

7. Pretend that you cannot completely extend your hip due to tight hip flexors. How might you compensate for this when standing?

Clinical Exercise Questions

1. While lying prone with your right knee flexed, raise your right leg straight upward, keeping your pelvis flat on the table. Describe what has occurred in terms of (a) hip joint motion, (b) whether stretching or strengthening is occurring, and (c) muscle(s) involved.

2. In the lunge position, move your right leg forward until your right knee is directly over your right ankle. Your left hip is hyperextended and your left knee is flexed and resting on the floor. Rock your weight

forward onto the front (right) leg without moving your right foot or right knee. Describe what has occurred at the left hip in terms of (a) joint

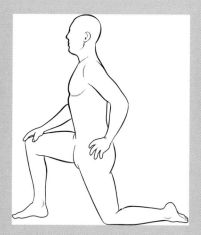

Figure 17-31.   The lunge position.

motion, (b) whether stretching or strengthening is occurring, and (c) muscle(s) involved (Fig. 17-31).

3. Sitting on the floor with your legs far apart; lean forward from the hips while keeping your back straight. Describe what has occurred in terms of (a) hip joint motion, (b) whether stretching or strengthening is occurring, and (c) muscle(s) involved.

4. Lying on your right side with your left hip and knee in extension, raise your left leg toward the ceiling about 2 feet.

   Describe what has occurred in terms of (a) joint motion, (b) whether stretching or strengthening is occurring, and (c) muscle(s) involved.

5. Repeat No. 4 with your left hip in approximately 30 degrees of flexion. Describe what has occurred in terms of (a) joint motion, (b) whether stretching or strengthening is occurring, and (c) muscle(s) involved.

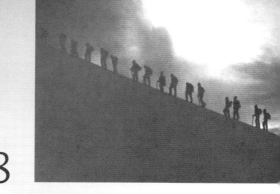

CHAPTER 18

Knee

Joint Structure and Motions

Bones and Landmarks

Ligaments and Other Structures

Common Knee Pathologies

Muscles of the Knee

Anterior Muscles

Posterior Muscles

Summary of Muscle Action

Summary of Muscle Innervation

Review Questions

General Anatomy Questions

Functional Activity Questions

Clinical Exercise Questions

Joint Structure and Motions

At first glance the knee joint appears to be a relatively simple joint; however, it is one of the more complex joints in the body. Because it is supported and maintained entirely by muscles and ligaments with no bony stability, and because it is frequently exposed to severe stresses and strains, it should be no surprise that it is one of the most frequently injured joints in the body.

The knee joint is the largest joint in the body and it is classified as a synovial hinge joint (Fig. 18-1). The motions possible at the knee are flexion and extension (Fig. 18-2). From 0 degrees of extension there are approximately 120 to 135 degrees of flexion. However, unlike the elbow, the knee joint is not a true hinge because it has a rotational component. This rotation is not a free motion but an accessory motion that accompanies flexion and extension.

All three types of arthrokinematic motion are used during knee flexion and extension. The convex femoral condyles move on the concave tibial condyles, or the other way around depending upon whether it is an open- or closed-chain activity. The articular surface of the femoral condyles is much greater than that of the tibial condyles. If the femur rolled on the tibia from flexion to extension, the femur would roll off the tibia before the motion was complete (Fig. 18-3A). Therefore, the femur must **glide** posteriorly on the tibia as it **rolls** into extension (Fig. 18-3B). It should also be noted that the articular surface of the femoral medial condyle is longer than that of the lateral condyle (Fig. 18-4A). As extension occurs, the articular surface of the femoral lateral condyle is used up while some articular surface remains on the medial condyle (Fig. 18-4B). Therefore, the medial condyle of the femur must also glide posteriorly to use all of its articular surface (Fig. 18-4C). It is

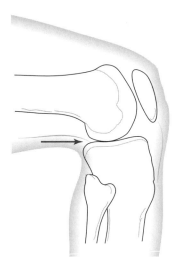

Figure 18-1.   The knee joint.

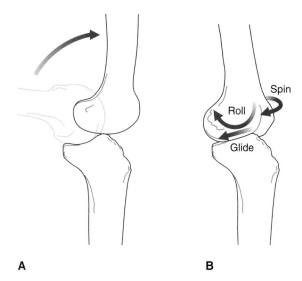

A   **B**

Figure 18-3.   Arthrokinematic movements of the knee joint surfaces in a closed-chain activity of knee extension in which the femur moves on the tibia, medial view. *(A)* Pure rolling of the femur would cause it to roll off the tibia as the knee extends. *(B)* Normal motion of the knee demonstrates a combination of rolling, gliding (posteriorly), and spinning (medially) in the last 20 degrees of extension.

this posterior gliding of the medial condyle during the last few degrees of weight-bearing extension (closed-chain action) that causes the femur to **spin** (rotate medially) on the tibia (see Fig. 18-3B).

Looking at the same spin, or rotational, movement during non–weight-bearing extension (open-chain action), the tibia rotates laterally on the femur. These last few degrees of motion lock the knee in extension, which is sometimes referred to as the *screw-home mechanism* of the knee. With the knee fully extended, an individual can stand for a long time without using muscles. The knee must be "*unlocked*" by the femur rotating laterally on the tibia for knee flexion to occur. It is this small amount of rotation of the femur on the tibia, or vice versa, that keeps the knee from being a true hinge joint. Because this rotation is not an independent motion, it will not be considered a knee motion.

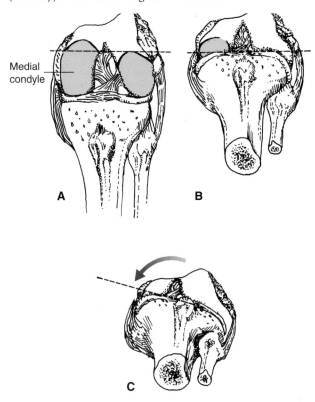

C

Figure 18-4.   The screw-home motion of the left knee. In the weight-bearing position (closed-chain activity), the femur rotates medially on the tibia as the knee moves into the last few degrees of extension.

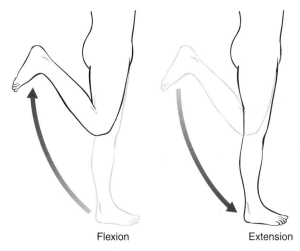

Flexion   Extension

Figure 18-2.   Knee motions.

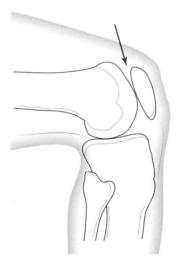

Figure 18-5.   The patellofemoral joint.

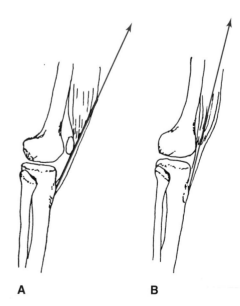

A   **B**

Figure 18-6.   Moment arm of the quadriceps muscles is greater with a patella *(A)*, than without a patella *(B)*.

The articulation between the femur and patella is referred to as the **patellofemoral joint** (Fig. 18-5). The posterior surface of the patella is smooth and glides over the patellar surface of the femur. The patella's main functions are to increase the mechanical advantage of the quadriceps muscle and to protect the knee joint. An increased mechanical advantage is achieved by lengthening the moment arm. As discussed in Chapter 7 on torque, moment arm is the perpendicular distance between the muscle's line of action and the center of the joint (axis). By placing the patella between the quadriceps tendon (also called the patellar tendon) and the femur, the action line of the quadriceps muscles is farther away (Fig. 18-6). Hence, the moment arm is lengthened, which allows the muscle to have greater angular force. Without the patella, the moment arm would be smaller and much of the force of the muscle would be a stabilizing force directed back into the joint.

The **Q angle,** or *patellofemoral angle,* is the angle between the quadriceps muscle, primarily the rectus femoris muscle, and the patellar tendon. It is determined by drawing a line from the anterior superior iliac spine (ASIS) to the midpoint of the patella and from the tibial tuberosity to the midpoint of the patella. Although the rectus femoris attaches to the anterior inferior iliac spine (AIIS), the ASIS lies just above the AIIS and is easier to palpate. The angle formed by the intersecting of these lines represents the Q angle (Fig. 18-7). This angle ranges from 13 to 18 degrees in normal individuals in knee extension, and tends to be greater in females (Magee, p 729). A greater angle in females is associated with the fact that females tend to have a wider pelvis. Many different knee and patellar problems such as patellofemoral

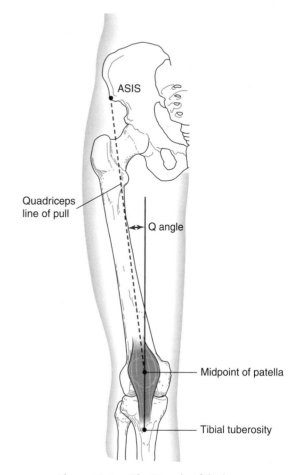

Figure 18-7.   The Q angle of the knee.

pain syndrome are associated with Q angles being greater or less than this range.

Bones and Landmarks

The knee is composed of the distal end of the femur articulating with the proximal end of the tibia. The significant landmarks for the femur were discussed in the previous chapter. The landmarks of the tibia significant to the knee are as follows (Fig. 18-8):

Intercondylar eminence
A double-pointed prominence on the proximal surface at about the midpoint, which extends up into the intercondylar fossa of the femur.

Medial condyle
The proximal medial end.

Lateral condyle
The proximal lateral end.

Plateau
The enlarged proximal end including the medial and lateral condyles and the intercondylar eminence.

Tibial tuberosity
Large projection at the proximal end on the anterior surface in the midline.

The **fibula** is lateral to, and smaller than, the tibia. It is set back from the anterior surface of the tibia, allowing a large space for muscle attachment (Fig. 18-9). This feature gives the lower leg its rounded circumference. The fibula is not part of the knee joint because it does not articulate with the femur. Although it does provide a point of attachment for some of the knee structures, it has a larger role at the ankle.

The **patella** is a triangular-shaped sesamoid bone within the quadriceps muscle tendon (Fig. 18-10). It has a broad superior border and a somewhat pointed distal portion.

The **calcaneus** (see Fig. 18-9) is the most posterior of the tarsal bones and is commonly known as the *heel*. It is identified here because it provides attachment for the gastrocnemius muscle.

Ligaments and Other Structures

As stated earlier, the knee is held together not by its bony structure but by ligaments and muscles. The cruciate and collateral ligaments are the two main

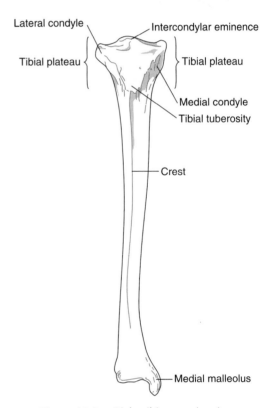

Figure 18-8. Right tibia, anterior view.

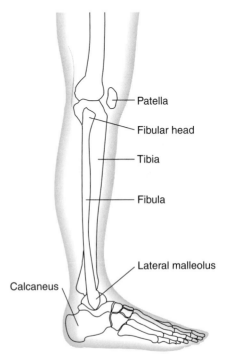

Figure 18-9. Right leg, lateral view.

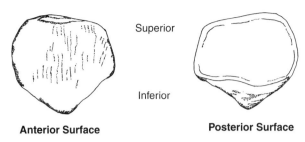

Anterior Surface   Posterior Surface

Figure 18-10.   The patella.

sets of ligaments for this task (Fig. 18-11). The cruciates are located within the joint capsule and are therefore called intracapsular ligaments. Located between the medial and lateral condyles, the cruciates cross each other obliquely (*cruciate* means "resembling a cross" in Latin). They are named by their attachment on the *tibia* (Fig. 18-12). The **anterior cruciate ligament** attaches to the anterior surface of the tibia in the intercondylar area just medial to the medial meniscus. It spans the knee laterally to the posterior cruciate ligament and runs in a superior and posterior direction to attach posteriorly on the lateral condyle of the femur. The **posterior cruciate ligament** attaches to the posterior tibia in the intercondylar area and runs in a superior and anterior direction on the medial side of the anterior cruciate ligament. It attaches to the anterior femur on the medial condyle. To summarize these attachments, the anterior cruciate runs from anterior tibia to posterior femur, and the posterior cruciate runs from posterior tibia to anterior femur.

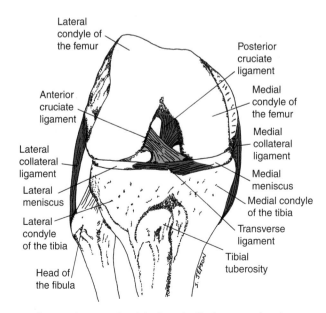

Figure 18-11.   The right knee in flexion, anterior view.

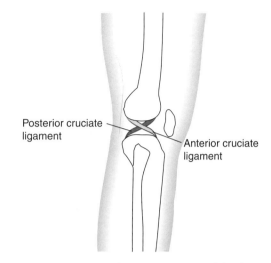

Figure 18-12.   Cruciate ligaments are named for their attachment on the tibia.

The cruciates provide stability in the sagittal plane. The anterior cruciate ligament keeps the femur from being displaced posteriorly on the tibia or, conversely, the tibia from being displaced anteriorly on the femur. It tightens during extension, preventing excessive hyperextension of the knee. When the knee is partly flexed, the anterior cruciate keeps the tibia from being moved anteriorly. Conversely, the posterior cruciate ligament keeps the femur from being displaced anteriorly on the tibia or the tibia from being displaced posteriorly on the femur. It tightens during flexion and is injured much less frequently than the anterior cruciate ligament.

Located on the sides of the knee are the collateral ligaments. The **medial collateral,** or **tibial collateral, ligament** is a flat, broad ligament attaching to the medial condyles of the femur and tibia. Fibers of the medial meniscus are attached to this ligament, which contributes to frequent tearing of the medial meniscus when there is excessive stress to the medial collateral ligament. On the lateral side is the **lateral collateral,** or fibular collateral, ligament. It is a round, cordlike ligament that attaches to the lateral condyle of the femur and runs down to the head of the fibula, independent of any attachment to the lateral meniscus. It protects the joint from stresses to the medial side of the knee. It is quite strong and not commonly injured.

The collateral ligaments provide stability in the frontal plane. The medial collateral ligament, providing medial stability, prevents excessive motion from a blow to the lateral side of the knee. The lateral collateral ligament provides stability to the medial side. Because their attachments are offset posteriorly and superiorly to the axis of flexion, the collateral ligaments

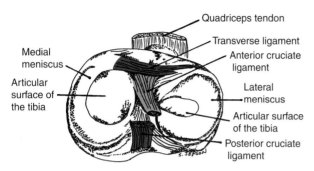

Figure 18-13. Right knee, superior view.

become tight during extension, contributing to the stability of the knee, and slack during flexion.

The **medial** and **lateral meniscus** are two half-moon, wedge-shaped fibrocartilage disks located on the superior surface of the tibia and are designed to absorb shock (Fig. 18-13). Because they are thicker laterally than medially and the proximal surfaces are concave, the menisci deepen the relatively flat joint surface. The medial meniscus, perhaps because of its attachment to the medial collateral ligament, is more frequently torn.

The purpose of a bursa is to reduce friction, and approximately 13 are located at the knee joint. They are needed because the many tendons located around the knee have a relatively vertical line of pull against bony areas or other tendons. Figure 18-14 illustrates many of the bursae around the knee as viewed from the medial side. The most commonly discussed bursae can be summarized as follows:

Name	Location
ANTERIOR	
Subcutaneous prepatellar	Between the patella and skin
Deep infrapatellar	Between proximal tibia and patellar ligament
Subcutaneous infrapatellar	Between tibial tuberosity and skin
Suprapatellar*	Between distal femur and quadriceps tendon
POSTERIOR	
Gastrocnemius*	Between lateral head of gastrocnemius muscle and capsule
Biceps	Between fibular collateral ligament and biceps tendon
Popliteal*	Between popliteus tendon and lateral femoral condyle
Gastrocnemius*	Between medial head of gastrocnemius muscle and capsule
Semimembranosus	Between tendon of semimembranosus muscle and tibia
LATERAL	
Iliotibial	Under the iliotibial band at its distal attachment
Fibular collateral ligament	Under the fibular collateral ligament next to the bone
MEDIAL	
Anserine	Under the sartorius, gracilis, and semitendinosus tendons

*Communicates with knee joint.

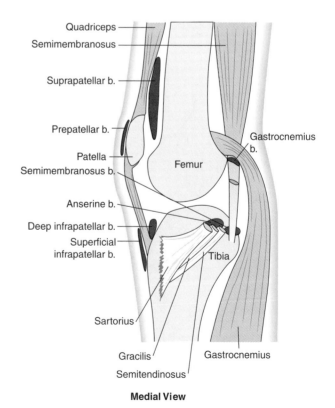

Medial View

Figure 18-14. Bursae around the knee joint.

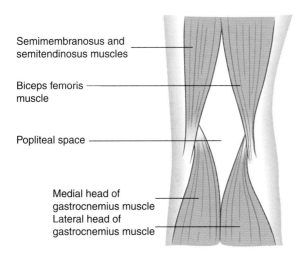

Semimembranosus and semitendinosus muscles

Biceps femoris muscle

Popliteal space

Medial head of gastrocnemius muscle
Lateral head of gastrocnemius muscle

Figure 18-15. The muscular boundaries of the right popliteal space, posterior view.

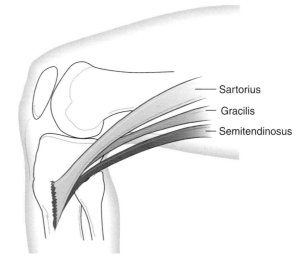

Sartorius

Gracilis

Semitendinosus

Figure 18-16. The three muscle attachments of pes anserine, medial view.

The **popliteal space** is the area behind the knee, and it contains important nerves (tibial and common peroneal) and blood vessels (popliteal artery). This diamond-shaped fossa is bound superiorly on the medial side by the semitendinosus and semimembranosus muscles and by the biceps femoris muscle on the lateral side (Fig. 18-15). The inferior boundaries are the medial and lateral heads of the gastrocnemius muscle.

The **pes anserine** (Latin, meaning "goose foot") **muscle group** is made up of the sartorius, gracilis, and semitendinosus (Fig. 18-16) muscles. Each has a different proximal attachment. The sartorius muscle arises anteriorly from the iliac spine, the gracilis muscle medially from the pubis, and the semitendinosus muscle posteriorly from the ischial tuberosity. They all cross the knee posteriorly and medially, then join together to have a common distal attachment on the anterior medial surface of the proximal tibia. Orthopedic surgeons sometimes alter this common attachment to provide for medial stability to the knee.

Common Knee Pathologies

Genu valgum, also called **"knock knees,"** is an alignment of the lower extremity in which the distal segments (ankles) are positioned more laterally than normal. The knees tend to touch while the ankles are apart. **Genu varum (bowlegs)** is the opposite alignment problem in which the distal segments are positioned more medially than normal. The ankles tend to touch while the knees are apart. Malalignment at one

joint often affects alignment at an adjacent joint. Therefore, coxa varus often results in genu valgus, while coxa valgus may cause genu varus. **Genu recurvatum,** also called, **"back knees"** is the positioning of the tibiofemoral joint in which range of motion goes beyond zero degrees of extension.

Jumper's knee, or **patellar tendonitis** is characterized by tenderness at the patellar tendon from the overuse stress or sudden impact overloading associated with jumping. It is commonly seen in basketball players, high jumpers, and hurdlers. **Osgood-Schlatter's disease** is a common overuse injury among adolescents. It involves the traction-type epiphysis on the tibial tuberosity of growing bone where the tendon of the quadriceps muscle attaches. **Baker's cyst (popliteal cyst)** is actually misnamed as a "cyst." This is a general term referring to any synovial hernia or bursitis involving the posterior aspect of the knee.

Although there is not universal agreement on terminology and causation, **patellofemoral pain syndrome** generally refers to a common problem causing diffuse anterior knee pain. It is generally considered the result of a variety of alignment factors, such as increased Q angle, patella alta (high riding patella), quadriceps weakness and/or tightness, and excessive foot pronation. **Chondromalacia patella** is the softening and degeneration of the cartilage on the posterior aspect of the patella causing anterior knee pain. Abnormal tracking of the patella within the patellofemoral groove causes the patellar articular cartilage to become inflamed leading to its degeneration. **Prepatellar bursitis (housemaid's knee)** occurs when there is constant pressure between the skin and the patella. It is commonly seen in carpet layers and is the result of repeated direct blows or sheering stresses on the knee.

Terrible triad is a term used to describe a knee injury involving tears to the anterior cruciate ligament, medial collateral ligament, and medial meniscus all resulting from a single blow to the knee. **Miserable malalignment syndrome** is an alignment problem of the lower extremity involving increased anteversion of the femoral head, associated with genu valgus, increased tibial torsion, and a pronated flat foot.

Muscles of the Knee

Many of the two-joint muscles of the knee were discussed with the hip. Further clarification of these muscles, however, does need to be made. Table 18-1 shows the muscles that cross the knee, although not all have a major function.

Anterior Muscles

The quadriceps muscles comprise four muscles that cross the anterior surface of the knee (Fig. 18-17). The **rectus femoris muscle** was described in Chapter 17 as originating from the anterior inferior iliac spine (AIIS) and superficially descending the thigh in the midline. The **vastus lateralis muscle** is located lateral to the rectus femoris muscle. It originates from the linea aspera of the femur, and spans the thigh laterally to join the other quadriceps muscles at the patella. The **vastus medialis muscle** also comes from the linea aspera, but spans the thigh medially. Located deep to the rectus femoris muscle is the **vastus intermedialis muscle.** It arises from the anterior surface of the femur and spans the thigh anteriorly. It blends together with the other vasti muscles along its length. All four quadriceps muscles attach to the base of the patella and the tibial tuberosity via the patellar tendon. Because all four muscles span the knee anteriorly, they all extend the knee. Because the rectus femoris muscle also spans the hip anteriorly, it flexes the hip.

Rectus Femoris Muscle

O	AIIS
I	Tibial tuberosity via patellar tendon
A	Hip flexion, knee extension
N	Femoral nerve (L2, L3, L4)

Table 18-1	Muscles of the Knee	
Area	**One-Joint Muscle**	**Two-Joint Muscle**
Anterior	Vastus lateralis Vastus medialis Vastus intermedialis	Rectus femoris
Posterior	Biceps femoris (short) Popliteus	Biceps femoris (long) Semimembranosus Semitendinosus Sartorius Gracilis Gastrocnemius
Lateral		Tensor fascia latae

Vastus Lateralis Muscle

O	Linea aspera
I	Tibial tuberosity via patellar tendon
A	Knee extension
N	Femoral nerve (L2, L3, L4)

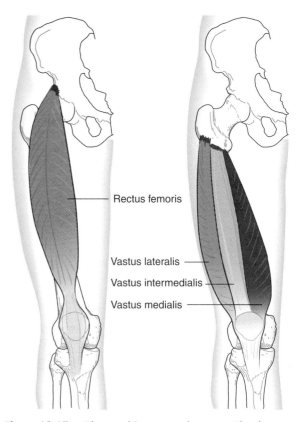

Figure 18-17.   The quadriceps muscle group. The three vasti muscles lie deep to the rectus femoris. The vastus medialis and lateralis attach proximally on the posterior femur but join the other two muscles to cross the knee anteriorly.

Vastus Medialis Muscle

O	Linea aspera
I	Tibial tuberosity via patellar tendon
A	Knee extension
N	Femoral nerve (L2, L3, L4)

Vastus Intermedialis Muscle

O	Anterior femur
I	Tibial tuberosity via patellar tendon
A	Knee extension
N	Femoral nerve (L2, L3, L4)

Posterior Muscles

Three muscles that are known collectively as the hamstring muscles cover the posterior thigh. They consist of the semitendinosus, the semimembranosus, and the biceps femoris muscles (Fig. 18-18). Because they were described in Chapter 17, they will only be summarized here.

Semimembranosus Muscle

O	Ischial tuberosity
I	Posterior surface of medial condyle of tibia
A	Extend hip and flex knee
N	Sciatic nerve (L5, S1, S2)

Semitendinosus Muscle

O	Ischial tuberosity
I	Anteromedial surface of proximal tibia
A	Extend hip and flex knee
N	Sciatic nerve (L5, S1, S2)

Biceps Femoris Muscle

O	Long head: ischial tuberosity Short head: lateral lip of linea aspera
I	Fibular head
A	Long head: extend hip and flex knee Short head: flex knee
N	Long head: sciatic nerve (L5, S1, S2) Short head: common peroneal nerve (L5, S1, S2)

Reference pg. 244 for correct Nerve Roots

The **popliteus muscle** is a one-joint muscle located posteriorly at the knee in the popliteal space deep to the two heads of the gastrocnemius muscles (Fig. 18-19).

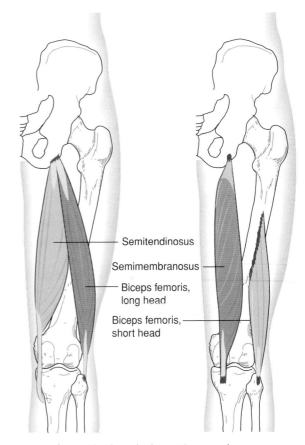

Figure 18-18.   The hamstring muscle group.

- Semitendinosus
- Semimembranosus
- Biceps femoris, long head
- Biceps femoris, short head

It originates on the lateral side of the lateral condyle of the femur and crosses the knee posteriorly at an oblique angle to insert medially on the posterior proximal tibia. Because it spans the knee posteriorly, it

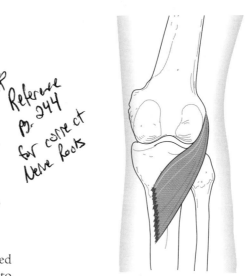

Figure 18-19.   The popliteus muscle.

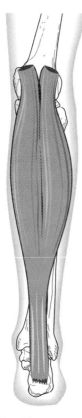

Figure 18-20.   The gastrocnemius muscle.

flexes the knee. It is credited with "unlocking" the knee, or initiating knee flexion.

Popliteus Muscle

O	Lateral condyle of femur
I	Posterior medial condyle of tibia
A	Initiates knee flexion
N	Tibial nerve (L4, L5, S1)

The **gastrocnemius muscle** is a two-joint muscle that crosses the knee and the ankle (Fig. 18-20). It is an extremely strong ankle plantar flexor but also has a significant role at the knee. It attaches by two heads to the posterior surface of the medial and lateral condyles of the femur. After descending the posterior leg superficially, it forms a common tendon with the soleus muscle and attaches to the posterior surface of the calcaneus. Although its major function is at the ankle, it does span the knee posteriorly, has a good angle of pull, and is a large muscle. Therefore, its contribution as a knee flexor cannot be overlooked. Its unusual contribution to knee *extension* has been demonstrated in individuals with no quadriceps muscle function (Fig. 18-21). In a

closed kinetic chain action with the foot planted on the ground so that the distal segment (leg) is stationary, the proximal segment (thigh) becomes the movable part. This is also a reversal of muscle action, in which the femur is pulled posteriorly, or into knee extension. This feature of the gastrocnemius muscle makes it possible for a person to stand upright without the use of quadriceps muscles.

Gastrocnemius Muscle

O	Medial and lateral condyles of femur
I	Posterior calcaneus
A	Knee flexion, ankle plantar flexion
N	Tibial nerve (S1, S2)

The gracilis, sartorius, and tensor fascia latae muscles span the knee joint posteriorly, but because of their angle of pull, size in relation to other muscles, and other such factors, they do not have a prime mover function. They do, however, provide stability to the joint.

The **tensor fascia latae muscle** spans the knee laterally essentially in the middle of the joint axis for flexion and extension. It contributes greatly to lateral stability. The **gracilis** and **sartorius muscles** span the knee medially, contributing greatly to medial stability. The gastrocnemius and hamstring muscles provide posterior stability both medially and laterally, and the quadriceps muscles provide anterior stability.

Table 18-2	Innervation of the Muscles of the Knee	
Muscle	**Nerve**	**Spinal Segment**
Quadriceps		
Rectus femoris	Femoral	L2, L3, L4
Vastus lateralis	Femoral	L2, L3, L4
Vastus intermedialis	Femoral	L2, L3, L4
Vastus medialis	Femoral	L2, L3, L4
Hamstrings		
Semimembranosus	Sciatic	L5, S1, S2
Semitendinosus	Sciatic	L5, S1, S2
Biceps femoris		
Long head	Sciatic	L5, S1, S2
Short head	Common peroneal	L5, S1, S2
Others		
Popliteus	Tibial	L4, L5, S1
Gastrocnemius	Tibial	S1, S2

Table 18-3	Segmental Innervation of the Knee					
Spinal Cord Level	**L2**	**L3**	**L4**	**L5**	**S1**	**S2**
Knee extensors						
Rectus femoris	X	X	X			
Vastus lateralis	X	X	X			
Vastus intermedialis	X	X	X			
Vastus medialis	X	X	X			
Knee flexors						
Popliteus			X	X	X	
Semitendinosus				X	X	X
Semimembranosus				X	X	X
Biceps femoris				X	X	X
Gastrocnemius					X	X

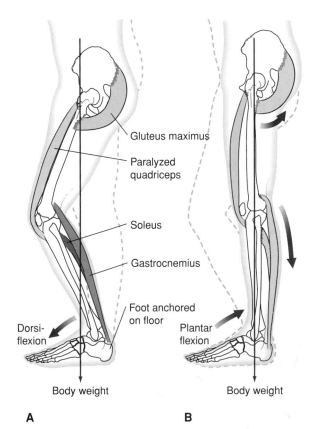

A   **B**

Figure 18-21. *(A)* With a paralyzed quadriceps unable to pull the knee into extension, the body weight line falls behind the knee causing flexion. However, in a combined reversal of muscle action of the gluteus maximus and gastrocnemius muscles, knee extension during stance is possible. *(B)* In the closed-chain position, they pull the knee into extension. The soleus assists by plantar flexing the dorsiflexed ankle into a neutral ankle position. This puts the body weight line in front of the knee and ankle axes and allows the knee to remain extended.

Summary of Muscle Action

The actions of the prime movers of the knee are summarized as follows:

Action	Muscle
Extension	Quadriceps group
	Rectus femoris
	Vastus medialis
	Vastus intermedialis
	Vastus lateralis
Flexion	Hamstring group
	Semimembranosus
	Semitendinosus
	Biceps femoris
	Popliteus

Summary of Muscle Innervation

The femoral and sciatic nerves play a major part in the innervation of the knee joint. The femoral nerve innervates the quadriceps muscle group, and the sciatic nerve innervates the hamstring muscle group. The only exception to this is the short head of the biceps femoris muscle, which receives innervation from the common peroneal nerve.

The other two knee flexors, the popliteus and gastrocnemius muscles, receive innervation from the tibial nerve. Not included in this discussion or in Table 18-2 are those two-joint hip muscles that span the knee but do not act as prime movers at the knee. As you can see, the knee extensors receive innervation from the femoral nerve, which comes off the spinal cord at a higher level than the knee flexors. This is significant when dealing with individuals with spinal cord injuries. Tables 18-2 and 18-3 summarize the innervation to the knee. It should be noted that there is some discrepancy among various sources regarding spinal cord level of innervation.

Review Questions

General Anatomy Questions

1. Describe the knee joints:
   a. Number of axes:
      Knee _____
      Patellofemoral _____
   b. Shape of joint:
      Knee _____
      Patellofemoral _____
   c. Type of motion allowed:
      Knee _____
      Patellofemoral _____

2. Describe knee joint motion in terms of planes and axes.

3. What is the "Q angle"? Why is it important?

4. Which bones make up the knee joint?

5. Why is the action of the popliteus muscle often described as "unlocking" the joint?

6. What is the pes anserine?

7. An individual with a spinal cord injury at L3 would be expected to have what knee motion.

8. Regarding Figure 18-21, what type of kinetic chain activity is being demonstrated?

9. Is it possible for these muscles to perform this function in either an open or closed kinetic chain?

10. Is either the gastrocnemius or gluteus maximus muscle working in a reversal of muscle action role?

Functional Activity Questions

1. Identify the sequence of knee motions (starting with the knee in extension) for kicking a ball.
   a. What is the knee motion when preparing to kick?
   b. Over what joints is the rectus femoris being elongated?
   c. What is the knee motion when making ball contact?
   d. What is happening to the rectus femoris at the knee during ball contact?
   e. What is the knee motion during follow-through?
   f. What is happening to the rectus femoris during follow-through?

2. What is the sequence of right knee motions when stepping up onto a curb leading with the right foot, starting with the right knee extended?
   a. Placing right foot up on curb ____
   b. Bringing left foot up on curb ____

3. What compensatory motions may occur when stepping up onto a curb if your right leg were in a long leg cast?
   a. Which would be the leading leg?
   b. What pelvic motion would assisting in getting the right leg up on the curb?

4. Analyze the two benches illustrated here to determine if one is more advantageous than the other when strengthening the hamstrings by doing leg curls. Note that the knees remain in extension during this analysis of hip position.
   a. What is the hamstring action at the hip and at the knee?
   b. What is the position of the hips in Figure 18-22A?
   c. What is the position of the hips in Figure 18-22B?
   d. In what position would the hamstrings be actively insufficient?
   e. Which bench position is better to more effectively work the hamstrings?
   f. Why?

5. Analyze the two benches illustrated here to determine if one is more advantageous than the other when strengthening the knee extensors. Knee extension is the motion being performed.
   a. What are the hip positions in Figures 18-23A and B?
   b. What are the names of the one-joint muscles performing the knee extension?
   c. What is the name of the two-joint muscle and what hip and knee motion does it perform?
   d. Describe the length-tension effect on these muscles in each position.
   e. Which bench position is better to more effectively work the rectus femoris?
   f. Which bench position is better to more effectively work the vasti muscles?

Clinical Exercise Questions

1. What types of exercises are occurring during a "wall sit": keeping the head, shoulders, and back against the wall with your feet shoulder-width apart, slowly

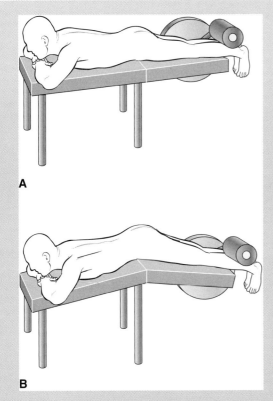

Figure 18-22. Hip positions during hamstring curl exercise.

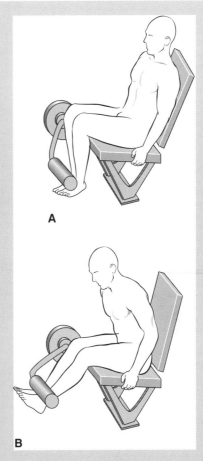

Figure 18-23. Hip positions during knee extension exercise.

slide down the wall until the thighs are almost parallel to the floor? Hold that position for the count of five. Return to the starting position.

During the slide down phase:
a. What is the knee motion?
b. What type of contraction is occurring? (isometric, concentric, eccentric)
c. What muscles are performing this action?

During the holding phase:
a. What type of contraction is occurring? (isometric, concentric, eccentric)
b. What muscles are performing this action?

During the return phase:
a. What is the knee motion?
b. What type of contraction is occurring? (isometric, concentric, eccentric)
c. What muscles are performing this action?

2. Sit on the edge of a table with right leg resting on the table, and the left leg over the side of the table with left foot on the floor. Keeping the back and right leg straight, lean forward at the right hip. See Figure 18-24 for starting position.
a. What are the right hip and knee motions?
b. Is stretching or strengthening occurring?

c. What are the muscles involved?

3. Lying supine, raise your right leg up toward the ceiling about 2 feet, keeping your right knee straight.
a. What are the right hip and knee motions?
b. Is stretching or strengthening occurring?
c. What are the muscles involved?
d. Is this an open- or closed-chain activity?

4. In a standing position, loop an elastic band around the back of your knee and anchor the other end around a heavy table leg or in a doorjamb. You may want to pad the back of the knee with a small towel. Face the anchor point and be far enough away so that there is sufficient tension in the elastic band (Fig. 18-25). From a partly flexed position, slowly straighten the knee, and keep the foot on the floor. Hold for the count of five, and then bend it (returning to starting position).

Straighten phase:
a. What is the knee motion that is occurring?
b. What type of contraction is occurring?

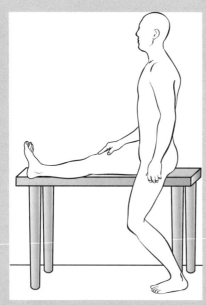

Figure 18-24. Starting position.

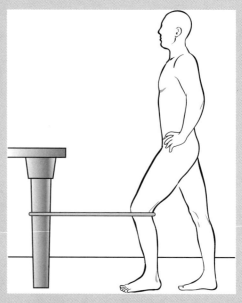

Figure 18-25. Starting position.

c. What are the muscles involved?
d. Is this an open- or closed-chain activity?

Holding phase:
a. What is the position of the knee?
b. What type of contraction is occurring?
c. What are the muscles involved?

Bending phase:
a. What is the knee motion that is occurring?

b. What type of contraction is occurring?
c. What are the muscles involved?

5. Standing on your left leg and holding on to something for balance, bend your right knee and grasp your right foot. Slowly pull your right heel toward your right buttock.
   a. What are the right hip and knee motions?
   b. Is stretching or strengthening occurring?
   c. What are the muscles involved?

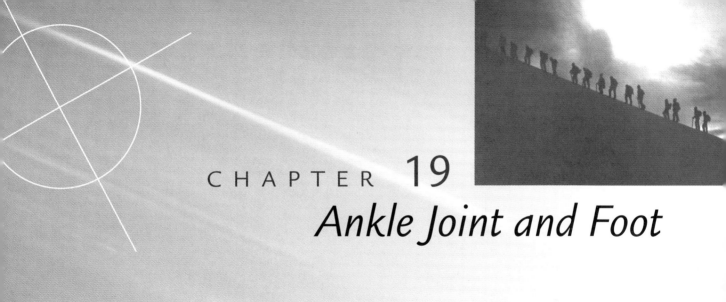

Bones and Landmarks

Functional Aspects of the Foot

Joints and Motions

Ankle Motions

Ankle Joints

Foot Joints

Ligaments and Other Structures

Arches

Common Ankle Pathologies

Muscles of the Ankle and Foot

Extrinsic Muscles

Intrinsic Muscles

Summary of Muscle Innervation

Points to Remember

Review Questions

General Anatomy Questions

Functional Activity Questions

Clinical Exercise Questions

The leg, that portion of the lower extremity extending from the knee to the ankle, is composed of the tibia and fibula. A strong interosseous membrane keeps the two bones together and provides a greater surface area for muscle attachment (Fig. 19-1).

Bones and Landmarks

The tibia, the larger of the two bones, is the only true weight-bearing bone of the leg. Triangular in shape, the tibia's apex (crest) is located anteriorly. The long, thin fibula is set back in line with the posterior surface of the tibia (Fig. 19-2). Laterally, this forms a gully, with the interosseous membrane as the floor, permitting attachment of several muscles without distorting the shape of the leg. Landmarks of the **tibia,** in addition to those discussed in Chapter 18, are as follows:

Crest
Anterior and most prominent of the three borders

Medial malleolus
The enlarged distal medial surface

The landmarks of the **fibula** are as follows:

Head
Enlarged proximal end of the bone

Lateral malleolus
Enlarged distal end

The bones of the foot include the tarsals, metatarsals, and phalanges. The seven **tarsal bones** and their landmarks consist of the following (see Fig. 19-3):

Calcaneus
Largest and most posterior tarsal bone.

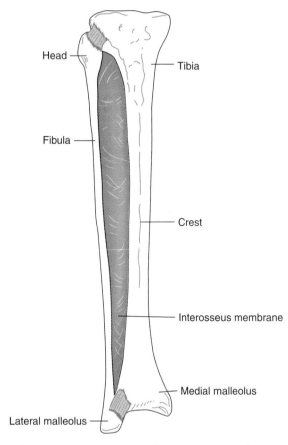

Figure 19-1.   Leg bones and interosseous membrane.

Calcaneal tuberosity

Projection on the posterior inferior surface of the calcaneus.

Sustentaculum tali

Medial superior part projecting out from the rest of the calcaneus, supporting the medial side of the talus. Three tendons loop around this projection, changing directions from the posterior leg to the plantar foot.

Talus

Sitting on the calcaneus, it is the second largest tarsal.

Navicular

On the medial side in front of the talus and proximal to the three cuneiforms.

Tuberosity of navicular

Projection on the medial side of the navicular; easily seen on the medial border of the foot.

Cuboid

On the lateral side of the foot proximal (superior) to the fourth and fifth metatarsals and distal (inferior) to the calcaneus.

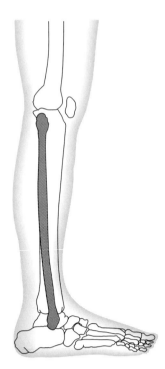

Figure 19-2.   Right leg, lateral view. Note the posterior position of the fibula.

Cuneiforms

Three in number; named the first through third, going from the medial toward the lateral side in line with the metatarsals. The first is the largest of the three.

The **metatarsals** are numbered 1 through 5, starting medially (see Fig. 19-3). Normally, the first and fifth metatarsals are weight-bearing bones and the second, third, and fourth are not. We tend to stand on a triangle. Weight is borne from the base of the calcaneus to the heads of the first and fifth metatarsals. The significant features and landmarks of the metatarsals are as follows:

Base

Proximal end of each metatarsal

Head

Distal end of each bone

First

Thickest and shortest metatarsal; located on the medial side of the foot

Second

The longest; articulates with the second cuneiform

Third

Articulates with the third cuneiform

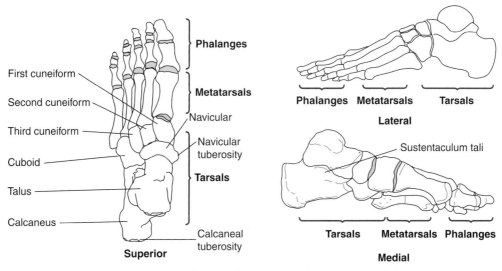

Figure 19-3. Bones of the left foot: superior, lateral, and medial views.

Fourth

With the fifth metatarsal, articulates with the cuboid

Fifth

Has prominent tuberosity located on the lateral side of its base

The **phalanges** of the foot have the same composition as those of the hand (Fig. 19-3). The first digit, the **great toe,** has a proximal and distal phalanx but no middle phalanx. The second through fifth digits, also called the four **lesser toes,** each have a proximal, middle, and distal phalanx.

Functional Aspects of the Foot

The foot can be divided into three parts (Fig. 19-4). The hindfoot is made up of the talus and calcaneus. In the gait cycle, the hindfoot is the first part of the foot that makes contact with the ground, thus influencing the function and movement of the other two parts. The midfoot is made up of the navicular, the cuboid, and the three cuneiform bones. The mechanics of this part provide stability and mobility to the foot as it transmits movement from the hindfoot to the forefoot. The forefoot is made up of the five metatarsals and all of the phalanges. This part of the foot adapts to the level of the ground. It is also the last part of the foot to be in contact with the ground during stance phase.

The ankle joint and foot perform three main functions: acting as a shock absorber as the heel strikes the ground at the beginning of stance phase; adapting to the level (or unevenness) of the ground; and providing a stable base of support from which to propel the body forward.

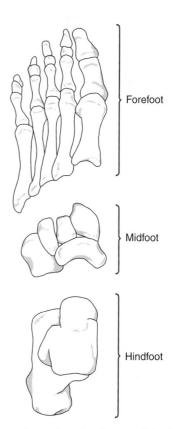

Figure 19-4. Functional areas of the foot.

Joints and Motions

Ankle Motions

Motions of the ankle joint and foot need to be defined because there is variation among authors. **Plantar flexion** is movement toward the plantar surface of the foot, whereas **dorsiflexion** is movement toward the dorsal surface of the foot. These motions occur in the *sagittal plane around the frontal axis.* The terms **flexion** and **extension** should not be used because of conflicting definitions. As a case in point, functionally speaking, plantar flexion is the same as extension, part of the general extension movement of the hip, knee, and ankle. However, anatomically speaking, dorsiflexion is the same as extension, meaning movement toward the extensor side of the foot.

Movement in the *frontal plane around the sagittal axis* is called inversion and eversion. **Inversion** is the raising of the medial border of the foot, or rotation at the tarsal joints turning the forefoot inward. **Eversion,** the opposite motion, is the raising of the lateral border of the foot, or rotation of the tarsal joints turning the forefoot outward. Movement in the transverse plane is called **adduction** and **abduction.** These motions occur primarily in the forefoot (Fig. 19-5), and accompany inversion and eversion, respectively.

In recent years, clinicians have begun using supination and pronation to describe ankle joint and foot motion. **Supination** describes a combination of plantar flexion, inversion, and adduction, and **pronation** describes a combination of dorsiflexion, eversion, and abduction. To avoid further confusion of terms, valgus and varus must be defined. These terms are more commonly used to describe a *position,* usually an abnormal one. **Valgus** refers to a position in which the distal segment is positioned away from the midline. Conversely, **varus** refers to a position in which the distal segment is positioned toward the midline. Therefore, a calcaneal valgus is a position in which the distal (inferior) part of the calcaneus is angled away from the midline (Fig. 19-6). These terms will not be used here because *motion,* not *position,* is the emphasis.

In summary, the terminology commonly used by clinicians to describe ankle and foot motions are dorsiflexion, plantar flexion, supination (combination of plantar flexion, inversion, and forefoot adduction), and pronation (combination of dorsiflexion, eversion, and forefoot abduction). These motions are illustrated in Figure 19-5. However, when describing muscle action, inversion and eversion are used in place of supination and pronation, respectively.

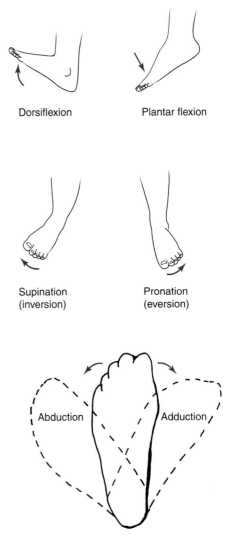

Figure 19-5.   Ankle joint and foot motions.

Two joints with little motion that are not part of the true ankle joint but play a small role in the proper function of the ankle are the tibiofibular joints (Fig. 19-7). The **superior tibiofibular joint** is the articulation between the head of the fibula and the posterior lateral aspect of the proximal tibia. It is a uniaxial plane joint. Being a synovial joint, it has a joint capsule. Ligaments reinforce the capsule. The gliding motion present is relatively small. It functions to dissipate the torsional stresses applied at the ankle joint. The **inferior tibiofibular joint** is a syndesmosis (fibrous union) between the concave distal tibia and the convex distal fibula. Because it is not a synovial joint, there is no joint capsule. However, there is fibrous tissue separating the bones and several ligaments holding the joint together. Much of the strength of the ankle joint is dependent

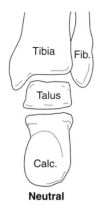

Tibia   Fib.

Talus

Calc.

Neutral

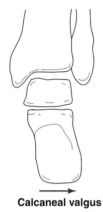

Calcaneal valgus

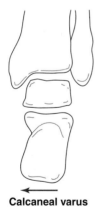

Calcaneal varus

Posterior View

Figure 19-6.   Calcaneal positions.

upon a strong union at this joint. The ligaments holding this joint together allow slight movement to accommodate the motion of the talus.

Subtalar	Supination
Midtarsal	Supination
Tarsometatarsal	Supination
Metatarsophalangeal	Full extension
Interphalangeal	Full extension

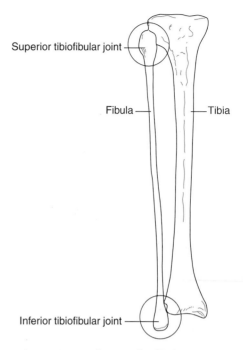

Superior tibiofibular joint

Fibula — — Tibia

Inferior tibiofibular joint

Figure 19-7.   The two tibiofibular joints.

Ankle Joints

The true **ankle joint** *(talocrural joint* or *talotibial joint)* is made up of the distal tibia sitting on the talus with the medial malleolus of the tibia fitting down around the medial aspect of the talus, and the lateral malleolus of the fibula fitting down around the lateral aspect. This type of joint often is described using a carpentry term as a *tenon and mortise joint.* A mortise is a notch cut in a piece of wood to receive a projecting piece (tenon) shaped to fit. Therefore, the malleoli of the tibia and fibula would be the mortise, and the talus would be the tenon (Fig. 19-8).

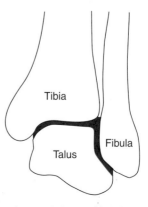

Tibia

Fibula

Talus

Figure 19-8.   Ankle joint.

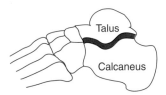

Figure 19-9.   Subtalar joint.

To summarize, the ankle is a uniaxial hinge joint consisting of articulation between the distal end and medial malleolus of the tibia and the lateral malleolus of the fibula with the talus. The ankle joint allows approximately 30 to 50 degrees of plantar flexion and 20 degrees of dorsiflexion. In the anatomical position, the ankle is in a neutral position. Because the axis of rotation is at an angle, it is considered **triplanar,** a term used to describe motion around an obliquely oriented axis that passes through all three planes. The close-packed position is maximum dorsiflexion.

The **subtalar,** or **talocalcaneal, joint** consists of the inferior surface of the talus articulating with the superior surface of the calcaneus. This joint has a primarily gliding motion (Fig. 19-9). The anterior surfaces of the talus and calcaneus articulating with the posterior surfaces of the navicular and the cuboid, respectively, make up the **transverse tarsal joint** (midtarsal joint) (Fig. 19-10). However, very little movement occurs between the navicular and the cuboid. Pronation and supination, which are motions between the hindfoot

and forefoot, occur at the transverse tarsal joint. These motions are triplanar motions.

Functionally, the subtalar and transverse tarsal joints cannot be separated. Therefore, supination and pronation are actually combinations of motions. Supination is a combination of inversion, adduction, and plantar flexion. Pronation is the reverse motion. It is a combination of eversion, abduction, and dorsiflexion. Remember, inversion/eversion is being used to describe motions occurring at the subtalar and transtarsal joints instead of supination/pronation, which also involves plantar flexion/dorsiflexion of the ankle joint.

Therefore, when the ankle is described as moving in plantar flexion and dorsiflexion, these motions are occurring at the talocrural joint. When the ankle moves in inversion and eversion, these motions are occurring at the subtalar and transverse tarsal joints.

The combined motions of these joints allow the foot to assume almost any position in space. This is quite useful in allowing the foot to adapt to irregular surfaces such as those found when walking on uneven ground. For example, think about the many foot positions needed when climbing about on rocks at the beach or mountains.

Foot Joints

The **metatarsophalangeal (MTP)** joints consist of the metatarsal heads articulating with the proximal phalanges (Fig. 19-11). Like the metacarpophalangeal joints of the hand, there are five joints allowing flexion, extension, hyperextension, abduction, and adduction (Fig. 19-12). The first MTP joint is much more mobile. It allows approximately 45 degrees of flexion and extension, and 90 degrees of hyperextension. The second through fifth MTP joints allow about 40 degrees of flexion and extension, and only about 45 degrees of hyperextension. This hyperextension is very important during the toe-off phase of walking. The point of reference for abduction and adduction is the second toe. Like the middle finger of the hand, the second toe abducts in both directions but adducts only as a return motion from abduction.

Also like the hand, there is a **proximal interphalangeal (PIP)** and **distal interphalangeal (DIP) joint** on each of the lesser toes (two through five). These joints individually are not as significant as in the hand because there is less dexterity required of the foot. The great toe has a proximal and distal phalanx but no middle phalange. Therefore, like the thumb, it has only one phalangeal joint, the **interphalangeal (IP) joint** (see Fig. 19-11).

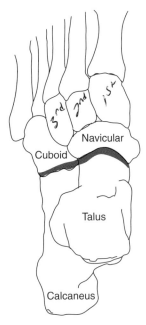

Figure 19-10.   Transverse tarsal joint.

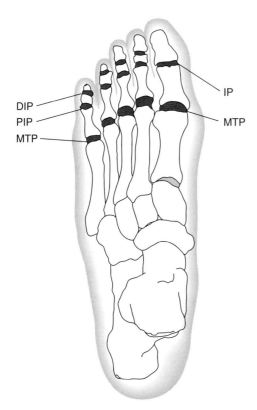

Figure 19-11. Joints of the phalanges of the foot. Note that the great toe has only two joints whereas the four lesser toes have three joints.

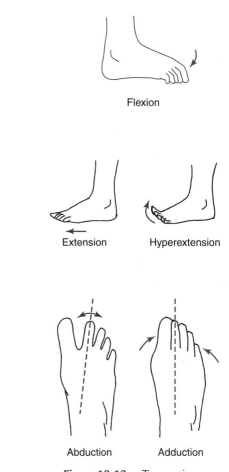

Figure 19-12. Toe motions.

Ligaments and Other Structures

The ankle joint, a synovial joint, has a joint capsule. This **capsule** is rather thin anteriorly and posteriorly but is reinforced by collateral ligaments on the sides. These collateral ligaments are actually groups of several ligaments. The collateral ligament on the medial side is a triangular-shaped **deltoid ligament** whose apex is located along the tip of the medial malleolus with a broad base spreading out to attach to the talus, navicular, and calcaneus in four parts (Fig. 19-13). The anterior fibers attach to the navicular (tibionavicular ligament). The middle fibers (tibiocalcaneal ligament) descend directly to the sustentaculum tali of the calcaneus. The posterior fibers (posterior tibiotalar ligament) run backward to the talus. The deep fibers (anterior tibiotalar ligament) can barely be seen from the medial side because they are deep to the tibionavicular portion. The deltoid ligament strengthens the medial side of the ankle joint, holds the calcaneus and navicular against the talus, and helps to maintain the medial longitudinal arch.

On the lateral side of the ankle joint is a group of three ligaments commonly referred to as the **lateral ligament** (Fig. 19-14). This ligament consists of three parts connecting the lateral malleolus to the talus and

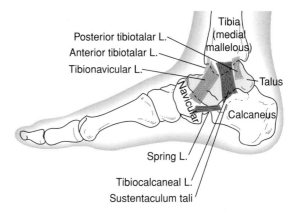

Figure 19-13. Ligaments of the right medial ankle. The four parts of the deltoid ligament. Note that the dotted lines show the outline of the talus under the ligaments.

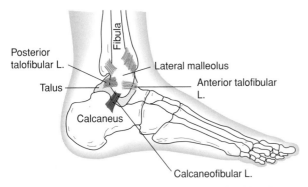

Figure 19-14.   Ligaments of the right lateral ankle. The three parts of the lateral ligament.

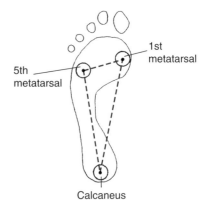

Figure 19-15.   The main weight-bearing surfaces of the right foot, plantar view.

calcaneus. The rather weak anterior talofibular ligament attaches the lateral malleolus to the talus. Posteriorly, the fairly strong posterior talofibular ligament runs almost horizontally to connect the lateral malleolus to the talus. In the middle is the long and fairly vertical calcaneofibular ligament that attaches the malleolus to the calcaneus. Numerous other ligaments attach the various tarsals to each other, to the metatarsals, and so on. They tend to be named for the bones to which they attach. Their individual names and locations will not be discussed here.

Arches

Because the foot is the usual point of impact with the ground, it must be able to absorb a great deal of shock, adjust to changes in terrain, and propel the body forward during movement. To allow these things to occur, the bones of the foot are arranged in arches. We tend to stand on a triangle with weight-bearing borne from the base of the calcaneus to the heads of the first and fifth metatarsals (Fig. 19-15). Between these three points we have two arches (medial and lateral longitudinal) (Fig. 19-16) at right angles to the third (transverse) arch (Fig. 19-17).

The **medial longitudinal arch** makes up the medial border of the foot, running from the calcaneus posteriorly through the talus, navicular, and three cuneiforms anteriorly to the first three metatarsals. The talus is at the top of the arch and often referred to as the *keystone* because it receives the weight of the body. A keystone is an essential part of an arch, usually the central or topmost, part. This arch depresses somewhat during weight-bearing and then recoils when the weight is removed. Normally, it never flattens or touches the ground.

The **lateral longitudinal arch** runs from the calcaneus anteriorly through the cuboid to the fourth and fifth metatarsals . It normally rests on the ground during weight-bearing.

The **transverse arch** runs from side to side through the three cuneiforms to the cuboid. The second cuneiform is the keystone of this arch.

These three arches are maintained by (1) the shape of the bones and their relation to each other; (2) the

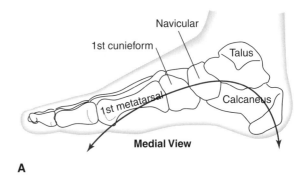

Medial View

A

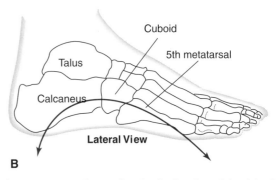

Lateral View

B

Figure 19-16.   The two longitudinal arches of the right foot: *(A)* Medial longitudinal arch, *(B)* lateral longitudinal arch.

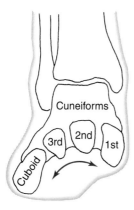

Figure 19-17.   Transverse arch of the foot, frontal view.

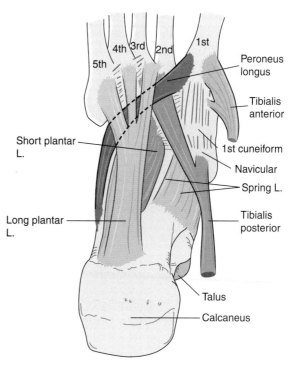

Figure 19-19.   Support structures of the right foot, inferior view.

plantar ligaments and aponeurosis (Figs. 19-18 and 19-19); and (3) muscles. The ligaments and aponeurosis are perhaps the most important features. The **spring ligament** (plantar calcaneonavicular) attaches to the calcaneus and runs forward to the navicular. It is short, wide, and most important because it supports the medial side of the longitudinal arch.

The **long plantar ligament,** the longest of the tarsal ligaments, is more superficial than the spring ligament. It attaches posteriorly to the calcaneus and runs forward to attach on the cuboid and bases of the third, fourth, and fifth metatarsals. It is the primary support of the lateral longitudinal arch. The long plantar ligament is assisted by the **short plantar ligament,** which also attaches the calcaneus to the cuboid. It mostly lies deep to the long plantar ligament. Both longitudinal arches are supported by the superficially located **plantar aponeurosis,** which runs from the calcaneus forward to the proximal phalanges. It acts as a tie rod, keeping the posterior segments (calcaneus and talus) from separating from the anterior portion (ante-

rior tarsals and metatarsal heads). This plantar fascia increases the stability of the foot and arches during weight-bearing and walking (Fig. 19-20).

The arches also are supported by muscles, mainly the invertors and evertors of the foot. The tibialis posterior,

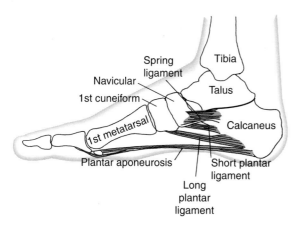

Figure 19-18.   Support structures of the right foot, medial view.

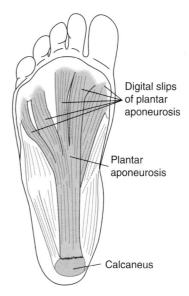

Figure 19-20.   Plantar aponeurosis.

flexor hallucis longus, and flexor digitorum longus muscles all span the ankle posteriorly on the medial side, passing under the sustentaculum tali of the calcaneus. Thus, they give some support to the medial side of the foot. The flexor hallucis longus and flexor digitorum longus muscles span the medial longitudinal arch and help support it. The peroneus longus muscle spans the foot from the lateral to the medial side providing support to the transverse and lateral longitudinal arches. The intrinsic muscles provide more support than the extrinsics because any motion will involve them. However, the total muscular support to the arches has been estimated to bear only about 15 to 20 percent of the total stress to the arches.

Common Ankle Pathologies

Shin splints is a general term given to exercise-induced pain along the medial edge of the tibia, usually in the lower half from a few inches above the ankle to midway up the tibia. Most commonly, inflammation of the periosteum causes the pain. The injury is an overuse injury and can be caused by running on hard surfaces, running on tiptoes, and in sports where a lot of jumping is involved. **Medial tibial stress syndrome** is a more specific term that includes anterior leg pain not associated with a stress fracture.

Deformities of the foot and toes often affect other joints of the lower extremity and trunk, especially during walking or running. A normal foot is defined as **plantigrade** in that the sole is at right angles to the leg when a person is standing. **Equinus foot** (horse's foot) means that the hindfoot is fixed in plantar flexion. A **calcaneus foot** is one that is fixed in dorsiflexion. **Pes cavus** refers to an abnormally high arch, while **pes planus** (flat foot) is the loss of the medial longitudinal arch. **Hallux valgus** is caused by pathological changes in which the great toe develops a valgus deformity (distal end pointed laterally). **Hallux rigidus** is a degenerative condition of the first MTP joint associated with pain and diminished range of motion. With the following lesser toe deformities, all MTP joints are hyperextended: with **hammertoe** the PIP is flexed and the DIP is extended. **Mallet toe** is just the opposite; it has an extended PIP joint and a flexed DIP joint. **Claw toe** has a flexed PIP joint and a flexed DIP joint.

Metatarsalgia is a general term referring to pain around the metatarsal heads. Often the individual describes the pain as a bruise, or "walking on pebbles." The pain usually becomes worse with increased activity. **Morton's neuroma** is caused by abnormal pressure on the plantar digital nerves commonly at the web space between the third and fourth metatarsals. This pressure can result in pain and numbness in the toe area that gets worse with activity, such as running. **Turf toe** is caused by forced hyperextension of the great toe at the MTP joint. It is commonly seen in football, baseball or soccer players.

The ankle is considered the most frequently injured joint in the body. **Ankle sprains** are probably the most common injury among recreation and competitive athletes and the lateral ligament is the most frequently injured ligament. Lateral or inversion sprains occur when the foot lands in a plantar-flexed and inverted position. One or more of the lateral ligament's three parts may be stretched or torn.

An **ankle fracture** often occurs when a person trips over an unexpected obstacle, or falls from a height, and usually involves a twisting component to the ankle. The lateral malleolus is most commonly involved. A **bimalleolar fracture** involves both malleoli, and a **trimalleolar fractures** involves both malleoli and the posterior lip of the tibia.

Plantar fasciitis is a common overuse injury resulting in pain in the heel. The plantar fascia helps maintain the medial longitudinal arch and acts as a shock absorber during weight-bearing. The site of pain is where the fascia attaches to the calcaneus on the plantar surface. **Achilles tendonitis,** an inflammation of the gastrocnemius-soleus tendon, is sometimes a precursor to a **ruptured Achilles tendon.** With a complete rupture, the individual has lost the ability to plantar flex the ankle. To determine if the tendon is intact, have an individual lie prone with the feet off the edge of the table. Squeeze on the muscle belly of the gastrocnemius muscle. If the tendon is intact, slight plantar flexion will occur, whereas no motion will occur if the tendon is ruptured.

A **triple arthrodesis** is a surgical procedure fusing the talocalcaneal, calcaneocuboid, and talonavicular joints. It provides medial-lateral stability of the foot, pain relief at the subtalar joint, but inversion and eversion at the ankle are lost. Ankle dorsiflexion and plantar flexion remain because the talotibial joint has not been involved.

Muscles of the Ankle and Foot

Extrinsic Muscles

There are extrinsic and intrinsic muscles in the ankle and foot as in the wrist and hand. The extrinsic muscles originate on the leg, and the intrinsic muscles

Table 19-1   Extrinsic Muscles of the Ankle and Foot

Muscle	Joint Crossing	Possible Actions
Posterior Group		
Superficial Posterior Group		
Gastrocnemius	Posterior	Plantar flexion
Soleus	Posterior	Plantar flexion
Plantaris	Posterior	Plantar flexion
Deep Posterior Group		
Tibialis posterior	Posterior, medial	Plantar flexion, inversion
Flexor digitorum longus	Posterior, medial	Plantar flexion, inversion, lesser toe flexion
Flexor hallucis longus	Posterior, medial	Plantar flexion, inversion, great toe flexion
Anterior Group		
Tibialis anterior	Anterior, medial	Dorsiflexion, inversion
Extensor hallucis longus	Anterior, medial	Dorsiflexion, inversion, great toe extension
Extensor digitorum longus	Anterior	Dorsiflexion, lesser toe extension
Lateral Group		
Peroneus longus	Posterior, lateral	Plantar flexion, eversion
Peroneus brevis	Posterior, lateral	Plantar flexion, eversion
Peroneus tertius	Anterior	Dorsiflexion, eversion

originate on the tarsal bones. The extrinsic muscles of the leg are found in groups of three or combinations of three and are located in three anatomical areas. All have proximal attachments on the femur, tibia, or fibula, and all cross the ankle joint. Table 19-1 summarizes these muscles. Assistive movers are the muscles indicated in parentheses. All other muscles listed are prime movers.

Superficial Posterior Group

The superficial posterior group includes the gastrocnemius, soleus, and plantaris muscles. Because the gastrocnemius muscle was described in Chapter 18, it will only be summarized here (Fig. 19-21). Its proximal attachment is posterior on the condyles of the femur, and its distal attachment is to the posterior calcaneus via the large Achilles tendon.

Gastrocnemius Muscle

O	Medial head: medial condyle of femur Lateral head: lateral condyle of femur
I	Posterior calcaneus
A	Knee flexion; ankle plantar flexion
N	Tibial nerve (S1, S2)

The **soleus** muscle is a large, one-joint muscle located deep to the gastrocnemius muscle (Fig. 19-22). Originating on the posterior tibia and fibula, it spans the posterior leg, blending with the gastrocnemius muscle to form the large, strong Achilles tendon that inserts on the posterior calcaneus. Because the soleus muscle spans the ankle in the midline, its only function is to plantar flex the ankle. The two heads of the gastrocnemius and soleus muscles make up what is sometimes referred to as the triceps surae muscle, meaning "three-headed calf muscle."

Soleus Muscle

O	Posterior tibia and fibula
I	Posterior calcaneus
A	Ankle plantar flexion
N	Tibial nerve (S1, S2)

The **plantaris** muscle is a long, thin, two-joint muscle with no significant function (see Fig. 19-22). It originates on the posterior surface of the lateral epicondyle of the femur, spans the posterior leg medially, and blends with the gastrocnemius and soleus muscles in the Achilles tendon. Theoretically, it should flex the knee and plantar flex the ankle. However, because of its size in relation to the prime movers of those actions, it is assistive at best.

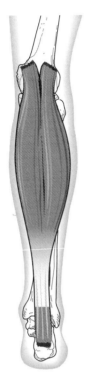

Figure 19-21.   The gastrocnemius muscle.

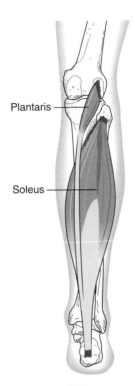

Figure 19-22.   The soleus and plantaris muscles.

Plantaris Muscle

O	Posterior lateral condyle of femur
I	Posterior calcaneus
A	Very weak assist in knee flexion and ankle plantar flexion
N	Tibial nerve (L4, L5, S1)

Deep Posterior Group

The deep posterior group is made up of the tibialis posterior, flexor hallucis longus, and flexor digitorum longus muscles. They all attach to the posterior tibia and/or fibula, and all terminate in the foot. Because they all cross the ankle posteriorly, they all can plantar flex it. However, because of their size in relation to the soleus and gastrocnemius muscles, their role is only assistive.

The **tibialis posterior** muscle is the deepest lying posterior muscle with its proximal attachment on the interosseous membrane and adjacent portions of the tibia and fibula (Fig. 19-23). It descends on the posterior aspect of the leg, looping around the medial malleolus to attach on the navicular with fibrous expansions to the cuboid, the three cuneiforms, sustentaculum tali of the calcaneus, and the bases of the

second through fourth metatarsals. Because the tibialis posterior muscle crosses the ankle medially and posteriorly, it can plantar flex and invert. Because of its size in relation to the other plantar flexors, it is assistive in this action.

Tibialis Posterior Muscle

O	Interosseous membrane, adjacent tibia and fibula
I	Navicular and most tarsals and metatarsals
A	Ankle inversion; assists in plantar flexion
N	Tibial nerve (L5, S1)

Situated mostly on the lateral side of the leg, the **flexor hallucis longus** muscle arises from the posterior fibula and interosseous membrane. It descends the leg posteriorly, loops around the medial malleolus through a groove in the posterior talus, and goes under the sustentaculum tali of the calcaneus. This muscle travels down the foot through the two heads of the flexor hallucis brevis muscle to attach at the base of the distal phalanx of the great toe (Fig. 19-24). This distal attachment is similar to the flexor digitorum profundus and superficialis muscles in the hand. The flexor

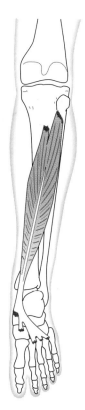

Figure 19-23. The tibialis posterior muscle. Note that the foot is in extreme plantar flexion.

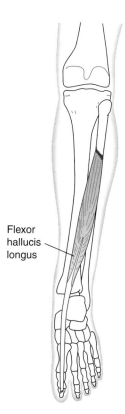

Flexor hallucis longus

Figure 19-24. The flexor hallucis longus muscle. Note that the foot is in extreme plantar flexion.

hallucis longus muscle flexes the great toe and assists in inversion and, to a lesser degree, assists in plantar flexion of the ankle.

Flexor Hallucis Longus Muscle

O	Posterior fibula and interosseous membrane
I	Distal phalanx of the great toe
A	Flexes great toe; assists in inversion and plantar flexion of the ankle
N	Tibial nerve (L5, S1, S2)

Situated mostly on the medial side of the leg, the **flexor digitorum longus** muscle arises from the posterior tibia (Fig. 19-25). It descends the leg posteriorly, loops around the medial malleolus, and runs down the foot, splitting into four tendons to insert into the distal phalanx of the second through fifth toes. This muscle passes through the split in the flexor digitorum brevis tendon in a similar fashion to the flexor digitorum profundus muscle, which goes through the split in the flexor digitorum superficialis muscle in the hand. It flexes the four lesser toes and assists in inversion and plantar flexion of the ankle.

Flexor Digitorum Longus Muscle

O	Posterior tibia
I	Distal phalanx of four lesser toes
A	Flexes the four lesser toes; assists in ankle inversion and plantar flexion of the ankle
N	Tibial nerve (L5, S1)

The relationships among the deep posterior muscles are interesting, crossing and intertwining with one another from their proximal to distal attachments. This feature provides added strength, much like a braided rope, which is stronger than one whose individual fibers run parallel to one another. Table 19-2 summarizes this changing relationship.

Table 19-2	Deep Posterior Group		
Location	**Relationship**		
Origin (medial to lateral)	FDL	TP	FHL
Medial malleolus (superior to inferior)	TP	FDL	FHL
Insertion (medial to lateral)	FHL	TP	FDL

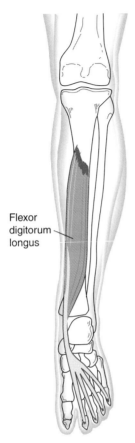

Figure 19-25.   The flexor digitorum longus muscle. Note that the foot is in extreme plantar flexion.

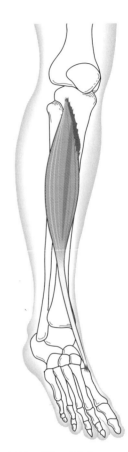

Figure 19-26.   The tibialis anterior muscle.

Anterior Group

The anterior muscle group is made up of the tibialis anterior, extensor hallucis longus, and the extensor digitorum longus muscles. They all attach proximally on the anterior lateral leg and cross the ankle anteriorly.

The **tibialis anterior** muscle originates on the lateral side of the tibia and interosseous membrane, then descends the leg to insert medially on the first cuneiform and base of the first metatarsal (Fig. 19-26). It makes up most of the bulk of the anterior lateral leg. Because the tibialis anterior muscle spans the ankle anteriorly and medially, it dorsiflexes and inverts the ankle.

Tibialis Anterior Muscle

O	Lateral tibia and interosseous membrane
I	First cuneiform and metatarsal
A	Ankle inversion and dorsiflexion
N	Deep peroneal nerve (L4, L5, S1)

The **extensor hallucis longus** muscle, a thin muscle lying deep to and between the tibialis anterior and the extensor digitorum longus muscles, originates on the fibula and interosseous membrane and inserts into the base of the distal phalanx of the great toe (Fig. 19-27). Its primary function is to extend the great toe, but this muscle also assists in dorsiflexing and inverting the ankle.

Extensor Hallucis Longus Muscle

O	Fibula and interosseous membrane
I	Distal phalanx of great toe
A	Extends first toe; assists in ankle inversion and dorsiflexion
N	Deep peroneal nerve (L4, L5, S1)

The most lateral of the anterior muscles, the **extensor digitorum longus** muscle attaches to most of the anterior fibula, interosseous membrane, and the lateral condyle of the tibia. It descends the leg to attach to the distal phalanx of the four lesser toes (Fig. 19-28). The extensor digitorum longus muscle functions primarily

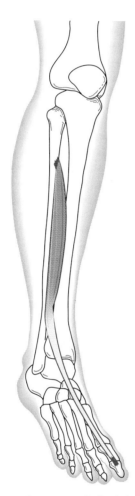

Figure 19-27.   The extensor hallucis longus muscle.

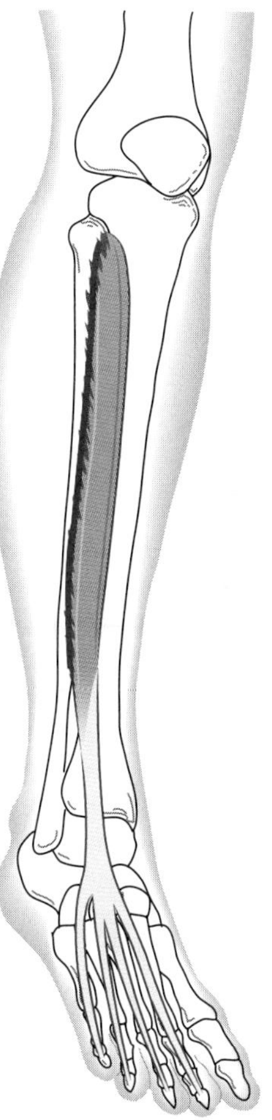

Figure 19-28.   The extensor digitorum longus muscle.

to extend the second through fifth toes, but it also assists in dorsiflexing the ankle. It does not have an inversion/eversion role because it crosses the joint through the middle of that axis.

Extensor Digitorum Longus Muscle

O	Fibula, interosseous membrane, tibia
I	Distal phalanx of four lesser toes
A	Extends four lesser toes, assists in ankle dorsiflexion
N	Deep peroneal nerve (L4, L5, S1)

Lateral Group

The lateral group of muscles consists of the peroneus longus, peroneus brevis, and peroneus tertius muscles. They all originate proximally on the fibula and run distally to the foot. Two cross the ankle joint posteriorly, and one crosses the ankle anteriorly.

The **peroneus longus** muscle is the more superficial of the peroneal muscles. Arising from the proximal end of the fibula and interosseous membrane, it descends the lateral leg and loops behind the lateral malleolus along with the peroneus brevis muscle. At this point the peroneus longus muscle goes deep to cross the foot obliquely from the lateral to the medial side of the foot to insert into the plantar surface of the first metatarsal and first cuneiform (Fig. 19-29). This distal attachment is very close to the attachment of the tibialis anterior muscle. Together, the peroneus longus and tibialis anterior muscles are sometimes referred to as the **stirrup of the foot** because the peroneus longus muscle vertically descends the leg laterally before crossing the foot medially to join the tibialis anterior muscle. The tibialis anterior muscle vertically descends the leg medially to meet the peroneus longus muscle, forming a "U" or stirrup. Crossing the foot as it does, the peroneus longus muscle provides some support to the lateral longitudinal

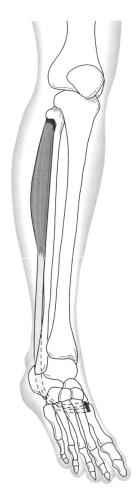

Figure 19-29. The peroneus longus muscle (dotted lines indicate location on plantar surface).

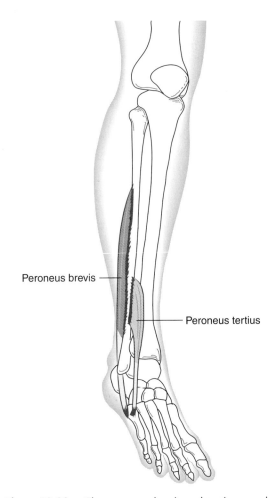

Figure 19-30. The peroneus brevis and tertius muscles.

and transverse arches of the foot. Its prime function is to evert the ankle, although this muscle is able to assist somewhat in ankle plantar flexion.

Peroneus Longus Muscle

O	Lateral proximal fibula and interosseous membrane
I	Plantar surface of first cuneiform and metatarsal
A	~~Ankle~~ eversion; assists in ankle plantar flexion
N	Superficial peroneal nerve (L4, L5, S1)

Mid-Foot

Deep to the peroneus longus muscle is the smaller, shorter **peroneus brevis** muscle. It attaches laterally on the distal fibula, descends the leg, and loops behind the lateral malleolus before coming forward to attach on the base of the fifth metatarsal (Fig. 19-30). The peroneus brevis muscle is superficial from the lateral malleolus

forward. Like the peroneus longus muscle, this muscle's prime function is to evert the ankle, although it is able to assist somewhat in plantar flexion.

Peroneus Brevis Muscle

O	Lateral distal fibula
I	Base of fifth metatarsal
A	Ankle eversion; assists in plantar flexion
N	Superficial peroneal nerve (L4, L5, S1)

The **peroneus tertius** muscle, not present in all people, is difficult to identify and often is confused as part of the extensor digitorum longus muscle. The muscle arises from the distal medial fibula and interosseous membrane, and crosses the ankle anteriorly to insert on the dorsal surface of the base of the fifth metatarsal, near the peroneus brevis muscle (see Fig. 19-30). Theoretically, this muscle should dorsiflex and evert the ankle, but due to its size, it is assistive at best.

Peroneus Tertius Muscle

O	Distal medial fibula
I	Base of fifth metatarsal
A	Assists in ankle eversion and dorsiflexion
N	Deep peroneal nerve (L4, L5, S1)

The following list summarizes the actions of the prime movers of the ankle.

Action	Muscle
Plantar flexion	Gastrocnemius, soleus
Dorsiflexion	Tibialis anterior
Inversion	Tibialis anterior, tibialis posterior
Eversion	Peroneus longus, peroneus brevis
Flexion of second through fifth toes	Flexor digitorum longus
Flexion of first toe	Flexor hallucis longus
Extension of second through fifth toes	Extensor digitorum longus
Extension of first toe	Extensor hallucis longus
No prime mover action	Plantaris, peroneus tertius

Intrinsic Muscles

Intrinsic muscles have both attachments distal to the ankle joint. Because we do not use these muscles in the foot to perform intricate actions, they do not tend to be as well developed as their counterparts in the hand. Their names tell a great deal about their location and action. All intrinsic muscles are located on the plantar surface, essentially in layers, except the extensor digitorum brevis and extensor hallucis brevis muscles, which are on the dorsal surface. Table 19-3 summarizes the intrinsic muscles according to surface location, depth location, function, and similar structure in the hand. Innervation of these muscles is summarized as follows:

Muscle	Nerve
DORSAL SURFACE	
Extensor digitorum brevis	Deep peroneal
Extensor hallucis brevis	Deep peroneal
PLANTAR SURFACE	
Abductor hallucis	Tibial
Flexor digitorum brevis	Tibial
Abductor digiti minimi	Tibial
Quadratus plantae	Tibial

Table 19-3	Intrinsic Muscles of the Foot	
Muscle	**Action**	**Comparable Hand Muscle**
Dorsal Surface		
Extensor digitorum brevis	Extends PIP joints of digits 2–5	None
Extensor hallucis brevis	Extends PIP joint of first digit	None
Plantar Surface		
First layer		
Abductor hallucis	Abducts; flexes IP of first toe	Abductor pollicis brevis
Flexor digitorum brevis	Flexes PIP of digits 2–5	Flexor digitorum superficialis
Abductor digiti minimi	Flexes; abducts fifth digit	Same name
Second layer		
Quadratus plantae	Straightens diagonal line of pull of flexor digitorum longus	None
Lumbricales	Flexes MPs; extends PIPs and DIPs	Same name
Third layer		
Flexor hallucis brevis	Flexes MP of first digit	Flexor pollicis brevis
Adductor hallucis	Adducts; flexes first digit	Adductor pollicis
Flexor digiti minimi	Flexes PIP of fifth digit	Same name
Dorsal Surface		
Fourth layer		
Dorsal interossei	Abducts second through fourth digits	Same name
Plantar interossei	Adducts second through fourth digits	Palmar interossei

[handwritten annotations:] Nerve — Deep peroneal — Deep peroneal; Tibial Nerve

Table 19-4	Innervation of the Muscles of the Leg and Foot	
Muscle	**Nerve**	**Spinal Segment**
Gastrocnemius	Tibial	S1, S2
Soleus	Tibial	S1, S2
Plantaris	Tibial	L4, L5, S1
Tibialis posterior	Tibial	L5, S1
Flexor digitorum longus	Tibial	L5, S1
Flexor hallucis longus	Tibial	L5, S1, S2
Peroneus longus	Superficial peroneal	L4, L5, S1
Peroneus brevis	Superficial peroneal	L4, L5, S1
Peroneus tertius	Deep peroneal	L4, L5, S1
Extensor digitorum longus	Deep peroneal	L4, L5, S1
Extensor digitorum brevis	Deep peroneal	L5, S1
Extensor hallucis longus	Deep peroneal	L4, L5, S1
Tibialis anterior	Deep peroneal	L4, L5, S1
Abductor hallucis	Medial plantar (tibial)	L4, L5
Flexor hallucis brevis	Medial plantar (tibial)	L4, L5, S1
Flexor digitorum brevis	Medial plantar (tibial)	L4, L5
Lumbricales (medial 1)	Medial plantar (tibial)	L4, L5
Lumbricales (lateral 3)	Lateral plantar (tibial)	S1, S2
Abductor digiti minimi	Lateral plantar (tibial)	S1, S2
Quadratus plantae	Lateral plantar (tibial)	S1, S2
Adductor hallucis	Lateral plantar (tibial)	S1, S2
Flexor digiti minimi	Lateral plantar (tibial)	S1, S2
Dorsal interossei	Lateral plantar (tibial)	S1, S2
Plantar interossei	Lateral plantar (tibial)	S1, S2

Lumbricales	Tibial
Flexor hallucis brevis	Tibial
Adductor hallucis	Tibial
Flexor digiti minimi	Tibial
Dorsal interossei	Tibial
Plantar interossei	Tibial

Summary of Muscle Innervation

The ankle and foot muscles fall into relatively tidy groupings according to innervation. Those muscles located on the posterior leg and plantar surface of the foot receive innervation from the **tibial nerve.** The plantar foot divides into two groups similar to the hand. The lateral plantar branch of the tibial nerve innervates muscles located on the lateral side, and the medial plantar branch innervates those on the medial side.

The **superficial peroneal nerve** innervates muscles on the lateral side of the leg (peroneals). The peroneus tertius muscle is the exception, because it crosses the ankle anteriorly to receive innervation with the other anterior muscles from the **deep peroneal nerve.**

Tables 19-4 and 19-5 summarize ankle and foot innervation. As has been noted in the previous chapters, there is some variation among sources regarding spinal cord level. *Gray's Anatomy* is used as the reference source when discrepancy occurs.

Points to Remember

- Stretching is performed on *relaxed* muscles, strengthening is occurring on *contracting* muscles.
- To stretch a two-joint muscle, stretch it over both joints at the same time within pain limits of that muscle.
- To stretch a one-joint muscle, select a joint position that stretches a two-joint muscle over only one joint.
- The excursion of a one-joint muscle will be greater than the range allowed by the joint.

Table 19-5	Segmental Innervation of the Ankle Joint and Foot			
Spinal Cord Level	L4	L5	S1	S2
Gastrocnemius			X	X
Soleus			X	X
Plantaris	X	X	X	
Tibialis posterior		X	X	
Flexor digitorum longus		X	X	
Flexor hallucis longus		X	X	X
Peroneus longus	X	X	X	
Peroneus brevis	X	X	X	
Peroneus tertius	X	X	X	
Extensor digitorum longus	X	X	X	
Extensor digitorum brevis		X	X	
Extensor hallucis longus	X	X	X	
Tibialis anterior	X	X		
Abductor hallucis	X	X		
Flexor hallucis brevis	X	X	X	
Flexor digitorum brevis	X	X		
Lumbricales	X	X	X	X
Abductor digiti minimi			X	X
Quadratus plantae			X	X
Adductor hallucis			X	X
Flexor digiti minimi			X	X
Dorsal interossei			X	X
Plantar interossei			X	X

- The excursion of a two-joint muscle is less than the combined range allowed by both joints.
- A muscle contraction is strongest if the muscle is stretched before it contracts.
- A muscle loses power quickly as it shortens.

- Two-joint muscles maintain their force of contraction for a longer period compared to a one-joint muscle. This is because they are able to elongate over one joint while shortening over the other joint.

Review Questions

General Anatomy Questions

1. Describe the ankle (talotibial) joint:
   a. Number of axes:
   b. Shape of joint:
   c. Type of action allowed:
   d. Bones involved:

2. What bones are involved in the subtalar joint? What are the bones involved in the transverse tarsal joint?

3. What are the functions of the interosseous membrane?

4. What ligaments provide medial stability to the ankle? What is their collective name?

5. What ligaments provide lateral stability to the ankle? What is their collective name?

6. What are the names of the two longitudinal arches?

7. List the bones involved in each longitudinal arch.

8. List the bones involved in the transverse arch.

9. What is the function of the arches?

10. Which muscles pass behind the medial malleolus?

11. Which muscles attach on the medial side of the foot?

12. Which muscles pass behind the lateral malleolus?

13. Which muscles attach on the lateral side of the foot?

14. Which muscles form the "stirrup" of the foot? Describe how the stirrup is formed.

15. Would an individual with an L4 spinal cord level injury be able to actively do ankle plantar flexion?

Functional Activity Questions

Identify the main ankle joint action or position in the following activities:

1. Pushing your foot down on the accelerator pedal while driving

2. Standing in high heels

3. Walking up a steep slope

4. Walking down a steep slope

5. Foot on floor with the heel as the pivot point, a "windshield swipe" motion of the foot

6. Walking on your heels

7. Taking off when jumping, hopping, or skipping

Clinical Exercise Questions

1. Answer the following questions:
   Gastrocnemius
   a. Number of joints crossed: 1 or 2
   b. Knee motion: flexion/extension/none
   c. Ankle motion: dorsiflexion/plantar flexion/none

   Soleus
   a. Number of joints crossed: 1 or 2
   b. Knee motion: flexion/extension/none
   c. Ankle motion: dorsiflexion/plantar flexion/none

2. Place your hands on the wall at shoulder level. Stand with your left foot 2 feet from the wall, and with your right foot about 1 foot from the wall (Fig. 19-31). Keeping your left leg straight and your right foot flat on the floor, lean in toward the wall leading with your pelvis and allowing your right knee to bend. In terms of what is occurring at the left knee and ankle, answer the following questions:
   a. What are the joint positions or motions that are occurring:
      at the left knee? _____
      at the left ankle? _____
   b. To be in the above position, is the left gastrocnemius contracting/stretching?
   c. To be in the above position, is the left soleus contracting/stretching?
   d. Which of these two muscles is being stretched more than the other?
   e. Why?

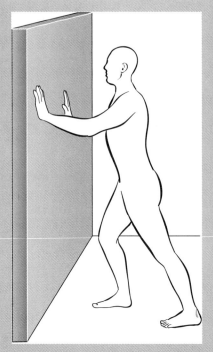

Figure 19-31.   Starting position.

3. Activity: Repeat the position of exercise No. 2, except this time bend your left knee as you lean into the wall.
   a. What are the joint positions or motions that are occurring:
      at the left knee? _____
      at the left ankle? _____
   b. In this new position, is the left gastrocnemius stretched or slack at the knee?
   c. In this new position, is the left gastrocnemius stretched or slack at the ankle?
   d. In this new position, is the left soleus stretched at the knee?
   e. In this new position, is the left soleus stretched at the ankle?
   f. Which of these two muscles is stretched more?
   g. Why?

4. Standing upright and holding on to the back of a chair for balance, rise up on your toes as high as possible.
   a. What are the joint positions or motions that are occurring:
      at the knee? _____
      at the ankle? _____.

b. Is the gastrocnemius shortening or elongating over the knee?

c. Is the gastrocnemius shortening or elongating over the ankle?

d. Does the soleus have an action at the knee?

e. Is the soleus shortening or elongating over the ankle?

f. Why is the gastrocnemius stronger than the soleus in this position?

5. Sitting with your knees bent, press the soles of your feet together (Fig. 19-32).

a. Is inversion or eversion the joint motion (or attempted joint motion) at the ankle?

b. What type of muscle contraction is occurring at the ankle (isometric, concentric, eccentric)?

c. What are the prime movers of this action?

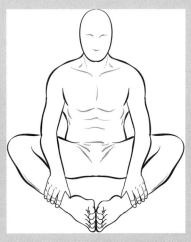

Figure 19-32. Starting position.

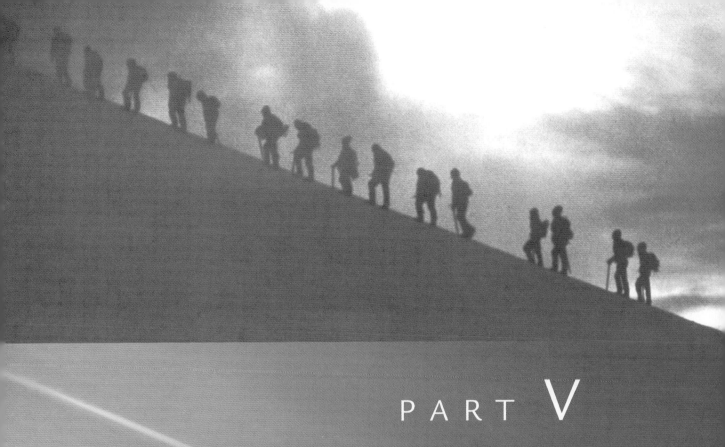

PART V

Clinical Kinesiology and Anatomy of the Body

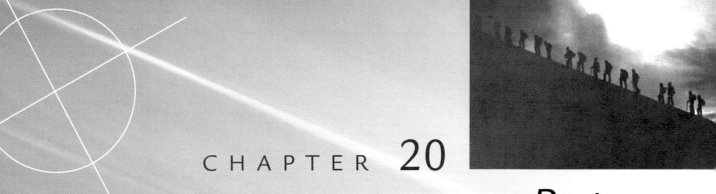

CHAPTER 20

Posture

Vertebral Alignment

    Development of Postural Curves

Standing Posture

    Lateral View

    Anterior View

    Posterior View

Sitting Posture

Supine Posture

Common Postural Deviations

Review Questions

    General Anatomy Questions

    Functional Activity Questions

    Clinical Exercise Questions

In general, posture is the position of your body parts in relation to each other at any given time. Posture can be static, as in a stationary position such as standing, sitting, or lying. It can be dynamic as the body moves from one position to another. Posture deals with alignment of the various body segments. These body segments can be compared to blocks. If you start stacking blocks one directly on top of the other, the column would remain relatively stable. However, if you stack them off center from each other, the column will remain upright only if the block, or blocks, above counter the block or blocks below, and remain within the base of support. In the human body, each joint involved with weight-bearing can be considered a postural segment.

Vertebral Alignment

The vertebral column can be compared to the column of blocks. It is not completely straight, but has a series of counterbalancing anterior-posterior curves. These curves, which must be maintained during rest and activity, act as shock absorbers and reduce the amount of injury. The thoracic and sacral curves counter the cervical and lumbar curves (Fig. 20-1). The thoracic and sacral curves are concave anteriorly and convex posteriorly. Conversely, the lumbar and cervical curves are convex anteriorly and concave posteriorly. Remember that a curve has two sides to it: a concave side and a convex. Therefore, whether a curve is concave or convex depends on to which side you are referring.

When one or more of these vertebral curves either increases or decreases significantly from what is considered good posture, poor posture results. For example, a "sway back" is an increased lumbar curve, whereas a "flat back" is a decreased thoracic curve. In most cases, if there is an increased lumbar curve, there is also an

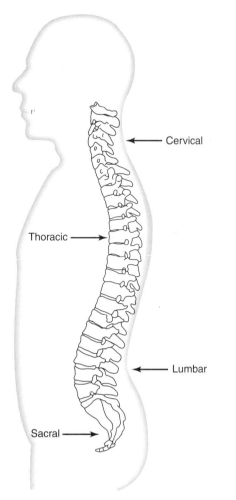

Figure 20-1.   The four major curves of the vertebral column.

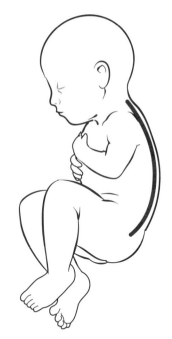

Figure 20-2.   The primary curve of a newborn.

increased thoracic curve. No lateral curves should exist. Any lateral curvature of the spine is a pathologic condition called scoliosis.

Development of Postural Curves

At birth, the entire vertebral column is concave anteriorly. This concave curve is called a **primary curve** (Fig. 20-2). The thoracic and sacral curves are considered primary curves for this reason. As the child grows, **secondary curves** develop. These are the anteriorly convex curves of the cervical and lumbar regions.

The position of the pelvis has great influence on the vertebral column, especially the lumbar region. The pelvis should be in a neutral position. This position is defined as (1) when the anterior superior iliac spine (ASIS) and posterior superior iliac spine (PSIS) are level with each other in a transverse plane; and (2) when the ASIS is in the same vertical plane as the symphysis pubis. When the pelvis is in a neutral position, the lum-

bar curve has the desired amount of curvature. When the pelvis is tilted anteriorly, there is an increased amount of lumbar curvature, or lordosis. When the pelvis is tilted posteriorly, there is a decreased amount of curve, or flat back. These positions are illustrated in Figure 16-13.

With weight evenly distributed on both legs, the pelvis should remain level from side to side, with both ASISs being at the same level. During walking, however, the pelvis dips from side to side as weight is shifted from stance to swing phase. This **lateral pelvic tilt** is controlled by the hip abductors, mainly the gluteus medius and gluteus minimus, and the trunk lateral benders, mainly the erector spinae and quadratus lumborum. If you bend your left knee and lift your foot off the ground, your pelvis on the left side becomes unsupported and will drop. Force couple action of the hip abductors and trunk lateral benders hold the pelvis level. The right hip abductors on the opposite side contract to pull the pelvis down on the right side while trunk lateral benders on the left (same side) contract to pull the pelvis up on the left side. These motions are illustrated in Figure 16-21. An abnormal lateral pelvic tilt can also occur if both legs are not of equal length. This will result in a lateral curvature, or scoliosis.

Muscle contractions are primarily responsible for keeping the body in the upright position in both static and dynamic posture. The muscles most involved are called **antigravity muscles** (Fig. 20-3). These muscles are the hip and knee extensors, and the trunk and neck

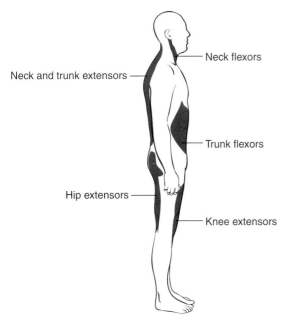

Figure 20-3.   Antigravity muscles.

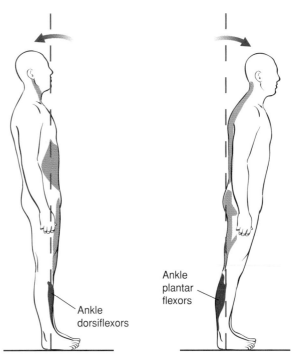

Figure 20-4.   Postural sway.

extensors. Other muscles, perhaps less involved, but also important in maintaining the upright position, are the trunk and neck flexors and lateral benders, hip abductors and adductors, and the ankle pronators and supinators. If all of these muscles were to relax, the body would collapse.

The ankle plantar flexors and dorsiflexors are important in controlling postural sway (Fig. 20-4). **Postural sway** is anterior-posterior motion of the upright body caused by motion occurring primarily at the ankles. This sway is the result of constant displacement and correction of the center of gravity within the base of support.

Stand upright with your feet slightly apart. Lean your entire body slowly forward by bending at the ankles. You will reach a point where you will need to either correct the forward lean or you will lose your balance forward. Notice that your ankle plantar flexors contract to bring you back to an upright position. Next, lean backward and notice what happens. Again, you will reach a point where you either need to correct the lean or lose your balance. Notice that your ankle dorsiflexors contract to bring you back to an upright position.

A high center of gravity and small base of support tend to increase the amount of postural sway. To demonstrate this, stand upright with your feet slightly apart. Notice how much your body tends to move back and forth. Next, observe the amount of sway when you stand on your toes in the upright position with your feet close together. You should notice much more motion in the latter position, because you have raised your center of gravity higher and made your base of support smaller.

Good posture, which means good alignment, is important because it decreases the amount of stress placed on bones, ligaments, muscles, and tendons. Good alignment also improves function and decreases the amount of muscle energy needed to keep the body upright. For example, if the knee is in full extension, little muscle contraction is needed to keep the knee from buckling. However, when the knee is partially flexed, the muscles at that joint (knee extensors) must contract to keep the knee from collapsing. Because standing is a closed-chain activity, muscles at the hip and ankle must also contract to keep the body's center of gravity over its base of support.

Standing Posture

Posture is easier to describe in a static standing position because, except for a slight amount of sway when standing, the body is not moving. However, many of the guidelines for static posture can be applied to dynamic posture. Assessing a person's posture can be done most accurately with the use of a plumb line suspended from the ceiling or a posture grid behind the person as a point of reference. A plumb line is a string or cord with a weight attached to the lower end. Because the string is weighted, it makes a perfectly straight vertical line of gravity.

Lateral View

In the standing position and viewed from the **lateral position,** the plumb line should be aligned so that it passes slightly in front of the lateral malleolus (Fig. 20-5). For ideal posture, the body segments should be aligned so that the plumb line passes through the landmarks listed below as follows:

Head
Through the earlobe

Shoulder
Through the tip of the acromion process

Thoracic spine
Anterior to the vertebral bodies

Lumbar spine
Through the vertebral bodies

Pelvis
Level

Hip
Through the greater trochanter (slightly posterior to the hip joint axis)

Knee
Slightly posterior to the patella (slightly anterior to the knee joint axis) with the knees in extension

Ankle
Slightly anterior to the lateral malleolus with the ankle joint in a neutral position between dorsiflexion and plantar flexion

Common postural deviations that can be detected from the side view are summarized in Table 20-1. Because standing is a closed kinetic chain activity, the position or motion of one joint will effect the position or motions of other joints.

Anterior View

In the standing position and viewed from the **anterior position,** the plumb line should be aligned to pass through the midsagittal plane of the body, thus dividing the body into two equal halves (Fig. 20-6). The body segments listed below should be aligned as follows:

Head
Extended and level, not flexed or hyperextended

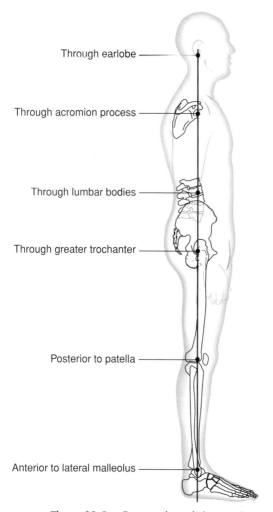

Through earlobe

Through acromion process

Through lumbar bodies

Through greater trochanter

Posterior to patella

Anterior to lateral malleolus

Figure 20-5. Posture, lateral view.

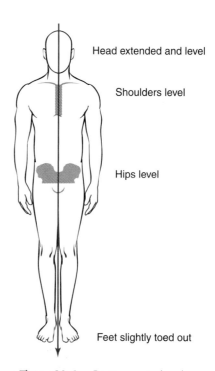

Head extended and level

Shoulders level

Hips level

Feet slightly toed out

Figure 20-6. Posture, anterior view.

Table 20-1	Summary of Common Postural Deviations			
	Lateral View		**Posterior View**	**Anterior View**
Head	Forward		Tilted	Tilted
			Rotated	Rotated
				Mandible asymmetrical
Cervical spine	Exaggerated curve			
	Flattened curve			
Shoulders	Rounded		Elevated	Elevated
			Depressed	Depressed
Scapulae			Abducted	
			Adducted	
			Winged	
Thoracic spine	Exaggerated curve		Lateral deviation	
Lumbar spine	Exaggerated curve		Lateral deviation	
	Flattened curve			
Pelvis	Anterior pelvic tilt		Lateral pelvic tilt	
	Posterior pelvic tilt		Pelvis rotated	
Hip				Medially rotated
				Laterally rotated
Knee	Genu recurvatum		Genu varum	External tibial torsion
	Flexed knee		Genu valgum	Internal tibial torsion
Ankle/foot	Forward posture			Hallux valgus
	Flattened longitudinal arch		Pes planus	Claw toe
	Exaggerated longitudinal arch		Pes cavus	Hammertoe
				Mallet toe

Shoulders
Level and not elevated or depressed

Sternum
Centered in the midline

Hips
Level with both ASISs in the same plane

Legs
Slightly apart

Knees
Level and not bowed or knock-kneed

Ankles
Normal arch in feet

Feet
Slight outward toeing

Posterior View

In the standing position and viewed from the **posterior position,** the plumb line should also be aligned to pass through the midsagittal plane of the body, dividing the body into two equal halves (Fig. 20-7).

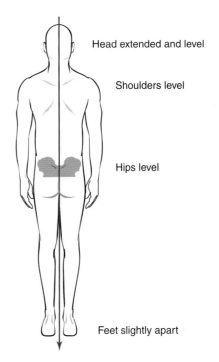

Head extended and level

Shoulders level

Hips level

Feet slightly apart

Figure 20-7. Posture, posterior view.

The following body segments should be aligned as follows:

Head
Extended, not flexed or hyperextended

Shoulders
Level and not elevated or depressed

Spinous processes
Centered in the midline

Hips
Level with both PSISs in the same plane

Legs
Slightly apart

Knees
Level and not bowed or knock-kneed

Ankles
Calcaneus should be straight

Sitting Posture

Good postural alignment while sitting is important because sitting is an activity that can place a great deal of pressure on the intervertebral disk. Studies have shown that disk pressure in the sitting position increases by slightly less than half of the amount of disk pressure in the standing position. To state the obvious, shifting weight on to the front part of the vertebrae will increase the amount of pressure placed on the intervertebral disks. As the person leans forward, disk pressure increases. As a person reaches, and/or picks up a weight, disk pressure further increases as the weight and/or length of the lever arm increases. Figure 20-8 illustrates disk pressure in various positions. Disk pressure is least when lying supine. It increases as you stand, and increases more as you sit. Leaning forward in these positions increases the disk pressure, and leaning forward with an object in your hand obviously also increases it.

If the lumbar curve is decreased, such as often happens when sitting with the back unsupported (Fig. 20-9), the pressure on the intervertebral disks and posterior structures increases. A chair with the seat inclined anteriorly, such as the kneeling stool (Fig. 20-10), can decrease disk pressure by tilting the pelvis forward slightly. This helps to maintain the lumbar curve. However, because the back is unsupported, increased and sustained muscle contraction is required to keep the body upright.

Shifting weight on to the front part of the vertebra is not always a problem. Although disk pressure increases in this position, the stresses placed on the posterior part of the vertebra, the facet joints, decreases. Therefore, if

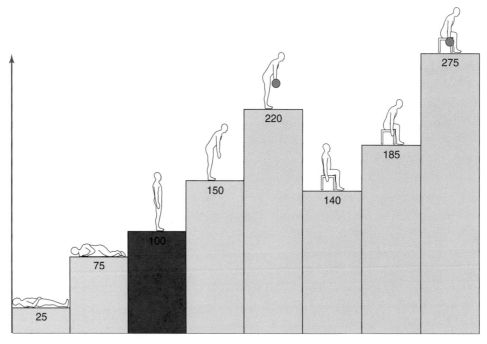

Figure 20-8. Disk pressures in various positions. (Adapted from Magee, DJ: Orthopedic Physical Assessment. WB Saunders, Philadelphia, 1987, p 378, with permission; original source, Nachemson, A: The lumbar spine: An orthopaedic challenge. Spine 1:59–71, 1976.)

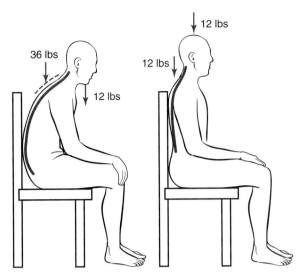

Figure 20-9. Slouched posture increases disk pressure.

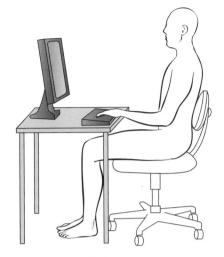

Figure 20-11. Sitting posture at computer.

a person has a facet joint problem, generally speaking, a flexed position is more desirable. Conversely, if a person has a disk problem, an extended position is usually more desirable.

With sitting postures, a chair that has a lumbar support that maintains the lumbar lordosis will place the least amount of pressure on the disks. Maintaining the vertebral curves, keeping the feet flat on the floor, having the low back supported, and keeping the upper body in good alignment are key elements of good sitting posture. Figure 20-11 demonstrates the best posture while working at a computer. The neck and trunk are upright, the trunk is supported, and the lumbar spine has a

support. The top of the monitor is at eye level. A person should not have to hyperextend the head to view the screen. The shoulders are relaxed. The elbows are flexed and close to the body. The hands, wrists, and forearms are straight and parallel to the ground. The chair should allow the hips and knees to be flexed. The thighs are parallel to the ground and the lower legs are vertical, allowing the feet to be flat on the floor or a footrest.

Supine Posture

Lying down is considered a resting position (Fig. 20-12). The least amount of intervertebral disk pressure occurs while lying supine (see Fig. 20-8). If you could run a plumb line horizontally, it would intersect many of the same landmarks as in the standing position. Good alignment in this position is also important. A good resting surface should be firm enough to avoid loss of the lumbar curve, yet soft enough to conform and give support to the normal curves of the body. In the side-lying position, the bottom leg is extended and the top leg is flexed. Placing a pillow between the legs can increase comfort by keeping the hips in good alignment. Lying prone is usually not recommended because of the

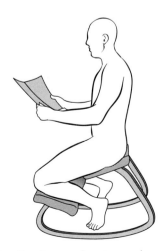

Figure 20-10. Kneeling stool posture reduces disk pressure.

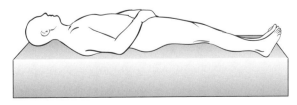

Figure 20-12. Lying posture.

increased pressure placed on the neck. In this position, using a pillow only increases the stresses on the neck.

When actively moving about and changing positions, whether vacuuming the rug, picking up a box from the floor, or raking leaves, keeping the body, especially the trunk, in good postural alignment is important. Most principles of good body mechanics involve avoiding stress to the trunk and maintaining the spinal curves, which involve maintaining good posture.

Common Postural Deviations

Table 20-1 is a summary of common postural deviations seen when assessing posture. It is not within the scope of this book to describe the individual causes and effects of postural problems. However, some general statements regarding cause and effect should be made.

Deviation from "good" posture is considered "poor" or "bad" posture. Causes of poor posture can be the result of structural problems. These structural problems may be the result of a congenital malformation such as a hemivertebra. The deviation may be an acquired deformity caused by trauma such as a com-

pression fracture. Postural deviations also may be the result of neurological conditions causing paralysis or spasticity. In addition, postural problems may also be functional, or nonstructural, in nature. A person who sits or stands for long periods of time will tend to slouch. This can result in a muscle imbalance.

Generally, if a person tends to maintain a posture in which a curve is increased, the muscles on the concave side will tend to tighten while the muscles on the convex side tend to weaken. For example, you would expect a person with a lumbar lordosis to have tight back extensors and weak abdominal muscles. Also, postures that tend to increase the lordotic curves (cervical and lumbar) will increase the pressure on the more posterior facet joints and decrease the pressure on the more anterior intervertebral disks. Conversely, an increase in the kyphotic curves (thoracic and sacral) will increase the pressure on the intervertebral disks while decreasing the pressure on the facet joints.

It should be noted that the terms "kyphotic" and "lordotic" can lead to confusion. They are used to describe both the normal amount of curvature, as well as the abnormal or excessive. Scoliosis is a term that refers to a lateral curvature. However, any amount of scoliosis is considered abnormal.

Review Questions

General Anatomy Questions

1. If a person had an excessive cervical lordosis, would you expect the cervical extensors or flexors to be tight?

2. Which position—the side, front, or back—would be best to assess the condition in question 1?

3. If a person had an anterior tilt of the pelvis, would you expect the hip flexors or hip extensors to be tight?

4. To assess the condition in question 3, which position—the side, front, or back—would be best?

5. What position should the shoulders be in relation to each other?

6. Which position—the side, front, or back—would be best to assess the position of the shoulders in relation to each other?

7. When assessing a person's posture in the lateral standing position and using a plumb line, you should begin by lining up the plumb line with what body structure?

8. For ideal posture (when viewed laterally), where should the plumb line pass on the following structures:
   a. Knee
   b. Hip
   c. Shoulder
   d. Head

Functional Activity Questions

1. Sitting in a chair with back and armrests, put with your hands together resting them between your thighs near your knees. Your shoulder girdles are in what position?

2. Sitting in the same position as in question 1, move from that position to one with your forearms resting on the arms of the chair. How does the position of your shoulder girdles change from their position in question 1?

3. Sitting slouched down in the chair, keeping your back in contact with the back of the chair, and sliding your buttocks forward. What position does your head assume?

4. Carry a heavy book bag on your right shoulder. By changing posture, how do you keep the strap from sliding off of your shoulder?

During pregnancy:

5. What direction does the woman's COG shift?

6. There would be a tendency for the pelvis to tilt in which direction in the sagittal plane?

7. What type of change would occur in the lumbar spine?

8. Those changes in the pelvic and lumbar positions could lead to:
   a. Which trunk muscle group becoming tight?
   b. Which trunk muscle group becoming stretched?

9. As compensatory posture, would you expect the hip flexors or extensors to become tight?

Clinical Exercise Questions

1. Sit in front of a computer screen. Pretend (if necessary) that you are wearing bifocals that require you to look through the bottom of the lenses for close-up work. This can be simulated by wrapping plastic wrap on the top half of a pair of clear or sunglasses. To read the screen, what position does the head and neck assume?

2. If the position in exercise No. 1 became a chronic posture
   a. Muscle groups on which side of the neck would become tighter?
   b. Muscle groups on which side of the neck would become stretched?

3. Stand upright on both feet with a 2- to 3-inch block under your left foot; stand upright with equal weight on both feet. Does your pelvis remain level? If not, which side of the pelvis is higher?

4. If the posture in exercise No. 3 became a permanent condition:
   a. Muscle groups on which side of the trunk would become tighter?

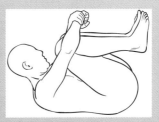

Figure 20-13.   Exercise position. Lie supine hugging knees to chest.

   b. Muscle groups on which side of the trunk would become stretched?

5. With exercise No. 3:
   a. Which side of the intervertebral disk would be compressed? Distracted?
   b. Which side of the intervertebral disk would be distracted?
   c. The intervertebral foramen on which side would be opened more?
   d. The intervertebral foramen on which side would be made smaller?

6. Lie supine hugging your knees close to your chest, and bring your knees and forehead together. Hug the knees close to your chest (Fig. 20-13).
   a. What trunk muscle group is being stretched?
   b. Which part of the intervertebral disk is being compressed?

7. Lie prone with your hips and knees extended. Rise up and rest on your elbows (Fig. 20-14).
   a. What trunk muscles are being stretched?
   b. Which part of the intervertebral disk is being compressed?

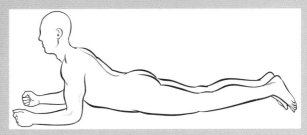

Figure 20-14.   Exercise position. Lie prone resting on elbows.

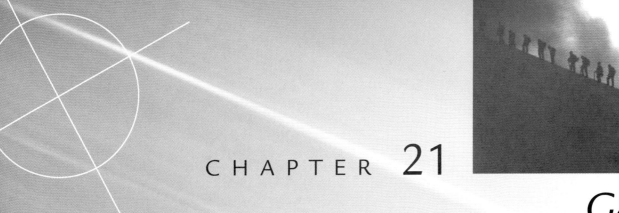

CHAPTER 21

Gait

Definitions

Analysis of Stance Phase

Analysis of Swing Phase

Additional Determinants of Gait

Age-Related Gait Patterns

Abnormal (Atypical) Gait

Muscular Weakness/Paralysis

Joint/Muscle Range of Motion Limitation

Neurological Involvement

Pain

Unequal Leg Length

Points to Remember

Review Questions

General Anatomy Questions

Functional Activity Questions

Clinical Exercise Questions

Walking is the manner or way in which you move from place to place with your feet. *Gait* is the process or components of walking. Each person has a unique style, and this style may change slightly with mood. When you are happy, your step is lighter, and there may be a "bounce" in your walk. Conversely, when sad or depressed, your step may be heavy. For some people, their walking pattern is so unique that they can be identified from a distance even before their face can clearly be seen. Regardless of the numerous different styles, the components of normal gait are the same.

In the most basic sense, walking requires balancing on one leg while the other leg is moved forward. This requires movement not only of the legs but also of the trunk and arms as well. To analyze gait, you must first determine what joint motions occur. Then, based upon that information, you must decide which muscles or muscle groups are acting.

Definitions

Certain definitions must be made to describe gait. **Gait cycle,** also called **stride,** is the activity that occurs between the time one foot touches the floor and the time the same foot touches the floor again (Fig. 21-1). A **stride length** is the distance traveled during the gait cycle.

A **step** is basically one-half of a stride. It takes two steps (a right one and a left one) to complete a stride or gait cycle. These steps should be equal. A **step length** is that distance between heel strike of one foot and heel strike of the other foot (see Fig. 21-1). With an increased or decreased walking speed, the step length will increase or decrease respectively. Regardless of speed, the step length of each leg should remain equal.

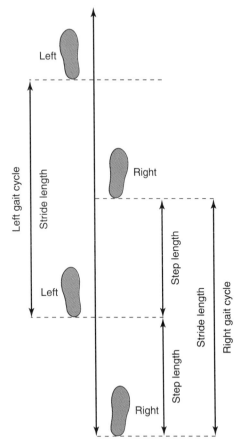

Figure 21-1.   Gait cycle terminology. A right and left step make up a gait cycle (also called stride).

Walking speed, or **cadence,** is the number of steps taken per minute, and can vary greatly. Slow walking may be as slow as 70 steps per minute. However, students on their way to an examination have been clocked at much slower speeds. Fast walking may be as fast as 130 steps per minute, although race walkers will walk much faster. Regardless of speed, the gait cycle is the same; that is, all parts occur in their proper place at the proper time.

There are two phases of the gait cycle (Fig. 21-2). **Stance phase** is the activity that occurs when the foot is in contact with the ground. It begins with heel strike of one foot and ends when that foot leaves the ground. This phase accounts for about 60 percent of the gait cycle. **Swing phase** occurs when the foot is not in contact with the ground. It begins as soon as the foot leaves the floor and ends when the heel of the same foot touches the floor. The swing phase makes up about 40 percent of the gait cycle.

Perry (1992) identifies three tasks that need to be accomplished during these phases of the gait cycle. Those tasks are (1) weight acceptance, (2) single leg support, and (3) leg advancement. They have been identified in Figure 21-2. **Weight acceptance** occurs at the very beginning of stance phase when the foot touches the ground and the body weight begins to be shifted onto that leg. **Single leg support** occurs next as the body weight shifts completely onto the stance leg so that the opposite leg can swing forward. The task of **leg advancement** occurs during swing phase.

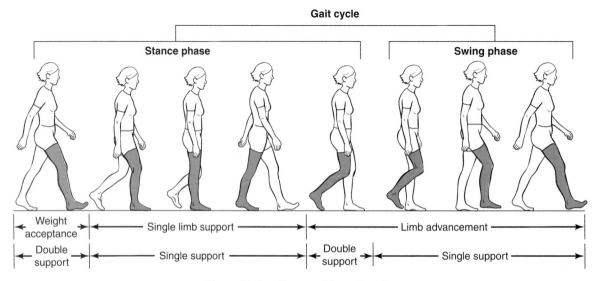

Figure 21-2.   Phases of the gait cycle.

The gait cycle has two periods of double support and two periods of single support. These periods have been identified in Figure 21-2. When both feet are in contact with the ground at the same time, this is a period of **double support.** This occurs as one leg is beginning its stance phase and the other leg is ending its stance phase. For example, the first period of double support occurs as the right leg is beginning stance phase and the left leg is ending stance phase. The second period of double support occurs as the right leg is ending its stance phase and the left leg is beginning its stance phase. Each period of double support takes up about 10 percent of the gait cycle at an average walking speed. If you increase your walking speed, you spend less time with both feet on the ground. Conversely, you spend more time in double support when you walk slowly.

A period of **nonsupport,** that is, a time during which neither foot is in contact with the ground, does not occur during walking. However, nonsupport does occur during running. Other than speed, this may be the biggest difference between running and walking. Other activities, such as hopping, skipping, and jumping, have a period of nonsupport but lose the order of progression that walking and running have. In other words, these activities do not include all the parts of stance and swing phase that walking and running have.

The period of **single support** occurs when only one foot is in contact with the ground (see Fig. 21-2). Thus, two periods of single support occur in a gait cycle: once when the right foot is on the ground as the left foot is swinging forward, then again when the left foot bears weight and the right leg swings forward. Each single support period takes up about 40 percent of the gait cycle.

Many sets of terms have been developed from the original, or traditional, terminology to describe the components of walking. In many cases, although the terminology may be accurate, it is often cumbersome. However, terminology developed by the Gait Laboratory at Rancho Los Amigos (RLA) Medical Center has been gaining in acceptance. Perhaps the biggest difference between the two sets of terms is that the traditional terms refer to *points in time* whereas RLA terms refer to *periods of time.* Traditional terminology accurately reflects key points within the gait cycle, whereas RLA periods accurately reflect the moving or dynamic nature of gait. It is best to be familiar with both sets of terms, because both terminologies will be seen in the literature. Table 21-1 provides the definitions of traditional terminology compared to the RLA terms. One can see that they are similar with a few exceptions. Table 21-2 describes the activities of each phase and the key points to observe. The reader is reminded of the slight differences between the two sets of terms. However, the key points are in the same sequence of the gait cycle, regardless of which terminology is used.

Analysis of Stance Phase

As defined earlier, *stance* is that period in which the foot is in contact with the floor. Traditionally, the stance phase has been broken down into five components consisting of (1) heel strike, (2) foot flat, (3) midstance, (4) heel-off, and (5) toe-off (Fig. 21-3). Some sources give stance phase only four components by combining heel-off and toe-off into one, and calling it "push-off." Because significantly different activities occur during these two periods, it is best to keep them separated.

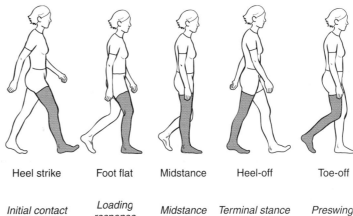

Traditional terminology	Heel strike	Foot flat	Midstance	Heel-off	Toe-off
RLA terminology	*Initial contact*	*Loading response*	*Midstance*	*Terminal stance*	*Preswing*

Figure 21-3.   The five components of stance phase.

Table 21-1	Comparison of Gait Terminology			
	Traditional		**Rancho Los Amigos**	
Term	**Definition**	**Term**	**Definition**	
Stance Phase				
Heel strike	Heel contacts the ground.	Initial contact	Same	
Foot flat	Plantar surface of the foot in contact with ground.	Loading response	Beginning: Just after initial contact when body weight is being transferred onto leg and entire foot makes contact with the ground. Ending: Opposite foot leaves the ground.	
Midstance	Point at which the body passes over the weight-bearing leg.	Midstance	Beginning: Opposite foot leaves the ground. Ending: Body is directly over the weight-bearing limb.	
Heel-off	Heel leaves the ground, while ball of the foot and toes remain in contact with the ground.	Terminal stance	Beginning: As the heel of weight-bearing leg rises. Ending: Initial contact of the opposite foot. The body has moved in front of the weight-bearing leg.	
Toe-off	Toes leave the ground, ending stance phase.	Preswing	Beginning: Initial contact and weight shifted onto the opposite leg. Ending: Just before toes of weight-bearing leg leave the ground.	
Swing Phase				
Acceleration	The swing leg begins to move forward.	Initial swing	Beginning: The toes leave the ground. Ending: The swing foot is opposite the weight-bearing foot and the knee is in maximum flexion.	
Midswing	The swing (non–weight-bearing) leg is directly under the body.	Midswing	Beginning: The swing foot is opposite the weight-bearing foot. Ending: The swing leg has moved in front of the body and the tibia is in a vertical position.	
Deceleration	The leg is slowing down in preparation for heel strike.	Terminal swing	Beginning: The tibia is in a vertical position. Ending: Just prior to initial contact.	

Heel strike signals the beginning of stance phase the moment the heel comes in contact with the ground (Fig. 21-4). At this point the ankle is in a neutral position between dorsiflexion and plantar flexion, and the knee begins to flex. This slight knee flexion provides some shock absorption as the foot hits the ground. The hip is in about 25 degrees of flexion. The trunk is erect and remains so throughout the entire gait cycle. The trunk is rotated toward the opposite (contralateral) side, the opposite arm is forward, and the same-side (ipsilateral) arm is back in shoulder hyperextension. At this point, body weight begins to shift onto the stance leg. In RLA, this is the period of *initial contact.*

The ankle dorsiflexors are active in putting the ankle in its neutral position. The quadriceps, which have been contracting concentrically, switch to contracting eccentrically to minimize the amount of knee flexion. The hip flexors have been active. However, the hip extensors are beginning to contract, keeping the hip from flexing more. The erector spinae are active in keeping the trunk from flexing. The force of the foot hitting the ground transmits up through the ankle, knee, and hip to the trunk. This would cause the pelvis to rotate anteriorly,

Table 21-2	Key Events of Normal Gait Cycle		
Traditional Terminology	RLA Terminology	Activity	Key Points to Observe
Stance Phase			
Heel strike* Foot touches the floor	*Initial contact* Foot touches the floor	• Stance phase begins • Task of weight acceptance begins • Double leg support begins • Body at lowest point in cycle	• Head and trunk are upright throughout cycle • Ankle dorsiflexed to neutral • Knee extended • Hip flexed • Leg in front of body • Pelvis rotated forward—ipsilateral side • Ipsilateral arm back, contralateral arm forward
Foot flat Entire foot in contact with ground	*Loading response* Begins with foot touching floor, continues until opposite foot leaves the floor	• Weight shift onto stance leg continues • Double leg support ends	• Ankle plantar flexes putting foot on ground • Knee partially flexed absorbing shock • Hip moving into extension • Body catching up with leg • Ipsilateral arm swinging forward
Midstance Body passes over stance leg	*Midstance* Begins with other leg leaving floor, continues until body is over stance leg	• Body at highest point in cycle • Single leg support begins	• Ankle slightly dorsiflexed • Knee and hip continue extending • Body passes over right foot • Pelvis in neutral position • Both arms parallel with body
Heel-off Heel rises off floor, beginning of push-off	*Terminal stance* Begins with heel rising, continues until other foot touches floor	• Body moves ahead of foot • Single leg support ends	• Ankle slightly dorsiflexed, then begins plantar flexion • Knee extending then beginning slight flexion • Hip hyperextending • Body ahead of stance leg • Pelvis rotating back – ipsilateral side • Ipsilateral arm swinging forward

(Continued)

Table 21-2	Key Events of Normal Gait Cycle (*continued*)		
Traditional Terminology	*RLA Terminology*	Activity	Key Points to Observe
Stance Phase			
Toe-off Toe leaves the floor	*Preswing* Begins with other foot touching floor, continues until toes leave floor	• Task of leg advancement begins • Double leg support begins and ends	• Ankle plantar flexed • Knee and hip are flexing • Lateral pelvic tilt on right side • Ipsilateral arm forward
Swing Phase			
Acceleration Leg is behind body, moving forward to catch up	*Initial swing* Begins with foot leaving floor, ends with swinging foot opposite stance foot	• Swing phase (non–weight-bearing) begins • Single leg support begins on contralateral side	• Ankle beginning to dorsiflex • Knee and hip continue flexing • Leg is behind body but moving forward • Pelvis beginning to rotate forward • Ipsilateral arm swinging backward
Midswing Foot swings under and past body	*Midswing* Begins with foot opposite stance foot, ends with tibia in vertical position	• Leg shortens to clear floor • Single leg support on contralateral side continues	• Ankle dorsiflexed • Knee at maximum flexion and begins to extend • Hip at maximum flexion • Leg passing under and moving in front of body • Pelvis in neutral position • Arms parallel with body and moving in opposite directions
Deceleration Leg slowing down, preparing to touch floor	*Terminal swing* Begins with vertical tibia, ends when foot touches floor	• Leg advancement task ends • Single support ends	• Ankle continuing in dorsiflexion • Knee extended • Hip flexed • Leg ahead of body • Pelvis rotated forward—ipsilateral side • Ipsilateral arm back, contralateral arm forward

Bold indicate Traditional terminology.
Italics indicates Rancho Los Amigos (RLA) terminology.

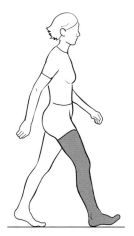

Figure 21-4.   Heel strike.

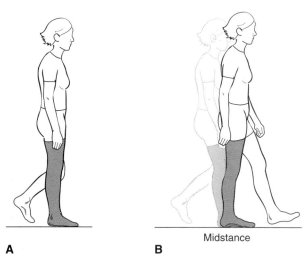

Midstance

A   **B**

Figure 21-6.   *(A)* Midstance. *(B)* Midstance period (RLA). The lighter tone shows the beginning of the loading response and the darker tone shows the ending of this period.

flexing the trunk somewhat, if it were not for the erector spinae counteracting this force.

Foot flat, when the entire foot is in contact with the ground, occurs shortly after heel strike (Fig. 21-5). The ankle moves into about 15 degrees of plantar flexion with the dorsiflexors contracting eccentrically to keep the foot from "slapping" down on the floor. The knee moves into about 20 degrees of flexion. The hip is moving into extension, allowing the rest of the body to begin catching up with the leg. Weight shift onto the stance leg continues. Foot flat is roughly comparable to the RLA period called *loading response,* which is

that period between the end of heel strike and the end of foot flat.

The point at which the body passes over the weight-bearing foot is called **midstance** (Fig. 21-6). In this phase, the ankle moves into slight dorsiflexion. However, the dorsiflexors become inactive. The plantar flexors begin to contract, controlling the rate at which the leg moves over the ankle. The knee and hip continue to extend, both arms are in shoulder extension essentially parallel with the body, and the trunk is in a neutral position of rotation. In RLA, *midstance* is the period between the end of foot flat and the end of midstance.

Following midstance is **heel-off,** in which the heel rises off the floor (Fig. 21-7). The ankle will dorsiflex slightly (approximately 15 degrees) and then begin to plantar flex. This is the beginning of the **push-off** phase, which is sometimes called the propulsion phase, because the ankle plantar flexors are actively pushing the body forward. The knee is in nearly full extension, and the hip has moved into hyperextension. The leg is now behind the body. The trunk has begun to rotate to the same side, and the arm is swinging forward into shoulder flexion. In RLA, *terminal stance* is that period between the end of midstance and the end of heel-off.

The end of the push-off portion of stance is **toe-off** (Fig. 21-8). The toes are in extreme hyperextension at the MP joints. The ankle moves into about 10 degrees of plantar flexion, and the knee and hip are flexing. The thigh is perpendicular to the ground. In RLA, *preswing* is

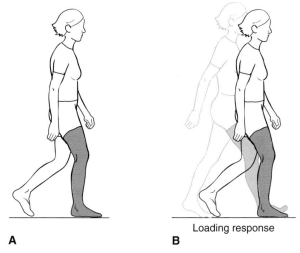

Loading response

A   **B**

Figure 21-5.   *(A)* Foot flat. *(B)* loading response period (RLA). The lighter tone shows the beginning of the loading response and the darker tone shows the ending of this period.

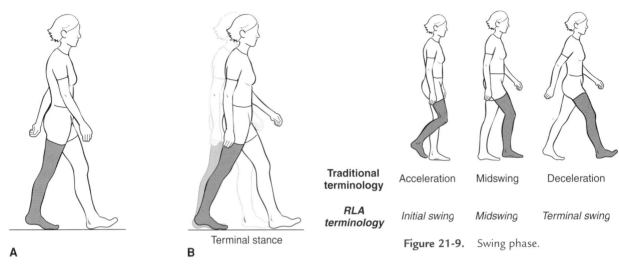

Figure 21-7. *(A)* Heel-off. *(B)* Terminal stance period (RLA). The lighter tone shows the beginning and the darker tone shows the ending of this period.

the period just before and including when the toes leave the ground, signaling the end of stance phase and the beginning of swing phase.

Analysis of Swing Phase

The swing phase consists of three components: acceleration, midswing, and deceleration (Fig. 21-9). These components are all non–weight-bearing activities. The first

part is **acceleration** (Fig. 21-10). The leg is behind the body and moving to catch up. The ankle is dorsiflexing, and the knee and hip continue to flex, which is moving the leg forward. In RLA, *initial swing* is that period between the end of toe-off and the end of acceleration.

At **midswing,** the ankle dorsiflexors have brought the ankle to a neutral position. The knee is at its maximum flexion (approximately 65 degrees) as is the hip (at about 25 degrees of flexion). These motions act to shorten the leg, allowing the foot to clear the ground as it swings through (Fig. 21-11). Further hip flexion moves the leg in front of the body and puts the lower leg in a vertical position. In RLA, *midswing* is that period between the end of acceleration and the end of midswing.

Figure 21-9.   Swing phase.

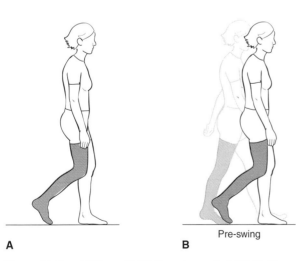

Figure 21-8. *(A)* Toe-off. *(B)* Preswing period (RLA). The lighter tone shows the beginning and the darker tone shows the ending of this period.

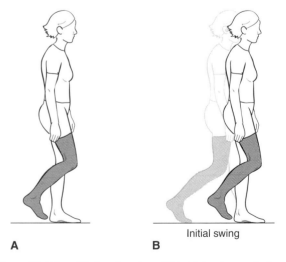

Figure 21-10. *(A)* Acceleration. *(B)* Initial swing period (RLA). The lighter tone shows the beginning and the darker tone shows the ending of this period.

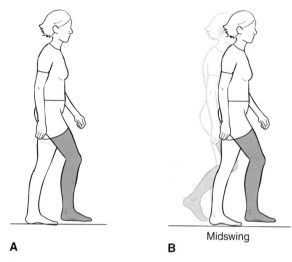

A   **B**
                                      Midswing

Figure 21-11. *(A)* Midswing. *(B)* Midswing period (RLA). The lighter tone shows the beginning and the darker tone shows the ending of this period.

In **deceleration,** the ankle dorsiflexors are active to keep the ankle in a neutral position in preparation for heel strike (Fig. 21-12). The knee is extending, and the hamstring muscles are contracting eccentrically to slow down the leg, keeping it from snapping into extension. The leg has swung as far forward as it is going to. The hip remains in flexion. In RLA, *terminal swing* is that period between the end of midswing and the end of deceleration.

Additional Determinants of Gait

To this point, the description of gait has centered mostly on the lower legs. However, other events are occurring in the rest of the body that must also be considered.

If you were to hold a piece of chalk against the blackboard and walk the length of the blackboard, you would see that the line drawn bobs up and down in wavelike fashion. This is described as the **vertical displacement** of the center of gravity (Fig. 21-13). The normal amount of this displacement is approximately 2 inches, being highest at midstance and lowest at heel strike *(initial contact)*. There is also an equal amount of **horizontal displacement** of the center of gravity as the body weight shifts from side to side. This displacement is greatest during the single support phase at midstance. In other words, this represents the distance the body must shift horizontally on to one foot so that the other foot can swing forward. This side-to-side displacement is usually about 2 inches.

When you walk, you do not place your feet one step in front of the other but slightly apart. If lines were drawn through the successive midpoints of heel contact *(initial contact)* on each foot, this distance would range from 2 to 4 inches. This is described as the **width of walking base** (Fig. 21-14).

If you were to walk across the room with your hands on your hips, you would notice that they move up and down as your pelvis on each side drops down slightly. This **lateral pelvic tilt** occurs when weight is taken off the leg at toe-off *(preswing)* (Fig. 21-15). This slight drop is sometimes referred to as the "Trendelenburg sign." This dip would be greater if it were not for the

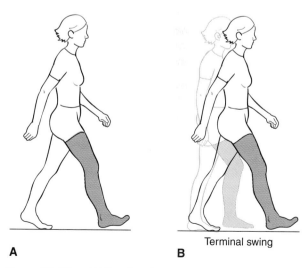

A   **B**
                                   Terminal swing

Figure 21-12. *(A)* Deceleration. *(B)* Terminal swing (RLA). The lighter tone shows the beginning and the darker tone shows the ending of this period.

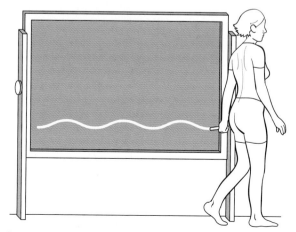

Figure 21-13. Vertical displacement of the body's center of gravity during the gait cycle.

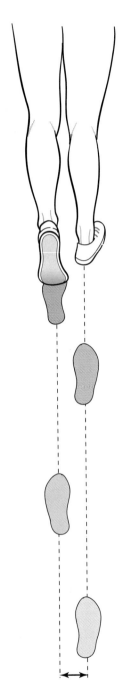

Figure 21-14. Walking base width.

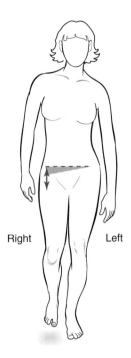

Figure 21-15. Lateral pelvic tilt.

muscle, which has attachment on the pelvis, contracts and "pulls up" on the side of the pelvis that wants to drop (Fig. 21-16).

In addition, step length should be equal in both distance and time. The arms should swing with the

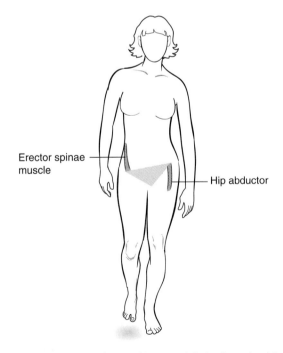

Figure 21-16. Muscles working to minimize lateral pelvic tilt. *(A)* Hip abductors. *(B)* Erector spinae muscles.

hip abductors on the opposite side (weight-bearing) and the erector spinae on the same side working together, keeping the pelvis essentially level. When the pelvis drops on the right side (non–weight-bearing side), the left hip (weight-bearing side) is forced into adduction. To keep the pelvis level, although it actually dips slightly, the left hip abductors contract to prevent hip adduction. At the same time the right erector spine opposite leg. The trunk rotates forward as the leg progresses through the swing phase. Arms swinging in opposition to trunk rotation control the amount of trunk rotation by providing counterrotation. The head should be erect, shoulders level, and trunk in extension.

When analyzing someone's gait, it is best to view the person from both the side and the front (and sometimes the back). Step length, arm swing, position of head and trunk, and the activities of the lower leg are usually best viewed from the side. Width of walking base, dip of the pelvis, and position of the shoulders and head should be viewed from the front or back.

Age-Related Gait Patterns

Not all gait patterns that don't comply with "normal" gait characteristics are the result of pathology. The walking patterns of young children and elderly adults have characteristic differences from the walking pattern of younger adults. These are considered age-related, not pathological, changes. The differences seen in young children tend to disappear as they get older. They tend to walk with a wider walking base, cadence is faster, and stride length is shorter. Initial contact with the floor is with a flat foot, as opposed to heel strike. Their knees remain mostly extended during stance phase. In other words, they tend to take more steps that are shorter and choppy in a faster period of time. They also have little or no reciprocal arm swing. This is easy to observe as a child walks with an adult.

Even in the absence of pathology, an elderly adult's walking pattern undergoes change. Although there is not universal agreement on the reasons for these changes, it is generally felt that security and fear of falling are major contributors. Typically, older adults lose muscle mass, are less active, and often have poorer hearing and vision. It should be recognized that the effects of age are relative to many factors such as health, activity level, and even attitude. Some 70-year-old people may appear "older" than others ten or more years their senior. Given all of these qualifiers, some general statements can be made regarding the changes in the walking pattern of elderly individuals. They tend to walk slower, spending more time in stance phase. Therefore, there are longer periods of double support. They take shorter steps, thus, vertical displacement is less. They walk with a wider base, and so have greater horizontal displacement. There are fewer, or slower, automatic movements, which may be another factor increasing the chance of stumbling or falling. In turn, this may contribute to increased toe-floor clearance.

Abnormal (Atypical) Gait

The causes of an abnormal gait are numerous. It may be temporary, due to a sprained ankle, or permanent, following a stroke. There can be great variation depending upon the severity of the problem. If a muscle is weak, how weak is it? If joint motion is limited, how limited is it? As with all causes of abnormal motion, severity or degree of involvement will always result in a range of variations from minor ones to major ones. There are many methods of classifying abnormal gait. The following is a listing of abnormal gaits based on general cause or basis for the abnormality:

Muscular weakness/paralysis
Joint muscle range-of-motion (ROM) limitation
Neurological involvement
Pain
Leg length discrepancy

Muscular Weakness/Paralysis

Depending upon the cause or severity of the condition, muscle weakness can range from slight weakness to complete paralysis, in which there is no strength at all. Generally speaking, with muscle weakness, the body tends to compensate by shifting the center of gravity over, or toward, the part that is involved. Basically, this reduces the moment of force (torque) on the joint, lessening the muscle strength required. Obviously, the portion of the gait cycle affected will be that portion in which the muscles or joints have a major role. Traditional terminology will be used with RLA terms in italics when there is a difference in terms.

In the case of the **gluteus maximus gait,** the trunk quickly shifts posteriorly at heel strike *(initial contact)*. This will shift the body's center of gravity (COG) posteriorly over the gluteus maximus, moving the line of force posterior to the hip joints (Fig. 21-17). With the foot in contact with the floor, this requires less muscle strength to maintain the hip in extension during stance phase. This shifting is sometimes referred to as a "rocking horse" gait because of the extreme backward-forward movement of the trunk.

With a **gluteus medius gait,** the individual shifts the trunk over the affected side during stance phase. In Figure 21-18, the left gluteus medius, or hip abductor, is weak causing two things to happen: (1) the body leans over the left leg during stance phase of the left leg, and (2) the right side of the pelvis will drop when the right leg leaves the ground and begins swing phase. This gait is also referred to as a "Trendelenburg" gait.

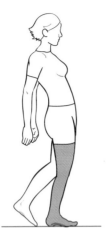

Figure 21-17. Gluteus maximus gait due to muscle weakness/paralysis on right side.

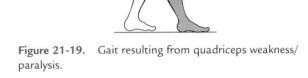

Figure 21-19. Gait resulting from quadriceps weakness/paralysis.

Do not confuse this with the normal amount of dipping of the pelvis. Shifting the trunk over the affected side is an attempt to reduce the amount of strength required of the gluteus medius to stabilize the pelvis.

When there is weakness in the **quadriceps** muscle group, several different compensatory mechanisms may be used. Depending upon whether only the quadriceps muscles are weak, or if there are additional weaknesses in the extremity, various compensatory maneuvers may be used. With quadriceps weakness, the individual may lean the body forward over the quadriceps muscles at the early part of stance phase, as weight is being shifted on to the stance leg. Normally, at this time, the line of force falls behind the knee, requiring quadriceps action to keep the knee from buckling. By leaning forward at the hip, the COG is

shifted forward and the line of force now falls in front of the knee. This will force the knee backward into extension. Another compensatory maneuver to use is the hip extensors and ankle plantar flexors in a closed-chain action to pull the knee into extension at heel strike *(initial contact)*. This reversal of muscle action can be seen in Figure 18-21. In addition, the person may physically push on the anterior thigh during stance phase, holding the knee in extension (Fig. 21-19).

If the **hamstrings** are weak, two things may happen. During stance phase, the knee will go into excessive hyperextension, sometimes referred to as "genu recurvatum" gait (Fig. 21-20). During the deceleration *(terminal swing)* part of swing phase, without the hamstrings to slow down the swing forward of the lower leg, the knee will snap into extension.

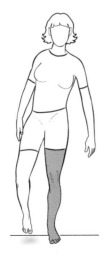

Figure 21-18. Gluteus medius gait.

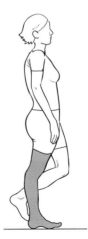

Figure 21-20. Genu recurvatum gait.

An individual may compensate in several ways depending on the amount of weakness of the **ankle dorsiflexors.** If there is insufficient strength to move the ankle into dorsiflexion at the beginning of stance phase, the foot will land with a fairly flat foot. However, if there is no ankle dorsiflexion, the toes will strike first, which is commonly referred to as an **equinnus gait** (Fig. 21-21A). Next, weak ankle dorsiflexors may not be able to support the body weight after heel strike moving toward foot flat *(loading response)* as they eccentrically contract. The result is **"foot slap."** With the dorsiflexors not being able to slow the descent of the foot, the foot slaps into plantar flexion as more weight is put on the leg. During swing phase, they may not be able to dorsiflex the ankle during swing phase. Gravity will cause the foot to fall into plantar flexion when it is off the ground. This is called **"drop foot."** As a result, the knee will need to be lifted higher for the dropped foot to clear the floor and **"steppage gait"** will result (Fig. 21-21B). The drum major in a marching band will utilize the elements of this gait when performing.

When the **triceps surae group** (the gastrocnemius and soleus) is weak, there is no heel rise at push off *(terminal stance)*, resulting in a shortened step length on the unaffected side. This is sometimes referred to as a "sore foot limp." Although this gait is noticeable on level ground, it becomes most pronounced when walking up an incline.

A **waddling gait** is commonly seen with muscular and other types of dystrophies because there is diffuse weakness of many muscle groups. The person stands with the shoulders behind the hips, much like a person

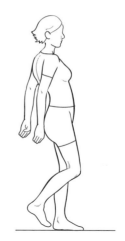

Figure 21-22.   Waddling gait.

with paraplegia would balance resting on the iliofemoral ligament of the hips (Fig. 21-22). There is an increased lumbar lordosis, pelvic instability, and Trendelenburg gait. Little or no reciprocal pelvis and trunk rotation occur. To swing the leg forward, the entire side of the body must swing forward. Normally, for example, as the right leg swings forward, the right arm swing backward. In this case, the right arm and leg swing forward together. Add this to the excessive trunk lean of Trendelenburg gait bilaterally, and one can see the waddling nature of the gait. A steppage gait is often present.

Joint/Muscle Range-of-Motion Limitation

In this grouping, the joint is unable to go through its normal range of motion because either there is bony fusion or soft tissue limitation. This limitation can be the result of contractures of muscle, capsule, or skin.

When a person has a **hip flexion contracture,** the involved hip is unable to go into hip extension and hyperextension during the midstance and push-off phases *(terminal stance)*. To compensate, the person will commonly assume the salutation or greeting position in which the hip is flexed and the person's trunk leans forward as if bowing (Fig. 21-23). The involved leg may also simultaneous flex the knee when it normally would be extended.

With a **fused hip,** increased motion of the lumbar spine and pelvis can greatly compensate for hip motion. A decreased lordosis and posterior pelvic tilt will allow the leg to swing forward (Fig. 21-24A), whereas an increased lordosis and anterior pelvic tilt will swing the leg posteriorly (Fig. 21-24B). This is

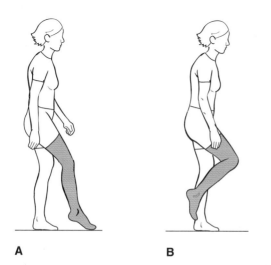

A   **B**

Figure 21-21.   Weakness, paralysis, or absence of ankle dorsiflexors results in *(A)* equinnus gait at heel strike *(initial contact—RLA),* and *(B)* steppage gait during swing phase.

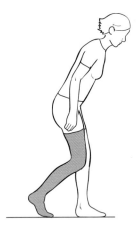

Figure 21-23. Salutation greeting resulting from hip flexion contracture.

sometimes referred to as a "bell-clapper gait." A bell swings back and forth causing the clapper inside to also move back and forth.

A **knee flexion contracture** will result in excessive dorsiflexion during midstance and an early heel rise during push-off *(terminal stance)*. There is also a shortened step length of the unaffected side. If a **knee fusion** is present, the lower leg will be at a fixed length. That length will depend on the position of the joint. If the knee is in extension, the leg will be unable to shorten during swing phase. Therefore, to compensate, the person (1) must rise up on the toes of the uninvolved leg in a **vaulting gait**

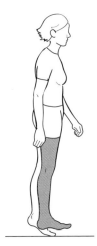

Figure 21-25. Vaulting gait resulting from a right knee fused in extension. The person must rise up her toes on the left side to allow the involved right leg to swing through.

(Fig. 21-25), (2) hike the hip of the involved side, (3) swing the leg out to the side, or (4) some variation of the three methods. With a **"circumducted gait,"** the leg begins near the midline at push-off *(terminal stance),* swings out to the side during swing phase, then returns to the midline for heel strike (Fig. 21-26). It is called an **"abducted gait"** if the leg remains in an abducted position throughout the gait cycle.

Depending on the severity of a **triceps surae contracture,** several things may result. The knee can be forced

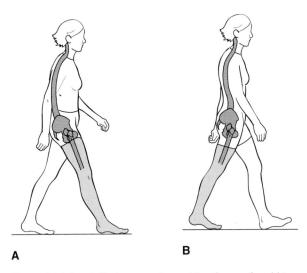

A   **B**

Figure 21-24. Bell-clapper gait resulting from a fused hip. In *(A)* the leg swings forward by flattening the lumbar lordosis and tilting the pelvis posteriorly. In *(B)* the leg swings backward by increasing the lumbar lordosis and tilting the pelvis anteriorly.

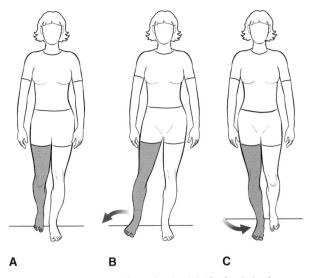

A   **B**   **C**

Figure 21-26. Circumducted gait. *(A)* The leg is in the normal position at the end of stance phase. *(B)* The leg then swings out and around during swing phase, *(C)* returning to the normal position for the beginning of stance phase.

into excessive extension during midstance because there is insufficient length of the plantar flexors to allow dorsiflexion. If the gastrocnemius does not have enough extensibility to be stretched over both the ankle and knee, something must give. Therefore, either there will be limited ankle dorsiflexion or the knee will be pulled into extreme extension. Remember that the gastrocnemius is a two-joint muscle that plantar flexes the ankle and flexes the knee. In weight-bearing, body weight may force a certain amount of dorsiflexion, thus forcing a tight gastrocnemius to pull the knee into extension. In addition, an early heel rise can occur during push-off *(terminal stance),* the knee will be lifted higher during swing phase, and the toes will land first during heel strike *(initial contact).* The latter is called a "steppage gait."

An **ankle fusion** is commonly called a triple arthrodesis because of fusion of the subtalar joint and the two articulations making up the transtarsal joint. This will result in loss of ankle pronation and supination. Plantar flexion and dorsiflexion will remain but will be limited. Usually, there is a shortened stride length. The person will have more difficulty walking on uneven ground because the ability to pronate and supinate the foot has been lost.

Neurological Involvement

As would be expected, the amount of gait disturbance will depend on the amount and severity of neurological involvement. For example, spasticity of the hip flexors affects moving the leg forward in mid- and terminal stance. Hamstring spasticity can keep the knee in a flexed position, which can interfere with moving the leg forward during stance, and limit the effectiveness of straightening the leg at the end of swing. Spasticity of the triceps surae can keep the ankle plantar flexed creating problems during both stance and swing phase. Spasticity tends to put the foot in a varus position, and flaccidity tends to put the foot in a valgus position.

A **hemiplegic gait** will vary depending on the severity of neurological involvement and the presence and amount of spasticity. Generally speaking, with spasticity, there is an extension synergy in the involved lower extremity. The hip goes into extension, adduction, and medial rotation. The knee is in extension, though often unstable. The ankle demonstrates a drop foot with ankle plantar flexion and inversion (equinovarus), which is present during both stance and swing phases. The involved upper extremity may typically be in a flexion synergy (Fig. 21-27). Usually, there will be no reciprocal arm swing. Step length tends to be lengthened on the involved side and shortened on the uninvolved side.

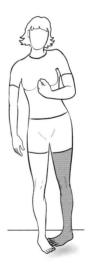

Figure 21-27. Hemiplegic gait.

Cerebellar involvement often results in an **ataxic gait.** Lacking coordination leads to jerky uneven movements. Balance tends to be poor, and the person walks with a wide base of support (abducted gait). The person usually has difficulty walking in a straight line, and tends to stagger. Reciprocal arm motion also appears to be jerky, and uneven. All movements appear exaggerated.

A **parkinsonian gait** demonstrates diminished movement. The posture of the lower extremities and trunk tends to be flexed. The elbows are partially flexed and there is little, or no, reciprocal arm swing. Stride length is greatly diminished and the forward heel does not swing beyond the rear foot. The person walks with a shuffling gait with the feet flat and weight mostly forward on the toes (Fig. 21-28). The person has difficulty initiating movements. This shuffling gait tends to start slowly and increase in speed, and the person

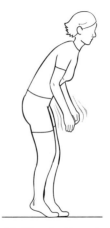

Figure 21-28. Parkinsonian gait.

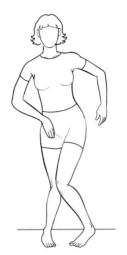

Figure 21-29. Scissors gait.

often has difficulty in stopping. It gives the appearance that the person's feet are trying to catch up to the forward leaning trunk. This is called a **festinating gait.**

Spasticity in the hip adductors results in a **scissors gait.** This gait is most evident during the swing phase in which the unsupported leg swings against or across the stance leg. Needless to say, the walking base is narrowed. The trunk may lean over the stance leg as the swing phase leg attempts to swing past it (Fig. 21-29).

A **crouch gait** describes the bilateral lower extremity involvement seen in spastic diplegia associated with cerebral palsy. There is often great variation in the gait from what is considered "typical." There is excessive flexion, adduction, and medial rotation at the hips, and flexion at the knees. The ankles are plantar flexed. The pelvis maintains an anterior pelvic tilt and there is an increased lumbar lordosis. To compensate, the reciprocal arm swing and horizontal displacement are exaggerated.

Pain

When a person has pain in any of the joints of the lower extremity, the tendency is to shorten the stance phase. In other words, if it hurts to stand on it, do not stand on it. A shortened, often abducted, stance phase on the involved side results in a rapid and shortened step length of the uninvolved side. Compensation in the reciprocal arm swing also is evident. Reciprocal arm swinging is shortened as the step length is shortened, exaggerated, and often abducted. This gait is often referred to as **antalgic gait.** If the pain is caused by a hip problem, the person will lean over that hip during weight-bearing. This will decrease the torque

placed on the joint and the amount of pressure placed on the femoral head. Magee (1997) stated that the amount of pressure will be decreased from more than twice the body weight to approximately that of the person's body weight.

Unequal Leg Length

We all have legs of unequal length, usually a discrepancy of approximately $1/4$ inch between the right and left legs. Clinically, these smaller discrepancies are often corrected by inserting heel lifts of various thicknesses into the shoe. When there is **minimal leg length discrepancy,** compensation occurs by dropping the pelvis on the affected side. Although this may not look abnormal, it does place added stress on the low back. The person may compensate by leaning over the shorter leg. Leg length discrepancies of up to 3 inches can be accommodated with these techniques.

When there is **moderate discrepancy,** approximately between 3 and 5 inches, dropping the pelvis on the affected side will no longer be effective. A longer leg is needed, so the person usually walks on the ball of the foot on the involved (shorter) side. This is called an **equinnus gait.**

A **severe leg length discrepancy** is usually any discrepancy of more than 5 inches. The person may compensate in a variety of ways. Dropping the pelvis and walking in an equinnus gait plus flexing the knee on the uninvolved side is often used. To gain an appreciation for how this may feel or look, walk down the street with one leg in the street and the other on the sidewalk.

Points to Remember

- Stance and swing are the two phases of the gait cycle.
- Using traditional terminology, there are five periods in stance phase: heel strike, foot flat, midstance, heel-off, and toe-off.
- In swing phase, there is acceleration, midswing, and deceleration.
- Using RLA terminology, stance phase also has five periods: initial contact, loading response, midstance, terminal stance, and preswing.
- RLA terms for the swing phase periods are initial swing, midswing, and terminal swing.
- Additional determinants of gait are vertical and horizontal displacement, walking base width, lateral pelvic tilt, equal step length, and opposite and equal arm swing.

Review Questions

General Anatomy Questions

1. Compare and contrast walking and running.

2. What are the main differences between the traditional terminology and terminology developed by Rancho Los Amigos?

3. What is the phase used for the period that occurs between heel strike and toe-off?

4. What is the time period called when both feet are in contact with the ground?
   a. What part of stance phase is each foot in during this period?

5. At what period of stance phase is a person's overall vertical height the greatest?

6. During which phase is the person's foot not in contact with the ground?

7. What will happen to the step length and cadence when a person increases their walking speed?

8. If unsteady, how does a person tend to adjust their walking?

9. If "foot drop," is present, which parts of the swing and stance phases of the person's gait will be altered?

10. If a person has an unrepaired ruptured Achilles tendon, which phase of the gait will be altered?

Functional Activity Questions

Identify the parts of gait that will change during the following:

1. Walking across the ice

2. Walking on a 4-inch wide beam

3. Walking down a railroad track with one foot on each side of the track (no train is coming!)

4. Walking in soft, dry sand (similar to running hard uphill)

5. Walking by taking long steps

6. Walking with a long leg brace

Clinical Exercise Questions

1. Stand upright as though you had bilateral knee flexion contractures of approximately 45 degrees. Identify how positions of other joints must change to maintain an upright posture.
   a. Ankle—
   b. Hip—
   c. Pelvis—
   d. Lumbar spine—

2. Identify the type of muscle contraction and muscle group involved during the following phases of walking:
   a. At the knee going into heel strike
      Type of contraction _____
      Muscle group involved _____
   b. At the ankle during foot flat
      Type of contraction _____
      Muscle group involved _____
   c. At the hip as the leg is moving into midstance
      Type of contraction _____
      Muscle group involved _____
   d. At the hip (in the frontal plane) during toe-off
      Type of contraction _____
      Muscle group involved _____
   e. At the knee during deceleration
      Type of contraction _____
      Muscle group involved _____

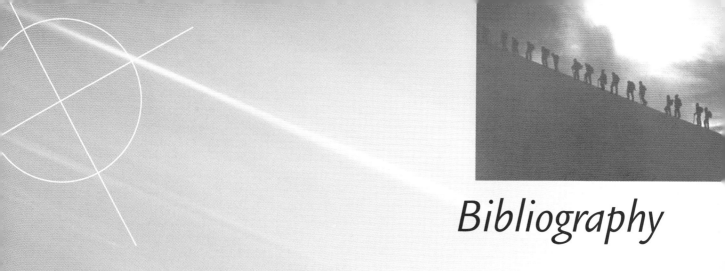

Bibliography

Anderson, MK: Fundamentals of Sports Injury Management, ed 1. Lippincott Williams & Wilkins, Philadelphia, 2002.

Anderson, MK and Hall, SJ: Fundamentals of Sports Injury Management, ed 2. Lippincott Williams & Wilkins, Philadelphia, 1997.

Anderson, MK, Hall, SJ, and Martin, M: Sports Injury Management, ed 2. Lippincott Williams & Wilkins, Philadelphia, 2002.

Basmajian, J and Blonecker, CE: Grant's Method of Anatomy, ed l. Williams & Wilkins, Baltimore, 1989.

Basmajian, J and DeLuca, C: Muscles Alive: Their Functions Revealed by Electromyography, ed 5. Williams & Wilkins, Baltimore, 1985.

Bertoti, DB: Functional Neurorehabilitation Through the Life Span, ed 1. FA Davis, Philadelphia, 2004.

Cailliet, R: Hand Pain and Impairment, ed 3. FA Davis, Philadelphia, 1982.

Cailliet, R: Hand Pain and Impairment, ed 4. FA Davis, Philadelphia, 1994.

Cailliet, R: Knee Pain and Disability, ed 3. FA Davis, Philadelphia, 1992.

Cailliet, R: Low Back Pain Syndrome, ed 4. FA Davis, Philadelphia, 1988.

Cailliet, R: Neck and Arm Pain, ed 3. FA Davis, Philadelphia, 1991.

Cailliet, R: Shoulder Pain, ed 3. FA Davis, Philadelphia, 1991.

Cailliet, R: Soft Tissue Pain and Disability, ed 3. FA Davis, Philadelphia, 1996.

Calais-Germain, B: Anatomy of Movement, ed 1. Eastland Press, Seattle, 1993.

Carlin, E: Human Anatomy and Biomechanics: Tapes 1–10 [Audio tape]. Audio-Learning, Norristown, PA, 1975.

Cooper, J and Glassow, R: Kinesiology, ed 3. CV Mosby, St. Louis, 1972.

Curtis, BA: Neurosciences: The Basics, ed 1. Lea & Febiger, Malvern, PA, 1990.

Cyriax, J and Cyriax, P: Illustrated Manual of Orthopaedic Medicine, ed 1. Butterworth-Heinemann, London, 1983.

Daniels, L and Worthingham, C: Muscle Testing: Techniques of Manual Examination, ed 5. WB Saunders, Philadelphia, 1986.

DesJardins, T: Cardiopulmonary Anatomy and Physiology, ed 4. Thomson Delmar Learning, Clifton Park, NY, 2002.

Donatelli, RA: The Biomechanics of the Foot and Ankle, ed 2. FA Davis, Philadelphia, 1996.

Ellis, H: Clinical Anatomy: A Revision and Applied Anatomy for Clinical Students, ed 10. Blackwell, Malden, MA, 2002.

Evjenth, O and Hamberg, J: Muscle Stretching in Manual Therapy: A Clinical Manual, vol. 1: The Extremities, ed 1. Alfta, Sweden, Chattanooga, 1984.

Gilman, S and Newman, SW: Essentials of Clinical Neuroanatomy and Neurophysiology, ed 10. FA Davis, Philadelphia, 2003.

Goldberg, S: Clinical Anatomy Made Ridiculously Simple, ed 1. MedMaster, Miami, FL, 1990.

Goss, CM (ed): Gray's Anatomy of the Human Body, American, ed 29. Lea & Febiger, Philadelphia, 1973.

Gould, J and Davies, G (eds): Orthopaedic and Sports Physical Therapy, ed 2. CV Mosby, St. Louis, 1985.

Hall, SJ: Basic Biomechanics, ed 3. McGraw-Hill, Boston, 1999.

Hamill, J and Knutzen, KM: Biomechanical Basis of Human Movement, ed 2. Lippincott Williams & Wilkins, Philadelphia, 2003.

Hay, J: Biomechanics of Sports Techniques, ed 1. Prentice-Hall, Englewood Cliffs, NJ, 1973.

Hinson, M: Kinesiology, ed 2. WC Brown, Dubuque, Iowa, 1981.

Hole, Jr. JW: Human Anatomy and Physiology, ed 5. WC Brown, Dubuque, Iowa, 1990.

Hoppenfeld, S: Physical Examination of the Spine and Extremities, ed 1. Appleton-Century-Crofts, New York, 1976.

Jacob, S and Francone, C: Elements of Anatomy and Physiology, ed 3. WB Saunders, Philadelphia, 1989.

Jenkins, DB: Hollinshead's Functional Anatomy of the Limbs and Back, ed 7. WB Saunders, Philadelphia, 1998.

Jenkins, DB: Hollinshead's Functional Anatomy of the Limbs and Back, ed 8. WB Saunders, Philadelphia, 2002.

Jones K and Barker, K: Human Movement Explained, ed 1. Butterworth-Heinemann, Oxford, 1996.

Kapandji, I: Physiology of the Joints: Upper Limbs, vol. 1, ed 2. Livingstone, Edinburgh, 1970.

Kessler, R and Hertling, D: Management of Common Musculoskeletal Disorders: Physical Therapy Principles and Methods, ed 1. Harper & Row, Philadelphia, 1983.

Kendall, FP and McCreary, EK: Muscles: Testing and Function, ed 3. Williams & Wilkins, 1983.

King, B and Showers, M: Human Anatomy and Physiology, ed 6. WB Saunders, Philadelphia, 1969.

Kingston, B: Understanding Joints: A Practical Guide to Their Structure and Function, ed 1. Stanley Thornes Ltd, Cheltenham, UK, 2000.

Kisner, C and Colby, LA: Therapeutic Exercise: Foundations and Techniques, ed 4. FA Davis, Philadelphia, 2002.

Lamport, NK, Coffey, MS, and Hersch, GI: Activity Analysis and Application, ed 4. Slack Inc, Thorofare, NJ, 2001.

Landau, BR: Essential Human Anatomy and Physiology, ed 2. Scott, Foresman, Glenview, IL, 1980.

Leeson, C and Leeson, T: Human Structure: A Companion to Anatomical Studies, ed 1. WB Saunders, Philadelphia, 1972.

Lehmkuhl, LD and Smith, LK: Brunnestrom's Clinical Kinesiology, ed 4. FA Davis, Philadelphia, 1983.

Lesh, SG: Clinical Orthopedics for the Physical Therapist Assistant, ed 1. FA Davis, Philadelphia, 2000.

Levangie, PK and Norkin, CC: Joint Structure and Function, ed 3. FA Davis, Philadelphia, 2001.

Levangie, PK and Norkin, CC: Joint Structure and Function, ed 4. FA Davis, Philadelphia, 2005.

Low, J and Reed A: Basic Biomechanics Explained, ed 1. Butterworth-Heinemann, Oxford, 1996.

MacConaill, M and Basmajian, J: Muscles and Movements: A Basis for Human Kinesiology, ed 1. Williams & Wilkins, Baltimore, 1969.

MacLeod, D, Jacobs, P, and Larson, N: The Ergonomics Manual, ed 1. The Saunders Group, Minneapolis, 1990.

Magee, D: Orthopedic Physical Assessment, ed 1. WB Saunders, Philadelphia, 1987.

Magee, KR and Saper, JR: Clinical and Basic Neurology for Health Professionals, ed 1. Year Book Medical, Chicago, 1981.

Manter, JT and Gatz, AJ: Essentials of Clinical Neuroanatomy and Neurophysiology, ed 8. FA Davis, Philadelphia, 1993.

McGinnis, Peter M: Biomechanics of Sport and Exercise, ed 1. Human Kinetics, Champaign, IL, 1999.

McKinnis, LN: Fundamentals of Musculoskeletal Imaging, ed 2. FA Davis, Philadelphia, 2005.

Melloni, J, et al: Melloni's Illustrated Review of Human Anatomy, ed 1. JB Lippincott, Philadelphia, 1988.

Miller, B and Keane, C: Encyclopedia and Dictionary of Medicine, Nursing, and Allied Health, ed 4. WB Saunders, Philadelphia, 1989.

Minor, MA, and Lippert, LS: Kinesiology Laboratory Manual for Physical Therapist Assistants, ed 1. FA Davis, Philadelphia, 1998.

Minor, M and Minor, S: Patient Evaluation Methods for the Health Professional, ed 1. Reston Publishing, Reston, VA, 1985.

Moore, K: Clinically Oriented Anatomy, ed 2. Williams & Wilkins, Baltimore, 1985.

Moore, K: Clinically Oriented Anatomy, ed 3. Williams & Wilkins, Baltimore, 1992.

Moore, K: Clinically Oriented Anatomy, ed 4. Williams & Wilkins, Baltimore, 2004.

Moore, K and Agur, A: Essential Clinical Anatomy, ed 2. Lippincott Williams & Wilkins, Philadelphia, 2002.

Netter, FH: Ciba Collection of Medical Illustrations: Musculoskeletal System: Part I, Anatomy, Physiology, and Metabolic Diseases, vol. 8: ed 1. Ciba-Geigy, Summit, NJ, 1987.

Netter, FH: Ciba Collection of Medical Illustrations: Nervous System, Part I, Anatomy and Physiology, ed 1. Ciba Pharmaceutical, West Caldwell, NJ, 1983.

Neumann, DA: Kinesiology of the Musculoskeletal System: Foundations for Physical Rehabilitation, ed 1. Mosby, St. Louis, 2002.

Nordin, M and Frankel, VH: Basic Biomechanics of the Musculoskeletal System, ed 3. Lippincott Williams & Wilkins, Baltimore, 2001.

Norkin, C and Levangie, P: Joint Structure and Function: A Comprehensive Analysis, ed 1. FA Davis, Philadelphia, 1983.

Norkin, C and Levangie, P: Joint Structure and Function: A Comprehensive Analysis, ed 2. FA Davis, Philadelphia, 1992.

Norkin, C and White, D: Measurement of Joint Motion: A Guide of Goniometry, ed 1. FA Davis, Philadelphia, 1985.

Oatis, CA: Kinesiology: The Mechanics and Pathomechanics of Human Movement, ed 1. Lippincott Williams & Wilkins, Philadelphia, 2004.

Oliver, J: Back Care: An Illustrated Guide. Butterworth–Heinemann, Oxford. 1994.

Olson, TR: ADAM: Student Atlas of Anatomy, ed 1. Williams & Wilkins, Baltimore, 1996.

Palastanga, N, Field, D, and Soames, R: Anatomy and Human Movement: Structure and Function, ed 2. Butterworth–Heinemann, Oxford, 1994.

Palmer, M and Epler, M: Clinical Assessment Procedures in Physical Therapy, ed 1. JB Lippincott, Philadelphia, 1990.

Palmer, M and Epler, M: Clinical Assessment Procedures in Physical Therapy, ed 2. JB Lippincott, Philadelphia, 1998.

Paris, SV and Patla, C: E-1 Course Notes: Introduction to Extremity Dysfunction and Manipulation. Institute Press, 1986.

Pedretti, LW: Occupational Therapy: Practice Skills for Physical Dysfunction, ed 4. CV Mosby, St. Louis, 1996.

Pedretti, LW and Early, MB: Occupational Therapy: Practice Skills for Physical Dysfunction, ed 5. CV Mosby, St. Louis, 2001.

Perry J: Gait Analysis: Normal and Pathological Function, ed 1. Slack Inc, Thorofare, NJ, 1992.

Perry JF, Rohe, DA, and Garcia, AO: The Kinesiology Workbook, ed 2. FA Davis, Philadelphia, 1996.

Pratt, NE: Clinical Musculoskeletal Anatomy, ed 1. JB Lippincott, Philadelphia, 1991.

Rasch, P: Kinesiology and Applied Anatomy, ed 7. Lea & Febiger, Philadelphia, 1989.

Richardson, JK and Iglarsh, ZA: Clinical Orthopaedic Physical Therapy, ed 1. WB Saunders, 1994.

Romanes, G (ed): Cunningham's Textbook of Anatomy, ed 10. Oxford University Press, New York, 1964.

Rothstein, JM, Roy, SH, and Wolf, SL: The Rehabilitation Specialist's Handbook, ed 1. FA Davis, Philadelphia, 1991.

Rothstein, JM, Roy, SH, and Wolf, SL: The Rehabilitation Specialist's Handbook, ed 2. FA Davis, Philadelphia, 1998.

Rothstein, JM, Roy, SH, and Wolf, SL: The Rehabilitation Specialist's Handbook, ed 3. FA Davis, Philadelphia, 2005.

Roy, S and Irvin, R: Sports Medicine: Prevention, Evaluation, Management, and Rehabilitation, ed 1. Prentice-Hall, Englewood Cliffs, NJ, 1983.

Rybski, M: Kinesiology for Occupational Therapy, ed 1, Slack Inc, Thorofare, NJ, 2004.

Scanlon, VC and Sanders, T: Essentials of Anatomy and Physiology, ed 3. FA Davis, Philadelphia, 1999.

Scanlon, VC and Sanders, T: Essentials of Anatomy and Physiology, ed 4. FA Davis, Philadelphia, 2003.

Shumway-Cook, A and Woollacott, M: Motor Control: Theory and Practical Applications, ed 1. Williams & Wilkins, Baltimore, 1995.

Sieg, K and Adams, S: Illustrated Essentials of Musculoskeletal Anatomy, ed 2. Megabooks, Gainesville, FL, 1985.

Smith, LK, Weiss, EL, and Lehmkuhl, LD: Brunnstrom's Clinical Kinesiology, ed 5. FA Davis, Philadelphia, 1996.

Soderberg, G: Kinesiology: Application of Pathological Motion, ed 1. Williams & Wilkins, Baltimore, 1986.

Somers, MF: Spinal Cord Injury–Functional Rehabilitation, ed 1. Appleton & Lange, Norwalk, CT, 1992.

Stanley, BG and Tribuzi, SM: Concepts in Hand Rehabilitation, ed 1, FA Davis, Philadelphia, 1992.

Starkey, C and Ryan, J: Evaluation of Orthopedic and Athletic Injuries, ed 2. FA Davis, Philadelphia, 2002.

Steindler, A: Kinesiology of the Human Body: Under Normal and Pathological Conditions, ed 1. Charles C Thomas, Springfield, IL, 1955.

Thibodeau, G: Anatomy and Physiology, ed 1. Times Mirror/Mosby College Publishing, St. Louis, 1986.

Tomberlin, JP and Saunders, HD: Evaluation, Treatment and Prevention of Musculoskeletal Disorders, vol 2: Extremities, ed 3. The Saunders Group, Minneapolis, 1994.

Tortora, G: Principles of Human Anatomy, ed 5. Canfield Press, San Francisco, 1990.

Tortora, G and Anagnostakos, N: Principles of Anatomy and Physiology, ed 3. Harper & Row, New York, 1981.

Tovin, BJ and Greenfield, BH: Evaluation and Treatment of the Shoulder: An Integration of The Guide to Physical Therapist Practice, ed 1, FA Davis, Philadelphia, 2001.

Tyldesley, B and Grieve, JI: Muscles, Nerves and Movement: Kinesiology in Daily Living, ed 1. Blackwell Scientific, Oxford, 1989.

Venes, D: Taber's Cyclopedic Medical Dictionary, ed 20, FA Davis, Philadelphia, 2005.

Vidic, B and Suarez, F: Photographic Atlas of the Human Body, ed 1. CV Mosby, St. Louis, 1984.

Warwick, R and Williams, P (eds): Gray's Anatomy, British ed 35. WB Saunders, Philadelphia, 1973.

Wells, K and Luttgens, K: Kinesiology: Scientific Basis of Human Motion, ed 7. WB Saunders, Philadelphia, 1982.

Whittle, MW: Gait Analysis: An Introduction, ed 4. Butterworth–Heinemann, Oxford, UK, 1996.

Williams, M and Lissner, H: Biomechanics of Human Motion, ed 1. WB Saunders, Philadelphia, 1962.

Yokochi, C: Photographic Anatomy of the Human Body, ed 1. University Park Press, Baltimore, 1971.

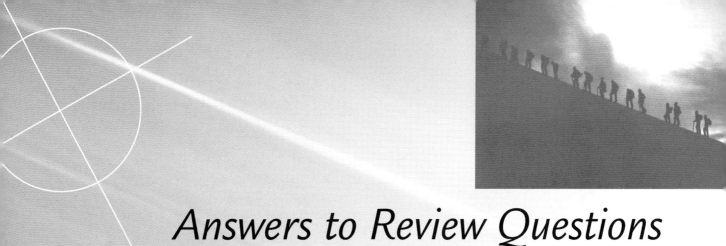

Answers to Review Questions

Chapter 1 • Basic Information

1. a. Anterior.
   b. Posterior.
   c. Inferior.
   d. Proximal.
   e. Lateral.

2. The football is demonstrating curvilinear motion, while the kicker's leg is demonstrating angular motion.

3. Neck hyperextension.

4. Shoulder medial rotation.

5. Trunk lateral bending.

6. Hip lateral rotation.

7. Anatomical position and fundamental position are the same except for the forearms, which are supinated in anatomical position and in neutral position (between supination and pronation) in the fundamental position.

8. Dorsal surface of dog, posterior surface of person.

Chapter 2 • Skeletal System

1. The axial skeleton contains no long or short bones, whereas the appendicular skeleton contains no irregular bones. The bones of the axial skeleton are particularly important in providing support and protection; the appendicular skeleton provides the framework for movement.

2. Compact bone is found in the diaphysis of long bones, and cancellous bone is found in the metaphysis and epiphysis. In other types of bone, can-

cellous bone is found sandwiched between layers of compact bone.

3. Compact bone is heavier than cancellous bone because it is less porous.

4. Most height growth is a result of growth in the epiphysis of long bones.

5. Sesamoid bones protect tendons from excess wear. The patella has the additional function of increasing the angle of pull of the quadriceps muscle.

6. a. Foramen, fossa, groove, meatus, sinus.
   b. Condyle, eminence, facet, head.
   c. Crest, epicondyle, line, spine, trochanter, tubercle, tuberosity.

7. *Bicipital groove:* Ditchlike depression.

8. *Humeral head:* Rounded articular projection that fits into a joint.

9. *Acetabulum:* Deep depression.

10. *Scapular spine:* Long thin projection to which tendons attach.

11. *Supraspinous fossa:* Depression or hollow.

Chapter 3 • Articular System

1. A joint that allows no motion is referred to as a fibrous joint. The three types of fibrous joints are synarthrosis, syndesmosis, and gomphosis.

2. A joint that allows a great deal of motion is called a synovial joint or diarthrosis.

3. Diarthrodial joints can be described by:
   a. the number of axes.
   b. the shape of the joint.
   c. the joint motion involved.

4. Tendon.

5. Bursa.

6. Hyaline cartilage is located on the bone ends of synovial joints and provides a smooth articulating surface. Fibrocartilage is thicker and is located between bones. Fibrocartilage provides shock absorption and spacing. Examples of fibrocartilage are the menisci of the knee and the disks of the vertebrae.

7. The joint motion involved is elbow flexion; it occurs in the sagittal plane around the frontal axis.

8. The joint involved is forearm pronation; it occurs in the transverse plane around the vertical axis.

9. The joint motion involved is finger (MP) adduction; it occurs in the frontal plane around the sagittal axis.

10. Shoulder = 3, elbow = 1, radioulnar = 1, wrist = 2, MCP = 2, PIP = 1, dip = 1.

Chapter 4 • Arthrokinematics

1. a. Osteokinematic.
   b. Arthrokinematic.

2. Soft tissue approximation.

3. a. Humerus is moving on scapula.
   b. Humerus is convex.
   c. Scapula is concave.
   d. Convex surface is moving on concave surface.
   e. Opposite direction.

4. a. Compression or approximation.
   b. Shear.
   c. Traction or distraction.

5. Close-packed position of TMJ is when teeth are clenched.

6. a. Convex.
   b. Concave.
   c. Concave.
   d. Convex.
   e. Sellar.

7. Roll.

8. Glide or slide.

9. a. Yes.
   b. Glide.

10. Spin.

Chapter 5 • Muscular System

1. a. Insertion.
   b. Origin.

2. Reversal of muscle action.

3. a. Agonists in wrist flexion.
   b. Antagonists in ulnar/radial deviation.

4. a. Gluteus maximus and hamstrings.
   b. Hip lateral rotation.
   c. Gluteus minimus.

5. Active insufficiency.

6. Eccentric.

7. a. Shoulder abduction.
   b. Concentric.
   c. Isometric.

8. a. Shoulder flexion.
   b. Concentric.
   c. Shoulder flexors during first 90 degrees.
   d. Eccentric.
   e. Shoulder extensors during second 90 degrees.

9. a. Wheelchair push-ups: Closed-chain activity.
   b. Exercises with weight cuffs: Open-chain activity.
   c. Overhead wall pulleys: Open-chain activity.

Chapter 6 • The Nervous System

1. L2.

2. Gray matter is unmyelinated tissue, and white matter is myelinated tissue.

3. The brain is protected from trauma by (1) the bony outer layer called the *skull;* (2) three layers of membrane called the *meninges;* and (3) shock absorption provided by cerebrospinal fluid.

4. The circle of Willis is a set of interconnecting arteries at the base of the brain. It is the source of the arteries that supply the brain. The interconnection of the arteries means that interruption of flow in one artery will not seriously decrease blood supply to all the regions of the brain.

5. Motor neurons that synapse above the level of the spinal cord's anterior horn are upper motor neurons. Those synapsing at the anterior horn or peripherally are lower motor neurons. Pathological conditions occurring to either upper or lower motor neurons have quite different clinical signs.

6. Thoracic nerves directly innervate the muscles near where they arise from the spinal cord. Cervical or lumbar nerves branch and/or divide, forming a plexus and innervate muscle quite distal from the level of the cord from which they originate.

7. Afferent nerve fibers transmit sensory impulses from the periphery toward the brain. Efferent fibers transmit motor impulses from the brain or spinal cord toward the periphery.

8. The involved nerve is the median nerve. The condition is referred to as *ape hand.*

9. The involved nerve is the peroneal nerve. The condition is referred to as *foot drop.*

10. The muscle group involved with claw hand is the intrinsics, which is mostly innervated by the ulnar nerve.

Chapter 7 • Basic Biomechanics

1. a. The wrist, because there is a longer resistance arm when the weight is around the wrist than when it is around the elbow.

2. b. The shorter person who is not on stilts, has a lower COG.

3. a.

b.

4. a. Scalar = 5 miles (magnitude only).
   b. Vector = 30 feet to the north (magnitude and direction).

5. More force is required when the hand truck is more horizontal. The force arm remains constant, while changing the angle of the hand truck lengthens or shortens the resistance arm. Lowering the load (angle becomes more horizontal) in effect lengthens the resistance arm and requires the person to exert more force. Raising the load (angle becomes more vertical) shortens the resistance arm and allows the person to use less force to move the hand truck.

6. This demonstrates the concept of the wheel and axle. The smaller push rim will require more force, but the distance the wheelchair will travel with a single push is greater.

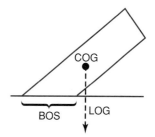

7. No, the object will fall because the LOG is outside the BOS.

8. The BOS of a wheelchair during a "wheelie" is very narrow. To maintain balance, the person must keep the body's COG within that BOS. However, the BOS is very wide when the wheelchair is resting on all four wheels and it is easy to keep the body's COG within it.

9. Linear force.

10. People need to get as close to the bed as possible as it shortens their lever arms; they need to move their legs apart, especially in the A/P direction as it increases their BOS; they need to bend their knees slightly as it lowers their COG.

Chapter 8 • Shoulder Girdle

General Anatomy Questions

1. The shoulder girdle includes the articulations between the scapula and clavicle. The shoulder joint includes the scapula and humerus. The shoulder complex includes the scapula, clavicle, humerus, sternum, and rib cage.

2. a. Use the inferior angle as a point of reference.
   b. When it moves away from the vertebral column, the motion is scapular upward rotation. When it moves toward the vertebral column, the motion is scapular downward rotation.

3. Elevation/depression and protraction/retraction are more linear.

4. Upward and downward rotation are more angular.

5. Scapulohumeral rhythm is the movement relationship between the shoulder girdle and shoulder joint. After the first 30 degrees, for every 2 degrees of shoulder joint flexion or abduction, the shoulder girdle rotates upwardly 1 degree.

6. Without this shoulder girdle movement, one cannot normally and completely raise the arm above the head.

7. a. Because the three different attachments of the trapezius muscle produce three different lines of pull, the three parts have different muscle actions.
   b. The rhomboid muscles, however, have the same line of pull and thus the same muscle action. There is no functional difference between the rhomboid muscles.

8. The serratus anterior plus the upper and lower trapezius muscles.

9. *Force couple:* a situation in which two or more muscles pull in different, often opposite, directions to accomplish the same motion.

10. The rhomboid muscles, the lower and middle trapezius muscles, the levator scapula muscle, and the upper trapezius muscle.

Functional Activity Questions

1. Downward rotation.
2. Upward rotation.
3. Elevation.
4. Upward rotation and retraction.
5. Protraction.

Clinical Exercise Questions

1. a. Scapular retraction.
   b. Middle trapezius, rhomboids.
   c. Open.

2. a. Scapular retraction.
   b. Sorratus anterior, pectoralis minor.

3. a. Scapular depression. Technically, there is a small amount of upward rotation due to the shoulder flexion from a hyperextended to extended position. This would result in some upward rotation of the scapula.
   b. Lower trapezius, pectoralis minor, upper trapezius, serratus anterior.

4. a. Scapular protraction and upward rotation.
   b. Serratus anterior, pectoralis minor, upper and lower trapezius.

5. a. Scapular retraction and downward rotation.
   b. Middle trapezius, rhomboids, levator scapula, pectoralis minor.

Chapter 9 • Shoulder Joint

General Anatomy Questions

1. a. In the frontal plane around the sagittal axis: Shoulder abduction/adduction.
   b. In the transverse plane around the vertical axis: Shoulder medial/lateral rotation, horizontal abduction/adduction.
   c. In the saggital plane around the frontal axis: Shoulder flexion/extension.

2. The circular arc of the upper extremity formed by a combination of the shoulder motions—flexion, abduction, extension, and adduction.

3. Subscapular fossa.

4. The supraspinous and infraspinous fossas.

5. With the humerus in the vertical position, the bicipital groove facing anteriorly, and head facing medially, the right humeral head faces toward the left.

6. The supraspinatus, infraspinatus, teres minor, and subscapularis muscles. They hold the head of the humerus in toward the glenoid fossa as it moves within the socket.

7. The subscapularis and coracobrachialis muscles and the short head of the biceps brachii muscle.

8. The teres major and minor, infraspinatus, supraspinatus, and posterior deltoid muscles.

9. The anterior deltoid, pectoralis major, and latissimus dorsi muscles.

10. a. Clavicular portion.
    b. First part of range—to approximately 60 degrees.
    c. Its vertical line of pull makes it more effective in the early part of the range.

Functional Activity Questions

1. a. Shoulder hyperextension and medial rotation.
   b. Scapular tilt, and protraction.

2. a. Shoulder abduction and lateral rotation.
   b. Scapular upward rotation and retraction.

3. a. Shoulder adduction and medial rotation.
   b. Scapular downward rotation and protraction.

4. a. Shoulder flexion.
   b. Scapular upward rotation and protraction.

5. a. Shoulder adduction.
   b. Scapular downward rotation.

Clinical Exercise Questions

1. a. Shoulder horizontal abduction.
   b. Concentric contraction of shoulder horizontal abductors.
   c. Posterior deltoid, infraspinatus, teres minor.

2. Flexing the elbow shortens the resistance arm.

3. a. Shoulder hyperextension.
   b. Concentric contraction of shoulder hyperextensors.
   c. Latissimus dorsi, posterior deltoid.

4. a. Shoulder flexion.
   b. Eccentric contraction of shoulder hyperextensors.
   c. Latissimus dorsi, posterior deltoid.

5. First part:
   a. Shoulder lateral rotation.
   b. Concentric.
   c. Shoulder lateral rotators: Infraspinatus, teres minor, posterior deltoid.

   Second part:
   a. Shoulder lateral rotation.
   b. Isometric.
   c. Shoulder lateral rotators.

   Third part:
   a. Shoulder medial rotation.
   b. Eccentric.
   c. Shoulder lateral rotators.

Chapter 10 • Elbow

General Anatomy Questions

1. a. *Bones in joint:*
      Forearm: Radius, ulna.
      Elbow: Humerus, radius, ulna.
   b. *Number of axes:*
      Forearm: 1
      Elbow: 1
   c. *Shape of joint:*
      Forearm: Pivot.
      Elbow: Hinge.
   d. *Type of motion allowed:*
      Forearm: Supination/pronation.
      Elbow: Flexion/extension.

2. The trochlear notch at the superior end faces anteriorly, the radial notch at the same end faces laterally, and the styloid process at the inferior end is on the medial side.

3. a. Lateral, or radial, collateral ligament.
   b. Medial, or ulnar, collateral ligament.
   c. Annular ligament.

4. The biceps and triceps muscles.

5. Radius, because it is the radius moving around the ulna that produces these motions.

6. The pronator quadratus and biceps muscles.

7. The biceps (to radius) and triceps (to ulna) muscles.

8. Anconeus, triceps, and brachialis muscles.

9. Long head of triceps.

10. a. Shoulder flexion, elbow flexion, forearm supination.
    b. Shoulder hyperextension, elbow extension, forearm pronation.

Functional Activity Questions

1. a. Elbow motion: Extension.
   b. Forearm motion: Supination.

2. a. Elbow motion: Flexion.
   b. Forearm motion: Supination.

3. a. Elbow motion: Extension.
   b. Forearm motion: Pronation.

4. a. Elbow motion: Flexion.
   b. Forearm motion: Supination.

5. a. Elbow motion: Extension.
   b. Forearm motion: Midposition.

Clinical Exercise Questions

1. a. Forearm supination.
   b. Pronator teres, pronator quadratus.

2. a. Elbow flexion.
   b. Triceps.

3. a. Elbow extension.
   b. Concentric.
   c. Triceps.
   d. Closed chain.

4. a. Ebow extension.
   b. Isometric.
   c. Triceps.

5. a. Elbow extension.
   b. Eccentric.
   c. Biceps, brachialis, brachioradialis.
   d. Open chain.

Chapter 11 • Wrist

General Anatomy Questions

1. Proximal row lateral to medial: Scaphoid, lunate, triquetrum, pisiform.

   Distal row lateral to medial: Trapezium, trapezoid, capitate, hamate.

2. a. Wrist flexion and extension.
   b. Wrist radial and ulnar deviation.
   c. No wrist motions occur in the transverse plane around the vertical axis.

3. a. *Number of axes:*
   Radiopcarpal joint: 2
   Intercarpal joint: 0
   b. *Shape of joint:*
   Radiocarpal joint: Condyloid
   Intercarpal joint: Plane or irregular
   c. *Joint motion allowed:*
   Radiocarpal joint: Flexion/extension, radial/ulnar deviation
   Intercarpal joint: Gliding

4. Flexor carpi ulnaris, flexor carpi radialis, palmaris longus.

5. Extensor carpi radialis longus and brevis, extension carpi ulnaris.

6. If the pisiform bone and "hook" of the hamate bone are visible, it would be the anterior side.

7. Extensor carpi radialis longus and flexor carpi radialis.

8. Extensor carpi ulnaris and flexor carpi ulnaris.

9. The palmaris longus located on the anterior surface in the middle of the wrist.

10. Flexor carpi ulnaris, palmaris longus (with flexor digitorum superficialis and profundus deep to it), flexor carpi radialis (abductor pollicis longus, extensor pollicis long and brevis, which are primarily thumb muscles but do cross the wrist), extensor carpi radialis longus and brevis (extensor digitorum, a finger extensor), and extensor carpi ulnaris.

Functional Activity Questions

1. a. Wrist position: Neutral.
   b. Wrist muscle group: Radial deviators.

2. a. Wrist position: Neutral.
   b. Wrist muscle group: Flexors.

3. a. Wrist position: Neutral/extension.
   b. Wrist muscle group: Flexors.

4. a. Wrist position: Neutral.
   b. Wrist muscle group: Extensors.

5. a. Wrist position: Neutral.
   b. Wrist muscle group: Flexors.

Clinical Exercise Questions

1. a. Wrist flexion.
   b. Concentric.
   c. Wrist flexors.

2. a. Wrist extensors
   b. Eccentric.
   c. Wrist flexors.

3. a. Wrist extension.
   b. Concentric.
   c. Wrist extensors.

4. a. Wrist flexion.
   b. Eccentric.
   c. Wrist extensors.

5. a. Wrist ulnar deviation.
   b. Concentric.
   c. Wrist ulnar deviators.

6. a. Wrist radial deviation.
   b. Eccentric.
   c. Elasticity of tubing would bring wrist back to neutral if ulnar deviators were not slowing down the motion.
   d. Wrist ulnar deviators.

Chapter 12 • Hand

General Anatomy Questions

1. a. *Finger:* MCP abduction/adduction.
   Thumb: MCP and IP flexion/extension.
   b. *Finger:* MCP, PIP, DIP flexion/extension.
   Thumb: CMP abduction/adduction.
   c. *Thumb:* Opposition/reposition.

2. Compare the thumb and fingers:
   a. Number of bones:
   Thumb: 3
   Finger: 4
   b. Number of joints:
   Thumb: 2
   Finger: 3
   c. Names of the joints:
   Thumb: MCP, IP
   Finger: MCP, PIP, DIP

3. Flexion, abduction, and rotation.

4. Rotation.

5. It holds the extrinsic tendons close to the wrist.

6. The floor of the carpal tunnel is made up of the carpal bones, and the ceiling is the transverse carpal ligament portion of the flexor retinaculum. The flexor digitorum superficialis and profundus muscles and the median nerve run through the carpal tunnel.

7. An extrinsic muscle has its proximal attachment above the wrist and its distal attachment below the wrist. The extrinsic muscles include the flexor digitorum superficialis and profundus, extensor digitorum, extensor digiti minimi, and extensor indicis muscles.

8. An intrinsic muscle has both attachments below the wrist; intrinsic muscles include the flexor and abductor pollicis brevis, opponens and adductor pollicis, flexor/abductor/opponens digiti minimi, interossei, and lumbricales.

9. Thenar muscles are intrinsic muscles on the thumb side (lateral) of the hand; hypothenar muscles are on the little finger side (medial). Any intrinsic muscle with "pollicis" in its name is a thenar muscle, whereas one with "digiti minimi" is a hypothenar muscle.

10. The indentation formed between the tendons of the abductor pollicis longus and extensor pollicis brevis laterally and extensor pollicis longus medially is referred to as the "anatomical snuffbox."

11. The lumbrical muscles; they attach proximally to the tendons of the flexor digitorum profundus muscle and distally to the tendons of the extensor digitorum muscle.

Functional Activity Questions

1. Holding the handle of a skillet: Cylindrical grip.
2. Pulling a little red wagon: Hook grip.
3. Picking up a CD: Pad-to-pad or pad-to-side prehension.
4. Fastening snaps or buttons: Tip-to-tip prehension.
5. Carrying a mug by its handle: Lateral prehension.
6. Holding a hand of cards: Lumbrical grip.
7. Holding an apple: Spherical grip.
8. Holding on to a barbell: Cylindrical grip.
9. a. Combination of cylindrical and lumbrical grip.
   b. Held in neutral position by wrist flexors and radial deviators.
   c. Flexor carpi ulnaris and radialis, extensor carpi radialis longus.

d. Elbow flexion in midposition.
e. Biceps, brachialis, especially brachioradialis.
f. Shoulder flexion and adduction.
g. Anterior deltoid, pectoralis major, teres major, and latissimus dorsi.
h. Shoulder girdle upward rotation and protraction.
i. Upper and lower trapezius, serratus anterior, pectoralis minor.

Clinical Exercise Questions

1. Joint motion: Finger MCP abduction followed by MCP adduction.

   Prime movers: Dorsal interossei, abductor digiti minimi followed by palmar interossei.

2. Joint motion: Thumb abduction.
   Prime movers: Abductor pollicis brevis and longus.

3. Joint motion: Thumb and little finger opposition.
   Prime movers: Opponens pollicis, opponens digiti minimi.

4. Joint motion: Finger MP flexion and IP extension
   Prime movers: Lumbricales.

5. Joint motion: Thumb CMC, MCP and IP flexion.
   Prime movers: Flexor pollicis longus and brevis.

Chapter 13 • Temporomandibular Joint

General Anatomy Questions

1. Zygomatic and temporal bones.
2. Synonymous terms are mandibular:
   a. Depression.
   b. Elevation.
   c. Retraction or retrusion.
   d. Protraction or protrusion.
   e. Lateral deviation.
3. Mandible and temporal bones.
4. Temporalis.
5. Masseter.
6. Diagastric.
7. Changes direction of the line of pull.
8. Fifth cranial (trigeminal) nerve.
9. Anterior rotation of the mandibular condyle on the disk.

10. The left condyle spins in the mandibular socket while the right condyle slides forward.

11. The thyroid cartilage.

Functional Activity Questions

1. Mandibular depression.

2. a. Mandibular elevation.
   b. Side opposite the bread.
   c. Same side as bread.

3. Side-to-side motion—lateral deviation.
   Anterior-posterior motion—protraction/retraction.

4. Motion: Mandibular elevation.
   Muscle: Temporalis, masseter, medial pterygoid.

Clinical Exercise Questions

1. a. Mandibular lateral deviation.
   b. Concentric.
   c. Right temporalis and masseter, left medial and lateral pterygoid.

2. a. Mandibular depression.
   b. Concentric.
   c. Lateral pterygoid.

3. a. Mandibular protraction.
   b. Isometric.
   c. Medial and lateral pterygoid.

Chapter 14 • Neck and Trunk

General Anatomy Questions

1. a. Neck and trunk lateral bending.
   b. Neck and trunk rotation.
   c. Neck and trunk flexion, extension, and hyperextension.

2. The cervical vertebra has a bifid spinous process, and there is a foramen in the transverse process. The thoracic vertebrae have a long slender, downward-pointing spinous process with rib facets on the body and transverse processes; the superior articular processes face posteriorly. The lumbar vertebra has a large spinous process pointing straight back; the superior articular processes face medially.

3. The front/back position of the superior and inferior articular processes.

4. The side-to-side position of the superior and inferior articular processes.

5. *From the occiput to C7:* Nuchal ligament.
   From C7 to the sacrum: Supraspinal ligament.

6. Ligamentum flavum.

7. Anterior and posterior longitudinal ligaments.

8. The muscle's line of pull is through or close to the center of the frontal axis of trunk flexion and extension, thus making it ineffective in this motion. To be effective in rotation, the muscle's line of pull would have to be horizontal or diagonal. The quadratus lumborum has a vertical line of pull.

9. The erector spinae.

10. A combination of trunk flexion and rotation to the right brought about by the rectus abdominis left external oblique and right internal oblique.

Functional Activity Questions

1. Neck rotation and possibly some hyperextension.

2. Neck lateral bending.

3. Neck hyperextension.

4. Neck flexion.

5. Neck hyperextension.

6. Trunk rotation to left.

7. Trunk rotation to right.

8. Trunk lateral bending.

9. Trunk flexion.

10. Trunk hyperextension.

Clinical Exercise Questions

Head and Neck:

1. a. Flexion of head on C1.
   b. Neck extension.
   c. Concentric.
   d. Isometric.
   e. Neck extensors + splenius capitis, splenius cervicis, and erector spinae.

2. a. Lateral bending of head and neck.
   b. Isometric.
   c. Right sternocleidomastoid, right splenius capitis, right splenius cervicis, right scalenes, and right erector spinae.

3. a. Neck lateral bending to the right.
   b. Left neck lateral benders.
   c. Left sternocleidomastoid, left scalenes, left splenius capitis and cervicis, and left erector spinae.

d. Right lateral benders.

e. Same as (c), except on right side.

4. Left sternocleidomastoid.

5. a. Flexion of head on C1.

b. Concentric.

c. Prevertebral muscles.

d. Neck flexion.

e. Concentric.

f. Sternocleidomastoid (bonus point if you included the longus colli of the prevertebral muscle group).

g. Isometric.

h. Sternocleidomastoid (another bonus point if you remembered the longus colli).

i. Neck extension.

j. Eccentric contraction.

k. Sternocleidomastoid and longus colli.

Trunk:

1. a. Trunk flexion—especially lumbar region.

b. Trunk extensors.

c. Erector spinae, transversospinalis, interspinales.

2. a. Trunk flexion.

b. Concentric.

c. Bilateral rectus abdominis, external and internal obliques.

3. a. Yes.

b. Flexing.

c. Origin-toward-insertion.

d. Reversal of muscle action.

e. Iliopsoas.

f. Holding down the feet makes the distal segment more stable and the proximal segment more movable. This allows the hip flexors to flex the hip (and trunk) in a reversal of muscle action.

4. a. Trunk flexion with rotation to the left.

b. Concentric.

c. Both rectus abdominis, right external oblique, and left internal oblique.

5. a. Flexion of head on C1.

b. Concentric.

c. Isometric.

d. Prevertebral muscle group.

e. Neck extension.

f. Isometric.

g. Splenius capitis and cervicis, erector spinae.

h. Trunk hyperextension.

i. Concentric.

j. Erector spinae, transversospinalis, intertransversarii.

Chapter 15 • Respiration

General Anatomy Questions

1. The sternum, ribs, and costal cartilages, and thoracic vertebrae.

2. The bodies and transverse processes of the thoracic vertebrae articulate with the tubercle and neck of the ribs.

3. Elevation and depression bringing about inspiration and expiration.

4. During inspiration the ribs elevate and the diaphragm lowers, and during expiration the ribs depress and the diaphragm muscle elevates.

5. The origin, or more stable attachment, is above the rib cage and in a position to pull the rib cage up.

6. No. While the line of pull does not change from front to back, the muscle moves 180 degrees around the rib cage giving the appearance of changing direction from front to back.

7. The origin, or more stable attachment, has a bony attachment, but the insertion attaches to a central tendon. When the muscle is relaxed, it is dome-shaped. When it contracts, the muscle flattens out, allowing more room in the thoracic cavity.

8. You talk only during expiration when air is moving out through the airway.

9. The accessory muscles of inspiration pull up on the sternum and rib cage while the accessory muscles of expiration pull down.

10. Rib cage movement is compared to bucket handle movement; thoracic cavity movement is compared to movement of a bellows.

11. The person with a C3 injury will not have an innervated diaphragm; therefore, they will need the assistance of a ventilator to breathe. A person with a C5 injury will have a neurologically intact diaphragm and can breath without mechanical assistance.

Functional Activity Questions

1. Forced inspiration followed by forced expiration.

2. Deep inspiration.

3. Forced expiration.

4. Forced expiration.

5. Quiet inspiration and expiration.

Clinical Exercise Questions

1. a. Chest breathing.
   b. Diaphragmatic breathing.

2. Anterior trunk muscles—rectus abdominis, external and internal oblique, and transverse abdominis.

3. a. Chest rose during sniffing.
   b. Muscles contracted.
   c. Sniffing requires deep inspiration. Accessory muscles of inspiration assisted by pulling up the rib cage in a reversal of muscle action. These muscles were the scalenes and sternocleidomastoid.

4. a./b. The pectoralis major is assisting in deep inspiration by pulling up on the ribs.
   c. This is a closed-chain activity.

Chapter 16 • Pelvic Girdle

General Anatomy Questions

1. a. Anterior/posterior pelvic tilt.
   b. Lateral tilt.
   c. Pelvic rotation.

2. To the left.

3. The hip joints.

4. a. Hip flexion.
   b. Hip extension.
   c. Hip abduction on the unsupported side and hip adduction on the weight-bearing side.

5. a. Right hip medial rotation/left hip lateral rotation.
   b. Right hip lateral rotation/left hip medial rotation.

6. a. Hyperextension.
   b. Flexion.
   c. Lateral bending to opposite side.

7. Back extensors, hip flexors.

Functional Activity Questions

1. Posterior pelvic tilt.

2. Anterior pelvic tilt.

3. Posterior pelvic tilt.

4. Left hip adducted and right hip abducted.

Clinical Exercise Questions

1. Motions: Posterior pelvic tilt, trunk flexion, hip extension.
   Muscles: Gluteus maximus and abdominals.

2. Motions: Left lateral pelvic tilt; left hip adduction and right hip abduction.
   Muscles: Right hip abductors (gluteus medius and minimus) and left quadratus lumborum.

Chapter 17 • Hip

General Anatomy Question

1. a. Two hip bones, the sacrum, and the coccyx.
   b. The fused bones of the ilium, ischium, and pubis.
   c. Acetabulum of the hip bone and head of the femur.
   d. The ilium, ischium, and pubis.
   e. The ischium and pubis.
   f. The ilium and ischium.

2. With the greater sciatic notch posterior and the body of pubis anterior, the acetabulum faces laterally. Therefore, if the acetabular opening is facing to the right in this position, it is a right hip bone.

3. With the femur in the vertical position, the linea aspera and lesser trochanter are posterior, and the head faces medially. Therefore, in this position the head of the right femur faces toward the left.

4. a. *Number of axes:* 3.
   b. *Shape of joint:* Ball and socket.
   c. *Type of motion allowed:* Flexion/extension, abduction/adduction, and rotation.

5. a. Medial and lateral rotation.
   b. Flexion/extension.
   c. Abduction/adduction.

6. The distal attachment of the iliofemoral ligament; because it splits into two parts, forming an upside-down Y.

7. The acetabulum forms a deep socket holding most of the femoral head, and the joint is surrounded by three very strong ligaments.

8. The line of attachment of the ligaments is a spiral. This arrangement causes the ligaments to become taut as the joint moves into extension and to slacken with flexion, thus limiting hyperextension without impeding flexion.

9. The rectus femoris, sartorius, gracilis, semitendinosus, semimembranosus, biceps femoris (longhead), and tensor fascia latae muscles.

10. The sartorius muscle is involved in hip flexion, abduction, and lateral rotation; the tensor fascia latae muscle is involved in flexion and abduction.

11. When you lift your right foot off the floor, the left hip abductors and right trunk extensors contract to keep the right side of the pelvis from dropping.

     A force couple exists when the hip abductors are pulling down while the trunk extensors are pulling up.

Functional Activity Questions

1. Hip extension and medial rotation, and maybe some adduction.

2. a. Greater hip flexion is required with a low surface.
   b. Medial rotation and adduction may accompany the increased flexion.

3. a. Adduction.
   b. Right hip adductors.

4. a. Swing phase includes hip flexion, extension, hyperextension.
   b. Greater hip flexion than walking.
   c. Hip flexion and abduction.
   d. Combination of hip hyperextension, abduction, flexion, adduction as you swing your leg over the bike, and maybe some rotation.

5. a. Posterior tilt.
   b. Anterior tilt with increased lumbar lordosis.

6. a. It maintains the pelvis in a posterior tilt.
   b. There is not sufficient length of the hip flexors to complete the range of motion.
   c. Iliopsoas.
   d. The anterior hip muscles are elongated more when the pelvis is in a posterior tilt position than when in the anterior tilt position.

7. You may compensate by standing with the lumbar spine in lordosis and the pelvis in anterior tilt, or by leaning forward in a slightly flexed hip position.

Clinical Exercise Questions

1. a. Hip hyperextension.
   b. Strengthening.
   c. Gluteus maximus.

2. a. Hip hyperextension.
   b. Stretching.
   c. Iliopsoas.

3. a. Hip abduction and flexion.
   b. Stretching.
   c. Adductors—pectineus, adductor longus, adductor brevis, adductor magnus.
      Extensors (hamstrings)—semimembranosus, semitendinosus, biceps femoris.

4. a. Hip abduction.
   b. Strengthening.
   c. Hip abductors—gluteus medius and gluteus minimus.

5. a. Combination of hip abduction and flexion.
   b. Strengthening.
   c. Tensor fascia latae.

Chapter 18 • Knee

General Anatomy Questions

1. a. *Number of axes:*
      Knee joint: 1
      Patellofemoral joint: 0
   b. *Shape of joint:*
      Knee joint: Hinge.
      Patellofemoral joint: Irregular.
   c. *Type of motion:*
      Knee joint: Flexion/extension.
      Patellofemoral joint: Gliding.

2. Knee flexion and extension occur in the sagittal plane around the frontal axis.

3. The Q angle is formed by the intersection of the line between the tibial tuberosity and middle of the patella and the line between the ASIS and the middle of the patella. The greater the angle, the higher the stress on the patellofemoral joint during knee flexion and extension.

4. Femur and tibia.

5. Because it initiates knee flexion, moving the knee out of the "locked" position of extension.

6. The distal attachments of the sartorius, gracilis, and semitendinosus muscles.

7. Weakened knee extension (quadriceps = L2–L4) and no knee flexion (hamstrings = L5–S2)

8. Closed kinetic chain.

9. No, this could only happen as a closed-chain action.

10. Yes, they both are.

Functional Activity Questions

1. a. Preparing to kick—bringing knee into flexion and hip into hyperextension.
   b. Rectus femoris is being stretched over both hip and knee.
   c. Point of ball contact—knee extension and hip extension.
   d. Rectus femoris is shortening at the knee but is still elongated at the hip.
   e. Follow-through—knee remains in extension, hip going into flexion.
   f. Rectus femoris is shortened over both joints and becoming actively insufficient.

2. a. Placing foot onto curb—knee flexion.
   b. Moving up onto curb—knee extension.

3. a. Left foot, not right foot, would lead.
   b. Hip hiking (Pelvic elevation on right side. Also called right trunk lateral bending in reversal action.)

4. a. Hamstring action: Hip extension and knee flexion.
   b. Hip position—(see Fig. 18-22A): Extension.
   c. Hip position—(see Fig. 18-22B): Partly flexed.
   d. Position of active insufficiency: Hip extension and knee flexion (of hamstrings).
   e. See Figure 18-22B: Hip partly flexed
   f. Keeping the hip in slight flexion keeps some elongation of the hamstrings while they are being shortened at the knee avoiding active insufficiency. Keeping the hip in extension has the hamstrings shortened over the hip while they are shortening over the knee. Thus, active insufficiency will be reached more quickly.

5. a. Hip position—See Figure 18-23A = partial hip flexion. See Figure 18-23B = greater hip flexion.
   b. Vasti muscle.
   c. Rectus femoris—Hip flexion and knee extension.
   d. The one-joint vasti muscles are elongated with knee flexion. Because they do not cross the hip, hip position has no effect on them. The two-joint rectus femoris is elongated in hip extension and knee flexion. Therefore, it is elongated more in position A. In position B, it is already shortened (on a slack) at the hip.
   e. If you want to strengthen the RF — use a more extended hip position (See Figure 18-23A).
   f. If you want to isolate and only strengthen the vasti muscles — use a more flexed hip position (See Figure 18-23B) where the rectus femoris is not as strong.

Clinical Exercise Questions

1. Slide down:
   a. Knee flexion.
   b. Eccentric contraction.
   c. Knee extensors (quadriceps).

   Hold position:
   a. Knee partly flexed but holding from going into more flexion.
   b. Isometric.
   c. Knee extensors (quadriceps).

   Return to standing:
   a. Knee extension.
   b. Concentric contraction.
   c. Knee extensors (quadriceps).

2. a. Hip flexion and knee extension
   b. Stretching of hamstrings, which extend hip and flex knee
   c. Hamstrings consist of semimembranosis, semitendinosis, biceps femoris

3. a. Hip flexion and knee extension
   b. Strengthening
   c. Hip flexors (rectus femoris, iliopsoas, and pectineus), and knee extensors (quadriceps group)
   d. Open chain

4. See Figure 18-25.
   Straighten knee:
   a. Knee extension.
   b. Concentric contraction.
   c. Knee extensors (quadriceps).
   d. Closed-chain activity.

   Hold position:
   a. Knee extension.
   b. Isometric contraction.
   c. Knee extensors (quadriceps).

   Bend knee:
   a. Knee flexion.
   b. Eccentric contraction.
   c. Knee extensors (quadriceps).

5. a. Hip extension and knee flexion.
   b. Stretching.
   c. Rectus femoris (which does hip flexion and knee extension).

Chapter 19 • Ankle Joint and Foot

General Anatomy Questions

1. a. 1
   b. Hinge.
   c. Dorsiflexion, plantar flexion.
   d. Tibia and talus (primarily).

2. The subtalar joint involves the talus and calcaneus; the transverse tarsal joint involves the talus and calcaneus with the navicular and cuboid bone.

3. The function of the interosseous membrane, which is located between the tibia and fibula, is to hold the two bones together and to provide a large area for muscle attachment.

4. The deltoid ligament, made up of the tibionavicular, tibiocalcaneal, and posterior tibiotalar ligaments.

5. The lateral ligament, made up of the posterior and anterior talofibular and calcaneofibular ligaments.

6. The medial and lateral longitudinal arches.

7. The longitudinal arch is made up of the calcaneus and the navicular, cuneiform, and first three metatarsal bones. The lateral longitudinal arch is made up of the calcaneus, cuboid, and fourth and fifth metatarsals.

8. The transverse arch, made up of the cuboid and three cuneiform bones.

9. Their function is to provide some shock absorption, adjusting to uneven terrain, and propelling the body forward.

10. Tibialis posterior, flexor digitorum longus, and flexor hallucis longus muscles.

11. Tibialis posterior, tibialis anterior, peroneus longus muscles.

12. Peroneus longus and peroneus brevis muscles.

13. Peroneus brevis and tertius muscles.

14. Tibialis anterior and peroneus longus muscles; together, the peroneus longus and tibialis anterior muscles are sometimes referred to as the stirrup of the foot because the peroneus longus muscle vertically descends the leg laterally before crossing the foot medially to join the tibialis anterior muscle. The tibialis anterior muscle vertically descends the leg medially to meet the peroneus longus muscle, forming a U or stirrup.

15. No, the strongest plantar flexors are the gastrocnemius and soleus, which are innervated at the S1–S2 levels. The posterior deep group is innervated at the L5–S1 level primarily.

Functional Activity Questions

1. Ankle plantar flexion
2. Ankle plantar flexion
3. Ankle dorsiflexion
4. Ankle plantar flexion
5. Ankle inversion/eversion
6. Ankle dorsiflexion
7. Ankle plantar flexion

Clinical Exercise Questions

1. Gastrocnemius:
   a. Number of joints crossed: 2 joints.
   b. Knee motion: Knee flexion.
   c. Ankle motion: Ankle plantar flexion.

   Soleus:
   a. Number of joints crossed: 1 joints.
   b. Knee motion: No knee motion.
   c. Ankle motion: Ankle plantar flexion.

2. a. Left knee: Extension
      Left ankle: Dorsiflexion.
   b. Left gastrocnemius is stretching.
   c. Left soleus is stretching
   d. Gastrocnemius
   e. The gastrocnemius is stretched more because it has to stretch over the combined range of both knee and ankle joints, while the soleus is being stretched over only one joint.

3. a. Left knee: Flexion.
      Left ankle: Dorsiflexion.
   b. The left gastrocnemius is slack at the knee.
   c. The left gastrocnemius is stretched at the ankle.
   d. The left soleus is not stretched at the knee because it doesn't cross the knee.
   e. Yes, the left soleus is stretched at the ankle.
   f. Soleus.
   g. The soleus is stretched more because there is more ankle ROM. With the gastrocnemius slack over the knee, more ankle motion is possible, which stretches the soleus more.

4. a. Left knee: Extension.
      Left ankle: Dorsiflexion.
   b. The left gastrocnemius is elongating.

c. Left gastrocnemius is shortening.
d. The left soleus is not acting over the knee.
e. The left soleus is shortening over the ankle.
f. The two-joint gastrocnemius is able to elongate over the knee while shortening over the ankle, thus keeping more tension in the muscle through a greater range. The one-joint soleus is shortening over the ankle and will lose tension quickly.

5. a. Inversion.
   b. Isometric.
   c. Tibialis anterior and tibialis posterior.

Chapter 20 • Posture

General Anatomy Questions

1. Cervical extensors.
2. The side view.
3. Hip flexors.
4. The side.
5. Level and not elevated or depressed.
6. From the front or back.
7. Slightly in front of the lateral malleolus.
8. a. Knee—slightly posterior to the patella.
   b. Hip—through the greater trochanter.
   c. Shoulder—through the tip of the acromion process.
   d. Head—through the earlobe.

Functional Activity Questions

1. Shoulder girdle protraction.
2. Shoulder girdle retraction, maybe some elevation.
3. Cervical flexion and possibly some forward head.
4. Right shoulder higher.
5. The woman's COG shifts anteriorly.
6. Anterior tilt.
7. Increased lordosis.
8. a. Posterior trunk—lumbar erector spinae and paraspinals become tight.
   b. Anterior trunk—abdominals become stretched.
9. Hip flexors.

Clinical Exercise Questions

1. Cervical hyperextension.
2. a. Cervical extensors—tighter.
   b. Cervical flexors—stretched.
3. Left side of pelvis is higher.
4. a. Left side muscles—tighter.
   b. Right side muscles—stretched.
5. a. Left side of disk more compressed.
   b. Right side more distracted.
   c. Intervertebral foramen—right side opened more.
   d. Intervertebral foramen on left made smaller.
6. a. Trunk extensors—posterior.
   b. Anterior part.
7. a. Trunk flexors—anterior.
   b. Posterior part.

Chapter 21 • Gait

General Anatomy Questions

1. Both have the same components and sequence of events. Walking has a period of double support while running does not. Running has a period of nonsupport that walking does not have.
2. Traditional terminology refers to single points in a time frame, whereas RLA terminology refers to periods in a time frame.
3. Stance phase.
4. Period of double support.
   a. Between heel-off and toe-off of one foot and heel strike and foot flat on the opposite foot.
5. During midstance of the stance phase.
6. Swing phase.
7. Step length lengthens, and cadence increases.
8. Walk with feet farther apart to widen the base of support.
9. Heel strike of stance phase and midswing of swing phase.
10. Push-off stance phase.

Functional Activity Questions

1. Shorter step length.
   Flatter foot during stance.
   Less arm swing.

2. Narrower walking base.

   Arms more out to side to help maintain balance.

3. Wider walking base.

   Greater horizontal displacement.

4. Increased forward lean.

5. Greater vertical displacement.

   Greater arm swing.

6. Circumducted gait during swing.

   Greater horizontal displacement during stance.

Clinical Exercise Questions

1. a. Ankle—dorsiflexion.
   b. Hip—flexion.

c. Pelvis—anterior pelvic tilt.

d. Lumbar spine—lordosis.

2. a. Type of contracture: Concentric contraction.

   Muscle group involved: Knee extensors.

   b. Type of contracture: Eccentric contraction.

   Muscle group involved: Ankle plantar flexors.

   c. Type of contracture: Concentric contraction.

   Muscle group involved: Hip extensors.

   d. Type of contracture: Isometric contraction.

   Muscle group involved: Contralateral hip abductors.

   e. Type of contracture: Eccentric contraction.

   Muscle group involved: Knee flexors.

Index

Note: Page numbers followed by "f" and "t" indicate figures and tables, respectively.

Abdominal muscles
    external oblique, 196–197, 196f
    internal oblique, 196f, 197
    rectus abdominis, 195–196, 196f
    transverse abdominis, 196–198, 196f
Abducted gait, 310
Abduction, 7
    of fingers, 146
    joint motions of, 8f
Abductor digiti minimi muscles, 155f, 156
Abductor pollicis brevis muscle, 155, 155f
Abductor pollicis longus muscle, 152, 152f, 154f
Acceleration, law of, 72
Accessory motion forces, 32–33
Accessory movement, 28
    of CMC joint, 144
Acetabular labrum, 236
Acetabulum, 234
Achilles tendon, 274
Achilles tendonitis, 274
Acromioclavicular joint, 96
    ligaments of, 96f
Acromion process, 95, 109
Action-reaction, law of, 72–73
Active insufficiency, 39–40
    of hamstring, 40f
Adam's apple (laryngeal prominence), 208
Adduction, 7
    of fingers, 146
    joint motions of, 8f
Adductor brevis muscle, 240–241, 241f
Adductor longus muscle, 240, 241f
Adductor magnus muscle, 241, 241f
Adductor pollicis muscle, 155–156, 155f
Adhesive capsulitis, of shoulder, 111
Ala, of sacrum, 220

Alveolus, 208
Anatomical position, 4
Anatomical snuff box, 153, 154f
Anconeus muscle, 128, 129f
Angular force, 76
Angular motion, 5, 6f
Ankle. *See also* Foot
    bones and landmarks of, 265–267
    dorsiflexors, gait and weakness in, 311, 311f
    fractures of, 274
    joints of
        inferior tibiofibular, 268–269, 269f
        subtalar, 270, 270f
        superior tibiofibular, 268, 269f
        talocrural (talotibial), 269–270, 269f
        transverse tarsal joint, 270, 270f
    ligaments of, 271
        right lateral, 272f
        right medial, 271f
    motions of, 268–269, 268f
    muscles of
        deep posterior group, 277t
        extensor digitorum longus, 278–279, 279f
        extensor hallucis longus, 278, 279f
        extrinsic, 275–281, 275t
        flexor digitorum longus, 277
        flexor hallucis longus, 276–277, 277f, 278f
        gastrocnemius, 260, 260f, 261f, 275, 276f
        intrinsic, 281–282
        peroneus brevis, 280–281, 280f
        peroneus longus, 279–280, 280f
        peroneus tertius, 280–281, 280f
        plantaris, 275–276, 276f
        soleus, 275, 276f
        tibialis anterior, 278, 278f
        tibialis posterior, 276, 277f

Ankle. *See also* Foot (*continued*)
  pathologies of, 273–275
  plantar flexion of, 7, 7f
  sprains of, 274
Ankle fusion (triple arthrodesis), 274, 313
Ankle joint (talocrural, talotibial joint), 269–270, 269f
Ankylosing spondylitis, 192
Annular ligament, of elbow, 125
Annulus fibrosus, 186
Antalgic gait, 314
Anterior longitudinal ligament, 190, 191f
Antigravity muscles, 290–291, 291f
Ape hand, 69
Aponeurosis, 22
Appendicular skeleton, 11, 12f
  bones of, 13t
Approximation (compression), 32, 32f
Arthrodesis, triple, 274, 313
Arthrokinematic motion (joint surface motion), 28–29
  definition of, 6
  of knee joint, 252f
  types of, 29–30
Arthrokinematics, 6, 71
Articular disk, of temporomandibular joint, 174, 174f
Articular system, 17–25
  planes and axes of, 23–24
Asthma, 214
Atlanto-occipital joint, 189
Atlantoaxial joint, 189, 189f
Atlas vertebra (C1), 187, 187f
Axes, 24, 24f
Axial skeleton, 11, 12f
  bones of, 13t
Axillary nerve, 63, 63f
Axis vertebra (C2), 187, 187f
  fracture of, 187
Axons, 49

Back knees (genu recurvatum), 257
Baker's cyst (popliteal cyst), 257
Ball-and-socket (triaxial) joints, 20, 21f
Basal ganglia, 52
Base of support (BOS), 78, 78f
  relationship with center of gravity, 79f, 80f
Basilar artery, 54
Bending force, 33, 33f
Biaxial joint motion, 19
Biceps brachii muscle, 126–127, 127f, 130f
  attachments, direction of movement, 36f
  attachments for, 123f
  as second- vs. third-class lever, 84f
  supination action of, 127f
Biceps femoris muscle, 243–244, 243f, 259, 259f
Biomechanics, 3
  force, 73–75
  laws of motion, 72–73

simple machines, 81–89
stability, 77–80
torque, 75–77
Bipennate muscles, 37f, 38
Body proportions, 78f
Bone(s), 14. *See also specific bones and body areas*
  composition of, 11–12
  of human body, 13t
  long, longitudinal cross section of, 12f
  markings on, 16t
  structure of, 12–14
  types of, 14f, 15t
    flat, 15
    irregular, 15
    long, 14
    sesamoid, 15
    short, 14–15
Bony end feel, 27
Boutonnière deformity, 148
Bowlegs (genu varum), 257
Brachial plexus, 60f, 62–63
  organization of, 62f
  terminal nerves of, 63–64
Brachialis muscle, 126, 126f
Brachioradialis muscle, 127–128, 127f
  as third-class lever, 84f
Brain, 50–54, 53f
  blood supply of, 54–55
  major arteries to, 55f
  protection of, 53–54
Brainstem, 52
Bronchioles, 208
Bronchitis, 214
Burner syndrome, 68–69
Bursae, 22–23, 22f
  of knee, 256, 256f
  of shoulder joint, 110
Bursitis
  prepatellar, 257–258
  trochanteric, 238

Cadence (walking speed), 300
Calcaneus, 254f, 255, 265
  positions of, 269f
Capitate bone, 134, 135f
Capitulum, 124
Capsular end feel, 27
Carotid arteries, 54
Carpal bones, 134–135
Carpal tunnel, 147f
Carpal tunnel syndrome, 69, 148
Carpometacarpal (CMC) joints, 29f, 133, 134f, 143–145, 144f, 145f
  structure of, 19–20
Carrying angle, 122f, 123
Cartilage, types of, 22

Cartilaginous joint, 18, 18f
Cauda equina, 55
Center of gravity (COG), 24, 24f, 77, 77f, 78f
  height of, relationship to stability, 79f
  relationship with base of support, 79f
  vertical displacement of, in gait cycle, 307f
Cerebellum, 53
Cerebrospinal fluid, 53–54
  circulation of, 54f
Cerebrum, 50–52
Cervical plexus, 60f, 62
Cervical sprains (whiplash), 191
Chest breathing, 212–213
Chondromalacia patella, 257
Circle of Willis, 54, 55f
Circumducted gait, 312, 312f
Circumduction, 8, 8f
Clavicle, 95, 95f
  fractures of, 111
Claw hand, 69
Close-packed position, 31, 31t
Cocontraction, 44
Collateral ligaments, 256
  of elbow, 124–125
  of knee, 255–256
Colles' fracture, 148
Component movements, 28
Compression (approximation), 32, 32f
Compression fractures, vertebral, 192
Concentric contraction, 42
  of quadriceps muscles, 42f
Condyle (condylar process), of mandible, 171
Condyloid (ellipsoidal) joints, 19, 20f
Congenital hip dislocation (dysplasia), 237
Congruency, joint, 31–32
Contraction, muscle, 41f, 44t
  concentric, 42
  eccentric, 42, 43
  isometric, 41
  isotonic, 41–42
Conus medullaris, 55
Convex-concave law, 30–31, 30f
Coracoacromial ligament, 96, 97f
Coracobrachialis muscle, 116–117, 117f
Coracohumeral ligament, 110
Coracoid process, 123
Coronoid process
  of mandible, 171
  of ulna, 124
Corticospinal tract, 57–58, 57f
Costoclavicular ligament, 96
Costovertebral joints, 206, 206f
Coxa plana, 237, 237f
Coxa vara, 237, 237f
Cranial nerves, 58–59, 58t, 59f
Crouch gait, 314

Cruciate ligaments, 254–255, 255f
Cuboid bone, tarsal, 266
Cuneiform bones, tarsal, 266
Curvilinear motion, 5, 6f

De Quervain's disease, 148
Deep rotator muscles, 242, 243f, 243t
Deltoid muscles, 111–112, 112f
  anterior and posterior, resultant force of, 75f
Dendrites, 49
Dens (odontoid process), 187
Dermatomes, 60, 61f
Diaphragm muscle, 209–210, 209f
  movement of, 209f
Diaphragmatic breathing, 212
Diaphysis, 13
Digastric muscle, 177–178, 178f
Disks, intervertebral. See Intervertebral disks
Dislocating force, 76
Dislocation, definition of, 23
Distal carpal arch, 147
Distal interphalangeal joint (DIP), 270, 271f
Distraction (traction), 32, 32f
Dorsal interossei muscles, 156f, 157, 157t
Dupuytren's contracture, 148
Dura mater, 53

Eccentric contraction, 42–43
Elastic cartilage, 22
Elbow joint, 121, 122f
  bones and landmarks of, 123–124
    capitulum, 124
    coracoid process, 123
    coronoid process, 124
    humerus, 123–124
    infraglenoid tubercle, 123
    lateral epicondyle, 125
    medial epicondyle, 125
    olecranon fossa, 124
    radial notch, 124
    radius, 124
    styloid process, 124
    supraglenoid tubercle, 123
    trochlea, 123
    trochlear notch, 124
    ulna, 124
    ulnar tuberosity, 124
  interosseous membrane, of forearm, 125
  joint capsule of, 125, 125f
  ligaments of, 124–125, 125f
    annular, 125
    lateral collateral, 125
    medial collateral, 124–125
  muscles of, 126–130
    anconeus, 128, 129f
    biceps brachii, 36f, 84f, 123f, 126–127, 127f, 130f

Elbow joint (*continued*)
 brachialis, 126, 126f
 brachioradialis, 84f, 127f
 innervation of, 130, 130t
 pronator teres, 129, 129f
 supinator, 129–130, 129f, 130f
 triceps brachii, 123f, 128, 128f
 pathologies of, 125–126
 structure and motions of, 121–123
Emphysema, 214
Empty end feel, 27–28
End feel, 27–28
Endosteum, 13
Epiphyseal lines, in hand bones, 14f
Epiphyses
 pressure, 13–14, 14f
 traction, 14, 14f
 types of, in immature bone, 14f
Equilibrium, states of, 78–79, 79f
Equinis foot (horse's foot), 274
Equinnus gait, 311, 311f
Erb's palsy, 68
Erector spinae muscles (sacrospinalis muscle group),
  198–199, 198f
Eversion, 9, 9f
Exercise
 isokinetic, 43–44
 terminology of, 46
Extension, 7
Extensor carpal ligament, 146
Extensor carpi radialis brevis muscle, 138, 138f
Extensor carpi radialis longus muscle, 137–138, 138f
Extensor carpi ulnaris muscle, 138–139, 139f
Extensor digiti minimi muscle, 151, 151f
Extensor digitorum longus muscle, 278, 279f
Extensor digitorum muscle, 150, 150f
Extensor expansion ligament, 147, 147f
Extensor hallucis longus muscle, 278, 279f
Extensor indicus muscle, 150–151, 151f
Extensor pollicis brevis muscle, 152–153, 153f
Extensor pollicis longus muscle, 153f
Extensor retinaculum ligament, 146, 147f
External oblique muscle, 196–197, 196f

Facet, vertebral, 184, 206, 206f
Facet joints, 189
Femoral nerve, 66, 66f
Femur, landmarks of, 234–235, 234f
 adductor tubercle, 235
 body, 234
 greater trochanter, 234
 head, 234
 lateral condyle, 235
 lateral epicondyle, 235
 linea aspera, 235
 medial condyle, 234
 medial epicondyle, 235

neck, 234
 patellar surface, 235
 pectineal line, 235
Festinating gait, 313–314
Fibrocartilage, 22
Fibula, 252
Fingers
 joints of, 145
  carpometacarpal joints, 145, 145f
  interphalangeal, 145–146
  metacarpophalangeal, 145–146, 145f
 motions of, 145, 145f
Flail chest, 214
Flat back, 191
Flat foot (pes planus), 274
Flexion, 6–7
Flexor carpi radialis muscle, 136, 137f
Flexor carpi ulnaris muscle, 136, 137f
Flexor digiti minimi muscles, 154f, 156
Flexor digitorum longus muscle, 277, 278f
Flexor digitorum profundus muscle, 149–150, 149f, 150f
Flexor digitorum superficialis muscle, 149, 149f
Flexor hallucis longus muscle, 276–277, 277f
Flexor pollicis brevis muscle, 154, 154f
Flexor pollicis longus muscle, 151–152, 152f, 154f
Flexor retinaculum ligament, 146, 146f
Foot. *See also* Ankle
 arches of, 271–273, 272f
  lateral longitudinal, 272, 272f
  medial longitudinal, 272, 272f
  transverse, 272, 273f
 bones of, 265–267, 267f
 eversion of, 9, 9f
 functional areas of, 267f
 inversion of, 9, 9f
 joints and motions of, 268f
 joints of, 270, 271f
  distal interphalangeal (DIP), 270, 271f
  metatarsophalangeal (MTP), 270, 271f
  proximal interphalangeal (PIP), 270, 271f
 ligaments of
  plantar, 273, 273f
  spring (plantar calcaneonavicular), 273, 273f
 main weight-bearing surfaces of, 272f
 muscles of
  deep posterior group, 277t
  extrinsic, 275–281, 275t
  innervation of, 282, 282t
  intrinsic, 281–282, 281t
  segmental innervation of, 283t
 plantar aponeurosis, 273, 273f
 stirrup of, 279–280
 support structures of
  inferior view, 273f
  medial view, 273f
 toe motions, 271f

Foot drop, 69
Foot flat, 305, 305f
Foot slap, 311
Force couple, 74–75, 75f
    causing anterior pelvic tilt, 226f
    causing level pelvis, 227f
    causing posterior pelvic tilt, 227f
    of deltoid/rotator cuff muscles, 117f
    of shoulder girdle, 103
Force(s), 71, 73–75
    accessory motion, 32–33
    concurrent system, 73f
Forearm
    interosseous membrane, 125
    muscles of, 126–130
        brachioradialis, 127–128
        pronator quadratus, 129, 129f
        pronator teres, 129, 129f
    oblique line of, 146
    pronation and supination of, 122f
Fracture(s), 23
    ankle, 274
    of hand/wrist, 148
    of shoulder bones, 111
    vertebral, 192
Freedom, degrees of, 24–25
Frontal axis, 24, 24f
Frontal plane, 23f, 24
Fundamental position, 4, 4f
Fusiform muscles, 37, 37f

Gait, 299
    abnormal, 309
        due to joint/muscle range of motion limitation,
            311–313
        due to muscular weakness/paralysis, 309–311, 310f
        due to neurological involvement, 313–314
        pain and, 314
        unequal leg length and, 314
    additional determinants of, 307–309
    age-related patterns, 309
    definitions, 299–300
Gait cycle (stride), 299, 300–301
    key events of, 303t–304t
    phases of, 300f
    stance phase, 301–302, 301f, 305–306, 305f, 306f
    swing phase, 306–307, 306f, 307f
    terminology of, 300f, 302t
    vertical displacement of center of gravity in, 307f
Gamekeeper's thumb, 148
Ganglion cyst, 148
Gastrocnemius muscle, 260, 260f, 261f, 275, 276f
Geniohyoid muscle, 177, 178
Genu recurvatum (back knees), 257
    gait in, 310f
Genu valgum (knock-knees), 257
Genu varum (bowlegs), 257

Glenohumeral joint, 117f
Glenohumeral ligament, 110
Glenohumeral subluxation, 111
Glenoid fossa, 95, 108
Glenoid labrum, 108, 110, 110f
Glide movement, 29, 29f
Gluteal nerves, 65
Gluteus maximus gait, 309, 310f
Gluteus maximus muscle, 242, 242f
Gluteus medius gait, 309–310, 310f
Gluteus medius muscle, 244–245, 244f
Gluteus minimus muscle, 244–245, 244f
Golfer's elbow, 125
Gomphosis, 18, 18f
Gomphosis (peg-in-socket joint), 18
Gracilis muscle, 242, 242f, 260
Gravity, 77
Gray matter, 50, 52f
    of spinal cord, 57, 57f
Greenstick fracture, 148

Hallux rigidus, 274
Hallux valgus, 274
Hamate bone, 134, 135f
Hamstring muscles, 243–244, 243f, 259, 259f, 260–261
    active insufficiency of, 40f
    gait due to weakness of, 310, 310f
    passive insufficiency of, 40f
    strain of, 238
Hand, 143
    bones of, 144f
        epiphyseal lines of, 14f
        metacarpals, 146
        phalanges, 146
    cylindrical grip, 162f
    extensor digitorum, 150, 150f
    extrinsic muscles of, 148–151
        abductor pollicis longus, 152, 152f, 154f
        extensor digiti minimi, 151, 151f
        extensor indicus, 150–151, 151f
        extensor pollicis brevis, 152–153, 153f
        extensor pollicis longus, 153, 153f
        flexor digitorum profundus, 149–150, 149f, 150f
        flexor digitorum superficialis, 149, 149f
        flexor pollicis longus, 151–152, 152f, 154f
    fractures of, 148
    function of, 160–161
    functional position of, 161f
    grip types, 161–164
    hook grip, 163f
    intrinsic muscles of, 154–158, 154t
        abductor digiti minimi, 155f, 156
        abductor pollicis brevis, 155, 155f
        adductor pollicis, 155–156, 155f
        deep palm, 154
        deep palm group, 157
        dorsal interossei, 156f, 157, 157t

Hand (*continued*)
    flexor digiti minimi, 154f, 156
    flexor pollicis brevis, 154, 154f
    hypothenar, 154
    lumbrical, 158, 158f, 159f
    palmar interossei, 157, 158f
    palmaris brevis, 156–157
    thenar, 154
  ligaments of
    extensor expansion, 147, 147f
    extensor retinaculum, 146, 147f
    flexor retinaculum, 146, 146f
    palmar carpal, 146, 146f
    transverse carpal, 146, 146f
  lumbrical grip, 164f
  muscle innervation of, 159–160, 160t
  pad-to-side grip, 164f
  palmar fascia, 136, 136f
  pathologies of, 148
  pinch grip, 163f
  power grip, 162f
  precision grip, 162f
  prime movers of, 159f
  segmental innervation of, 161t
  sensory innervation of, 161f
  side-to-side grip, 164f
  spherical grip, 163f
  three-jaw chuck grip, 163f
Hangman's fracture, 192
Heel-off, 305f
Heel strike, 302, 305, 305f
Hemiplegic gait, 313, 313f
Hiccups, 214
Hinge joints, 19, 20f
Hip bone (os coxae), 231, 232–233
  landmarks of
    acetabulum, 234
    greater sciatic notch, 234
    obturator foramen, 234
   lateral view, 233f
   medial view, 221f
Hip flexion contracture, 311, 312, 312f
Hip joint
  adductor brevis, 240–241, 242f
  angle of inclination, 237, 237f
  angle of torsion, 237, 238f
  anteversion of, 237, 238f
  associated motions with pelvic girdle, 227t
  bones and landmarks of, 232–235
  fused, abnormal gait and, 311–312, 312f
  joint capsule of, 235f, 236f
  ligaments of, 235–237, 236f
    iliofemoral, 235
    ischiofemoral, 235–236
    ligamentum teres, 236
    pubofemoral, 235
  muscle actions of, 245–246

  muscles of, 238–246, 239t
    adductor longus, 240, 241f
    deep rotator, 242, 243f, 243t
    gluteus maximus, 242, 242f
    gracilis, 242, 242f, 260
    iliopsoas, 238–239, 239f
    innervation of, 246t
    pectineus, 240, 241f
    rectus femoris, 239, 240f, 258, 259
    sartorius, 240, 240f, 260–261
    segmental innervation of, 247t
    tensor fascia latae, 245, 245f, 260
  pathologies of, 237–238
  retroversion of, 237, 238f
  structure and motions, 231–232, 232f
Horizontal abduction, of shoulder, 7, 8f
Horizontal adduction, of shoulder, 7, 8f
Horizontal displacement, 307
Horse's foot (equinis foot), 274
Housemaid's knee (prepatellar bursitis), 257–258
Humerus, 109f
  fractures of, 111
  landmarks of, 109, 123f
  rotator cuff attachments, 116
Hyaline (articular) cartilage, 22
Hyoid bone, 173, 173f
  muscles of, 195t
Hyperextension, definition of, 7
Hyperreflexia (autonomic dysreflexia), 62
Hyperventilation, 214
Hypothalamus, 52
Hypothenar muscles, 154

Iliac crest, 220, 233f
Iliac fossa, 233f
Iliocostalis muscles, 198
Iliofemoral ligament, 235, 236f
Iliolumbar ligament, 223
Iliopsoas muscle, 238–239, 239f
Iliotibial band, 237, 245f
Iliotibial band syndrome, 238
Ilium, 220
  landmarks of, 233, 233f
    anterior inferior iliac spine, 233
    anterior superior iliac spine, 233
    iliac crest, 233
    iliac fossa, 233
    posterior inferior iliac spine, 220, 233
    posterior superior iliac spine, 220, 233
Impingement syndrome, 111
Inchworm effect, 112
Inclined plane, 89, 89f
Inertia, law of, 72
Infraglenoid tubercle, 123
Infrahyoid muscles, 178, 179f
Infraspinatus fossa, 115
Infraspinatus muscle, 115, 115f

Intercarpal joints, 133, 134f
Interclavicular ligament, 96
Intercondylar eminence, 252
Intercostal muscles, 210–211
    external, 210f
    internal, 210f
Internal oblique muscle, 196f, 197
Interosseous membrane, of forearm, 125, 125f
Interphalangeal joints (IP)
    of fingers, 146
    of great toe, 270, 271f
Interspinal ligaments, 190, 191f
Interspinalis muscles, 199, 199f
Intertransversarii muscles, 199f, 200f
Intervertebral disks, 186–187, 186f, 187f
    herniation of, 192
    landmarks of
        annulus fibrosus, 186
        nucleus pulposus, 186
    lumbar, herniation of, 190
    pressure in various positions, 294f
Intervertebral foramen, 56, 57f
Intraspinous fossa, 108
Inversion, of foot, 9, 9f
Ischial tuberosity, 233
Ischiofemoral ligament, 235–236, 236f
Ischium, landmarks of, 233–234, 233f
    body, 233
    ischial tuberosity, 233
    ramus, 233
    spine, 234
Isokinetic contraction, 43–44
Isometric contraction, 41, 41f
Isotonic contraction, 41–42

Joint capsule, 21, 21f
    of ankle joint, 271
    of elbow, 125, 125f
    of hip, 235f
    of radiocarpal joint, 136
    of shoulder, 109–110, 110f
    of temporomandibular joint, 174, 174f
Joint mobilization, 28
Joint play movements, 28
    in open-packed positions, 31–32
Joint(s). See also specific joints
    classification of, 19t
    close-packed positions of, 31, 31t
    congruency, 31–32
    loose-packed positions of, 31, 32t
    motion, by plane and axis, 25t
    structure of, 20–23
    surface shapes, 28–29
        ovoid, 28–29, 28f
        sellar, 29, 29f
    types of
        cartilaginous joint, 18, 18f

diarthrodial, 18
fibrous, 17, 18f
gomphosis, 18, 18f
nonaxial, 18, 20f
saddle, 20, 21f
synarthrosis, 17, 18f
syndesmosis, 17–18, 18f
synovial, 18, 18f, 21f
triaxial, 20
Jumper's knee (patellar tendonitis), 257

Kienböck's disease, 148
Kinematics, 3, 71
Kinesiology, 3
Kinetic chains, 45–46
    closed, 45f
    open, 46f
Kinetics, 3
Knee/knee joint, 29–30, 252f
    arthrokinematic motion of, 252f
    bones and landmarks of, 253–254
        calcaneus, 254, 254f
        fibula, 254
        intercondylar eminence, 254
        lateral condyle, 254
        medial condyle, 254
        patella, 254, 255f
        plateau, 254
        tibial tuberosity, 254
    bursae around, 256f
    extension of, 261f
    in flexion, 255f
    ligaments of, 255–257
        collateral, 255–256
        cruciate, 254–255
    muscle action of, 261
    muscles of, 258–261, 258t
        biceps femoris, 243–244, 243f, 259, 259f
        gastrocnemius, 260, 260f, 275, 276f
        innervation of, 260t, 261
        popliteus, 259–260, 259f
        rectus femoris, 239, 240f, 258
        segmental innervation of, 261t
        semimembranosus, 243f, 244, 259
        semitendinosus, 243, 243f, 244, 259, 259f
        tensor fascia latae, 245, 245f, 260
        vastus intermedialis, 258f, 259
        vastus lateralis, 258
        vastus medialis, 258f, 259
    pathologies of, 257–258
    pes anserine muscle group, 257, 257f
    popliteal space, 257, 257f
    right, superior view, 256f
    screw-home motion of, 252f
    structure and motions of, 251–253, 252f
Knock-knees (genu valgum), 257
Kyphosis, 191–192

Labrum, 22, 22f
Laryngeal prominence (Adam's apple), 208
Larynx, 208
Lateral epicondyle, of elbow, 125
Lateral epicondylitis (tennis elbow), 125
Lateral longitudinal arch, 272, 272f
Lateral malleolus, 265
Lateral meniscus, 256
Lateral pelvic shift, 290
Lateral pelvic tilt, 307, 308f
    muscles minimizing, 308f
Lateral pterygoid muscle, 177, 177f
Latissimus dorsi muscle, 114, 114f
Leg. See also Ankle; Hip joint; Knee/knee joint
    bones and interosseous membrane, 266f
    extrinsic muscles of, 275-281
    gait and unequal length of, 314
    innervation of muscles of, 282t
    lateral view, 254f, 266f
Legg-Calvé-Perthes disease, 237
Levator costarum muscles, 212f
Levator scapula muscle, 100-101, 101f
Levers, 81
    classes of, 81-83
        factors changing, 83-84
    first class, 81f, 82f
    mechanical advantage of, 84-86, 85f, 86f
    second class, 81f, 82f, 83f
    third class, 82f, 83f
Ligamentous joint (syndesmosis), 17-18
Ligaments, 20-21. See also specific ligaments
Ligamentum teres, 236, 236f
Linea alba, 195
Linear force, 73, 74f
Linear motion, 5, 6f
Little league elbow, 125-126
Longissimus muscle group, 198
Longitudinal arch
    of foot, 272, 272f
    of hand, 147, 148f
Lordosis (swayback), 191
Lower extremity, bones of, 232f, 232t
Lower respiratory infection (LRI), 214
Lumbosacral angle, 223, 223f
Lumbosacral joint, 217, 222-223
    ligaments of, 222-223
        iliolumbar, 223
        lumbosacral, 223
Lumbosacral plexus, 60f, 64-66
    terminal nerves of, 66-68
Lumbrical muscles, 158, 158f
    side view, 159f
Lunate bone, 134, 135f
Lungs, 208

Malleolar fracture, 274
Mallet finger, 148

Mandible (mandibular bone), 170-171
    joint motion during depression of, 175f
    landmarks of, 171f
        angle, 170
        body, 170
        condyle, 171
        coronoid process, 171
        mental spine, 171
        neck, 171
        notch, 171
        ramus, 171
    motion during lateral deviation of, 175f
Manubrium, 95, 95f, 206
Mass, 71-72, 72
Masseter muscle, 176, 176f
Maxilla (maxillary bone), 172f, 173
Mechanical advantage, 84
Mechanics, 71
Medial epicondyle, of elbow, 125
Medial epicondylitis (golfer's elbow), 125
Medial longitudinal arch, 272, 272f
Medial malleolus, 265
Medial meniscus, 256
Medial pterygoid muscle, 176, 177f
Medial tibial stress syndrome, 274
Median nerve, 64, 65f
Medulla oblongata, 52
Medullary canal, definition of, 13
Metacarpal bones, 28f
Metacarpophalangeal (MCP) joints, 28f, 145-146
Metatarsal bones, 266-267, 267f
Metatarsalgia, 274
Metatarsophalangeal joints (MTP), 270, 271f
Midbrain, 52
Midcarpal joint, 133, 133f
Midstance, 305, 305f
Miserable malalignment syndrome, 258
Moment arm, 76, 76f
    effect on torque, 76F
    of quadriceps muscle, 77f, 253f
Morton's neuroma, 274
Motion
    angular, 5, 6f
    curvilinear, 5, 6f
    laws of, 72-73
    linear, 5, 6f
    rectilinear, 5, 5f
    types of, 5-6
Mouth
    muscles of, 195t
    opening of, against slight pressure, 181f
Multipennate muscles, 37f, 38
Muscle guarding, 28
Muscle(s). See also specific muscles
    angle of pull, 44-45, 45f
    attachment of, 35-36
    contraction, types of, 41-44, 41f, 44t

fiber arrangement, 37–38, 37f
naming of, 36–37
role of, 44
stretching of, 40
tendon action of, 40–41
tissue
    functional characteristics of, 38
    length-tension relationship in, 38–41, 39f
Musculocutaneous nerve, 63, 64f
Myelin, 49–50
Mylohyoid muscle, 17f, 177, 178f

Nasal cavity, 207
Navicular bone, 266
Neck
    motions of, 184f
    muscles of, 192–200, 192t
        actions of, 200
        erector spinae group, 194–195
        innervation of, 201
        prevertebral, 193–194, 194f, 194t
        scalene, 193, 193f, 211
        splenius capitus, 194–195, 196f
        splenius cervicis, 194–195, 196f
        sternocleidomastoid, 37, 37f, 193, 193f, 211f
        suboccipital, 194, 194t
Nervous system, 49, 50f
    central, 50–58
    peripheral, 58
        cranial nerves, 58–59
        pathologies of, 68–69
        spinal nerves, 59–60
Neurons, 49–50
    motor, upper and lower, 58
        clinical differences between lesions in, 58t
    structure of, 51f
Nonaxial joints, 18–19, 20f
Nuchal ligament (ligamentum nuchae), 190, 191f
Nucleus pulposus, 186

Oblique muscle fibers, 37
Obturator foramen, 234
Obturator nerve, 65, 66, 67f
Occipital bone, 185
Olecranon fossa, 124
Olecranon process, 124
Omohyoid muscle, 179, 179f
Open-packed (loose-packed) position, 31, 32t
Opponens digiti minimi muscles, 156
Opponens pollicis muscle, 155, 155f
Oral cavity, 207
Osgood-Schlatter's disease, 257
Osteoarthritis, 238
Osteoclasts, 13
Osteokinematic motion (joint motion), 27–28
Osteokinematics, 6–9, 71

Osteoporosis, 192
Ovoid joint, 28–29, 28f

Palmar carpal ligament, 146
Palmar fascia (palmar aponeurosis), 136, 136f
Palmar interossei muscles, 157, 158f
Palmaris brevis muscle, 156–157
Palmaris longus muscle, 137, 137f
Palmer flexion, 7, 7f
Parallel force, 73, 74f
Parallel muscle fibers, 37
Parallelogram, in demonstration of force, 73, 75f
Parkinsonian gait, 311, 311f
Passive insufficiency, 40
    of hamstring, 40, 40f
Patella, 255, 255f
Patellar tendonitis (jumper's knee), 257
Patellofemoral angle (Q angle), 253–254, 253f
Patellofemoral joint, 253, 253f
Patellofemoral pain syndrome, 257
Pathological terms, 23
Pectineus muscle, 240, 241f
Pectoralis major muscle, 113–114, 113f, 211f
Pectoralis minor muscle, 102–103, 103f
Pelvic girdle (pelvis)
    bones of, 233f
    false pelvis, 217, 218f
    ligaments of, 221–222
        posterior view, 222f
    lumbosacral joint, 222–223
    male vs. female, 218f
    motions of, 223–226, 224f
        anterior tilt, 223
        associated vertebral column/hip joint motions, 227t
        force couple causing anterior tilt, 226f
        in frontal plane, 224f
        lateral tilt, 224–225, 225f
        posterior tilt, 223
        rotation, 225–226, 226f
    muscle control of, 226–227
    points of, 218f
    sacroiliac (SI) joints, 219–222
    structure and function, 217
    symphysis pubis, 222f
    true pelvis, 218, 218f
Periosteum, definition of, 13
Peroneal nerve, 67, 68f
Peroneus brevis muscle, 280, 280f
Peroneus longus muscle, 279–280, 280f
Peroneus tertius muscle, 280–281, 280f
Pes anserine muscle group, 257, 257f
Pes cavus, 274
Pes planus (flat foot), 274
Phalanges
    of foot, 267, 267f
        joints of, 271f
    of hand, 144f, 146

Pharynx, 207–208
Pia mater, 53
Pisiform bone, 134, 135f
Plane joint, 20f
Planes of action, 23–24, 23f
Plantar aponeurosis, 273f
Plantar calcaneonavicular ligament (spring ligament), 273, 273f
Plantar fasciitis, 274
Plantar flexion, 7, 7f
Plantar ligaments, 273
Plantaris muscle, 275–276, 276f
Pleurisy, 214
Plexus formation, 62
  brachial, 62–63, 62f
  cervical, 62
  lumbosacral, 62–66, 62f
    anterior view of, 66f
Pneumonia, 214
Pneumothorax, 214
Popliteal cyst (baker's cyst), 257
Popliteal space, 257
  muscular boundaries of, 257f
Popliteus muscle, 259–260, 259f
Positions
  anatomical, 4, 4f
  backswing motion, 202f
  descriptive, 4f
  fundamental, 4, 4f
  hip
    during hamstring curl exercise, 263f
    during knee extension exercise, 263f
  of hip when beginning to stand, 248f
  intervertebral disk pressure and, 294f
  lunge, 251f
Posterior longitudinal ligament, 190, 191f
Postural sway, 291, 291f
Posture, 289
  common deviations, 293t, 296
  intervertebral disk pressure and, 294f
  kneeling stool, 295f
  lying, 295f
  sitting, 294–295, 295f
  slouched, 295f
  standing, 291–294
    anterior view, 292–293, 292f
    lateral view, 292, 292f
    posterior view, 293–294, 293f
  supine, 295–296, 295f
  vertebral alignment, 289–291
Prepatellar bursitis (housemaid's knee), 257–258
Pressure epiphyses, 13–14
Prevertebral muscles, 193–194, 194t
Pronation
  definition of, 9
  of forearm, 122f
Pronator quadratus muscle, 129, 129f

Pronator teres muscle, 129, 129f
Protraction, 9, 9f
Proximal carpal arch, 147, 148f
Proximal interphalangeal joint (PIP), 270, 271f
Pubic ligaments, 222
Pubic symphysis, 222, 222f
Pubis, 234
  landmarks of
    body, 234
    inferior ramus, 234
    superior ramus, 234
    symphysis pubis, 234
    tubercle, 234
Pubofemoral ligament, 235, 236f
Pulleys, 86–87, 86f, 87f
  fixed, 87f
  movable, 87f

Q angle (patellofemoral angle), 253–254, 253f
Quadratus lumborum muscle, 200, 200f
Quadriceps muscles, 258–259
  gait due to weakness/paralysis of, 310f
  moment arm of, 253f
  paralysis of, 261f

Radial nerve, 63, 64f
Radial notch, 124
Radiocarpal joint, 133, 134f
Radiocarpal ligament
  dorsal, 135–136, 135f
  palmar, 135, 135f
Radioulnar joint, 121, 122f
Radius, 122f, 124
  right, anterior view, 125f
Ramus
  of ischium, 233
  of pubis, 234
  of skull, 171
Rectilinear motion, 5, 5f
Rectus abdominis muscle, 195, 196f, 211f
Rectus femoris muscle, 239, 240f, 258, 258f
Respiration
  diaphragmatic vs. chest, 212–213
  mechanics of, 208, 208f
  muscles of, 209–212
    diaphragm, 209–210, 209f
    innervation of, 213
    intercostal, 210–211, 210f
    levator costarum, 212, 212f
    serratus anterior, 212f
    serratus posterior, 212f
  phases of, 209, 213t
Respiratory system, 205–215
  conditions/pathologies of, 214
  structures of, 207–208, 207f
Resting position. See Open-packed (loose-packed) position

Retraction, 9, 9f
Reversal of muscle action, 35
  in shoulder girdle, 104
Reversal of muscle function, of gluteal muscles, 245, 245f
Rhomboid muscle, 101, 101f
Rhomboidal muscles, 37, 37f
Rib cage, 205
Rib dislocation, 214
Rib separation, 214
Roll movement, 29, 29f
Rotary force, 33, 33f
Rotation
  joint, 9f
  medial vs. lateral, 8
Rotator cuff, 110
  humoral attachment, 116f
  tear of, 111

Sacroiliac (SI) joint, 217, 219
  bones and landmarks of, 219–221
    ala, 220
    articular surface, 220
    base, 219
    foramina, 220
    greater sciatic foramen, 220
    greater sciatic notch, 220
    iliac crest, 220
    ischium, 220–221
    lesser sciatic notch, 221
    pelvic surface, 220
    posterior inferior iliac spine, 220, 233
    posterior superior iliac spine, 220, 233
    promontory, 219
    sacrum, 219, 220f
    spine, 221
    superior articular process, 219
    tuberosity, 220, 221
  cross section of, 221f
  ligaments of, 221–222, 222f
    anterior sacroiliac, 221
    iliolumbar, 222
    interosseous sacroiliac, 221
    long posterior sacroiliac, 221–222
    sacrospinous, 222
    sacrotuberous, 222
    short posterior sacroiliac, 221
  structure and motions of, 219, 219f
Sacrum, 219
  lateral view, 220f
  posterior view, 220f
Saddle joints, 20, 21f
Sagittal axis, 24, 24f
Sagittal plane, 23f, 24
Sartorius muscle, 240, 240f, 260–261
Scalene muscles, 193, 193f, 211
Scaphoid bone, 134, 134f
  fracture of, 148

Scapula, 109f
  bony landmarks of, 94f
  motion during upward rotation, 97f
  muscular force couple
    producing downward rotation, 103f
    producing upward rotation, 103f
  resting position of, 94f
  rotational movement of, 100f
  winging of, 102f
Scapular winging, 69
Scapulohumeral rhythm, 98
Scapulothoracic articulation, 93
Sciatic nerve, 66–67, 67f
Sciatic notch/foramen, 220
Sciatica, 191
Scissors gait, 314, 314f
Sellar (saddle-shaped) joint, 29, 29f
Semimembranosus muscle, 242, 243f, 244, 259
Semitendinosus muscle, 243, 243f, 244, 259, 259f
Serratus anterior muscle, 36f, 102, 102f, 212f
Serratus posterior muscles, 212f
Sesamoid bones, 15
Shear force, 32, 33f
Shin splints, 274
Shoulder
  fractures of, 111
  horizontal abduction of, 7, 8f
  horizontal adduction of, 7, 8f
  labrum of, 22
  protraction of, 9, 9f
  retraction of, 9, 9f
Shoulder complex, 93, 94f
  glenohumeral joint, 117f
  scapulothoracic articulation, 93
  sternoclavicular joint, 95–96
Shoulder girdle, 93
  bones and landmarks of, 94–95
    clavicle, 95, 95f
    scapula, 94–95, 94f
  companion motions with shoulder joint, 98
  force couples of, 103
  joint motions of, 96–98, 97F
  joints of
    acromioclavicular, 96
    sternoclavicular, 95–96
  ligaments of
    coracoacromial, 96, 97f
    coracoclavicular, 96
    costoclavicular, 96
    interclavicular, 96
  motions of, 97f
  muscles of, 98–104
    innervation of, 104f, 104t
    levator scapula, 100–101, 101f
    pectoralis minor, 102–103, 103f
    rhomboid, 101, 101f
    segmental innervation of, 104f

Shoulder girdle (*continued*)
    serratus anterior, 36f, 102, 102f
    trapezius, 99–100, 99f, 100f
  reversal of muscle action, 104
  sternoclavicular joint, 95–96, 96f
Shoulder joint (glenohumeral joint), 93–94
  bones and landmarks of, 108–109
    glenoid fossa, 95
    glenoid labrum, 108
    infraspinatus fossa, 115
    subscapular fossa, 108
    supraspinous fossa, 108
  joint motions of, 107–108, 108f
  ligaments of, 109–111
    coracohumeral, 110, 110f
    glenohumeral, 110
  movement of, 117–118
  muscles of, 111–117
    biceps brachii, 36f, 84f, 123f, 126–127, 127f, 130f
    coracobrachialis, 116–117, 117f
    deltoid, 75f, 111–112, 112f
    infraspinatus, 115, 115f
    innervation of, 118t
    latissimus dorsi, 114, 114f
    pectoralis major, 113–114, 113f, 211f
    segmental innervation of, 119t
    subscapularis, 116f
    supraspinatus, 112–113, 113f
    teres major, 114–115, 115f, 116f
    teres minor, 115–116, 115f, 116f
    triceps brachii, 123f, 128, 128f
  pathologies of, 11
Skeleton
  appendicular, 11, 12f
  axial, 11, 12f
  functions of, 11
Skier's thumb, 148
Skull, 53f
  bones of, 169–170, 171f, 185, 185f
    mandible, 170–171, 171F, 175F
    maxilla, 172f, 173
    occipital, 185
    sphenoid, 172, 172f
    temporal, 171–172, 185
    zygomatic, 172, 172f
Slipped capital femoral epiphysis, 237
Smith's fracture, 148
Soft tissue approximation, 28
Soleus muscle, 275, 276f
Sphenoid bone, 172, 172f
  landmarks of
    greater wing, 172
    lateral pterygoid plate, 172
    spine, 172
Sphenomandibular ligament, 173, 174f
Spin rotation, 29, 30f
Spinal cord, 55–58, 56f

  cross section of, 52f, 57f
  level, functional significance of, 60–62
  sensory and motor pathways in, 52f
Spinal nerves, 60f
  branches of, 59–60, 60f
  positions and muscle innervations, 61f
Spinal stenosis, 192
Spinalis muscle group, 198
Spine, 56f. *See also* Vertebrae; Vertebral column
Splenius capitus muscles, 194–195, 196f
Splenius cervicis muscles, 194–195, 196f
Spondylolisthesis, 192
Spondylolysis, 192
Spondylosis (spinal osteoarthritis), 192
Sprain(s), 23
  ankle, 274
  cervical, 191
Spring ligament (plantar calcaneonavicular), 272, 272f
Stability, 77–80
Stance phase, 300
  analysis of, 301–302, 305–306
Standing posture, 291–294
Statics, 71
Stenosing tenosynovitis (trigger finger), 148
Step/step length, 299
Sternoclavicular joint, 95–96
  ligaments of, 96f
Sternocleidomastoid muscle, 37, 37f, 193, 193f, 211f
Sternohyoid muscles, 178–179, 179f
Sternum, 95, 95f, 205
Stinger syndrome, 68–69
Stirrup of the foot, 279
Stitch, 214
Strain, 23
Strap muscles, 37, 37f
Stride. *See* Gait cycle
Stride length, 299
Stylohyoid ligament, 173–174, 173f
Stylohyoid muscle, 178, 178f
Styloid process, of elbow, 124
Stylomandibular ligament, 173–174, 174f
Subluxation, 23
Suboccipital muscles, 194, 194f, 195t
Subscapular fossa, 108
Subscapularis muscle, 116f
Subtalar joint (talocalcaneal joint), 270, 270f
Supination, 8
  of forearm, 122f
Supinator muscle, 129–130, 129f, 130f
Supraglenoid tubercle, 123
Suprahyoid muscles, 177
Supraspinal ligament, 190, 191f
Supraspinatus muscle, 112–113, 113f
Supraspinous fossa, 108
Sustentaculum tali, 266
Swan neck deformity, 148
Swayback (lordosis), 191

Swimmer's shoulder, 111
Swing phase, 306f
    analysis of, 306–307
Symphysis pubis, 222f, 234
Synapses, 50
Synarthrosis (suture joint), 17, 18f
Syndesmosis (ligamentous joint), 17–18, 18f
Synovial fluid, 21
Synovial joints (diarthrodial joints), 18, 18f
    classification of, 19t
    longitudinal cross section, 21f
Synovial membrane, 21

Talus, 266
Tarsal bones, 265–266, 267f
    calcaneal tuberosity, 265
    calcaneus, 265, 269f
    cuboid, 266
    cuneiforms, 266
    navicular, 266
    sustentaculum tali, 266
    talus, 266
    tuberosity of navicular, 266
Temporal bone, 171
    landmarks of, 172f
        articular fossa, 171
        articular tubercle, 171
        external auditory meatus, 172
        mastoid process, 172
        postglenoid tubercle, 172
        zygomatic process, 172
Temporal fossa, 173, 173f
Temporalis muscle, 175–176, 176f
Temporomandibular joint (TMJ), 170f
    joint capsule of, 174, 174f
    joint structure and motions, 169
    lateral view of, 174f
    ligaments of, 173–174
        sphenomandibular, 173
        stylohyoid, 174, 174f
        stylomandibular, 173–174
        temporomandibular, 173
    mechanics of movement of, 174–175
    motions of, 170f
    muscles of, 175–179
        actions of, 179
        digastric, 177–178, 178f
        infrahyoid, 178, 179f
        innervation of, 179–180, 180t
        lateral pterygoid, 177f
        masseter, 176, 176f
        medial pterygoid, 176, 177f
        mylohyoid, 177, 177f, 178f
        omohyoid, 179, 179f
        sternohyoid, 178–179, 179f
        stylohyoid, 178, 178f
        suprahyoid, 177–178
        temporalis, 175–176, 176f
        thyrohyoid, 179, 179f
Temporomandibular ligament (lateral ligament), 173, 174f
Tendons, 22
Tennis elbow, 125
Tenodesis, 40–41
    of finger flexor and extensor muscles, 41f
Tenon and mortise joint, 269, 269f
Tenosynovitis, 23, 148
Tension. *See* Traction
Tensor fascia latae muscle, 245, 245f, 260
Teres major muscle, 114–115, 115f, 116f
Teres minor muscle, 115–116, 115f, 116f
Terminology
    accessory motion, 28
    of common pathologies, 23
    descriptive, 4–5, 4f
        for quadrupeds, 5f
    exercise, 46
    of gait cycle, 300f, 302t
Terrible triad, 258
Thalamus, 51–52, 53f
Thenar muscles, 154
Thoracic cage, 205–206, 206f
Thoracic nerves, 60
Thoracic outlet syndrome, 191
Thoracolumbar fascia, 110
Thorax
    joints and articulations of, 206–207
    movements of, 206–207, 207f
Thumb
    extrinsic muscles of, 151–153
    joints of, 143–145, 144f
        carpometacarpal (CMC), 19–20, 29f, 133, 134f,
            143–145, 144f, 145f
    motions of, 143–145, 144f
Thyrohyoid muscle, 179, 179f
Tibia, 235
    anterior view, 235f
    landmarks of, 265
        crest, 265
        head, 265
        intercondylar eminence, 254
        lateral condyle, 254
        lateral malleolus, 265
        medial condyle, 254
        medial malleolus, 265
        plateau, 254
        tibial tuberosity, 235, 254
    lateral view, 254f
Tibial nerve, 67, 68f
Tibial tuberosity, 254
Tibialis anterior muscle, 278, 278f
Tibialis posterior muscle, 276, 277f
Tibiofibular joints, 268, 269f
Toe, motions of, 271f
Toe off, 305, 306f

Torque, 75–77
　　moment arm effect on, 76F
Torticollis, 191
Trachea, 208
Traction, 32, 32f
Traction epiphyses, 14, 14f
Transverse abdominis muscle, 196f, 197
Transverse arch, 272, 273f
Transverse carpal ligament, 146, 147f
Transverse plane, 23f, 24
Transverse tarsal joint, 270, 270f
Transversospinalis muscle group, 199, 199f
Trapezium bone, 134, 135f
Trapezius muscle, 99–100, 99f, 100f
Trapezoid bone, 134, 135f
Trendelenburg gait, 245, 309
Trendelenburg sign, 307–308
Triangular muscles, 37, 37f
Triaxial (ball-and-socket) joints, 20, 21f
Triceps brachii muscle, 128, 128f
　　attachments for, 123f
Triceps surae contraction, 312–313
Trigger finger, 148
Triple arthrodesis, 274, 313
Triquetrum bone, 134, 135f
Trochanteric bursitis, 238
Trochlea, 123
Trochlear notch, of elbow, 124
Trunk
　　motions of, 184f
　　muscles of, 192t, 195–200
　　　actions of, 200
　　　erector spinae, 198–199, 198f
　　　external oblique, 196–197, 196f
　　　iliocostalis, 198
　　　internal oblique, 196f, 197
　　　interspinalis, 199, 199f
　　　intertransversarii, 199f, 200f
　　　line of pull and action of, 197f
　　　longissimus group, 198
　　　posterior, 198t
　　　quadratus lumborum, 200, 200f
　　　rectus abdominis, 195, 196f, 211f
　　　spinalis group, 198
　　　transverse abdominis, 196f, 197
　　　transversospinalis group, 199, 199f
Tuberosity
　　of ilium, 220
　　of ischium, 221, 233
　　of navicular bone, 266
　　tibial, 254
　　ulnar, 124
Turf toe, 274

Ulna, 124
　　movement of radius around, 122f
　　right, lateral view, 124f

Ulnar drift, 148
Ulnar nerve, 64, 65f
Ulnar tuberosity, 124
Uniaxial joints, 19
Unipennate muscles, 37–38, 37f
Upper respiratory infection (URI), 214

Valgus position, 301
Valsalva's maneuver, 213–214
Varus position, 301
Vastus intermedialis muscle, 258f, 259
Vastus lateralis muscle, 258, 258f
Vastus medialis muscle, 258f, 259
Vaulting gait, 312, 312f
Vector, 71
　　force and, 73
Vertebrae, 56, 57f
　　arrangement of, 183
　　atlas (first cervical), 187, 187f
　　axis (second cervical), 187, 187f
　　C7 (vertebra prominens), 187
　　cervical, 188f
　　costal facets, 187, 188f
　　demifacets of, 188f
　　dens (odontoid process), 187
　　fractures of, 192
　　lumbar, 188f
　　of lumbosacral joint, 222–223
　　parts of, 186, 186f, 189f
　　　articular process, 186
　　　body, 186
　　　intervertebral opening, 186
　　　lamina, 186
　　　neural arch, 186
　　　pedicle, 186
　　　spinous process, 186
　　　transverse process, 186
　　　vertebral foramen, 186
　　　vertebral notches, 186
　　thoracic, 188f
　　　costal facets of, 188f
　　　facets/demifacets on, 206f
　　transverse foramen, 188f
Vertebral column. See also Intervertebral disks
　　alignment of, 289–291
　　associated motions with pelvic girdle, 227t
　　cervical, muscles of, 193–195
　　curves of, 183, 184f
　　　major, 290f
　　　postural , development of, 290–291
　　　primary, of newborn, 290f
　　joint motions of, 184–185, 184f
　　joints of, 189–190
　　　atlanto-occipital, 189
　　　atlantoaxial, 189, 189f
　　　facet, 189
　　ligaments of, 190, 191f

anterior longitudinal, 190, 191f
interspinal, 190, 191f
ligamentum flavum, 190
nuchal, 190, 191f
posterior longitudinal, 190, 191f
supraspinal, 190, 191f
muscles of, 192t
cervical spine, 193–195
posterior trunk, 197–200, 198f
pathologies of, 191–192
segments of, 184f
Vertebral foramen, 56
Vertical axis, 24, 24f
Vertical displacement, 307, 307f

Waddling gait, 311, 311f
Walking base width, 307, 308f
Walking speed (cadence), 300
Wheel and axle, 87–88, 88f
upper extremity acting as, 89f
Whiplash (cervical sprain), 191
White matter, 50, 52f
of spinal cord, 57, 57f
Wrist drop, 69
Wrist, fractures of, 148
Wrist joint
bones and landmarks of, 134–135, 135f
capitate, 134, 135f
hamate, 134, 135f

lunate, 134, 135f
pisiform, 134, 135f
scaphoid, 134, 134f
trapezium, 134, 135f
triquetrum, 134, 135f
functional position of, 161f
ligaments of, 135
dorsal radiocarpal, 135–136, 135f
palmar radiocarpal, 135, 135f
radial collateral, 135, 135f
ulnar collateral, 135, 135f
motions of, 134, 134f
muscles of, 136–139
extensor carpi radialis brevis, 138, 138f
extensor carpi radialis longus, 137–138, 138f
extensor carpi ulnaris, 138–139, 139f
flexor carpi radialis, 136, 137f
flexor carpi ulnaris, 136, 137f
innervation of, 139, 139t
palmaris longus, 137, 137f
pathologies of, 148
structure of, 133–134
terminology, 134f

Xiphoid process, 95, 95f, 206

Zygomatic bone, 172
landmarks of, 172f
temporal process, 172